Alfredo Guglielmi • Andrea Ruzzenente • Calogero Iacono

Surgical Treatment of Hilar and Intrahepatic Cholangiocarcinoma

In cooperation with
Luigi Marchiori
Silvia Pachera
Luca Bortolasi
Riccardo Manfredi
Paola Capelli

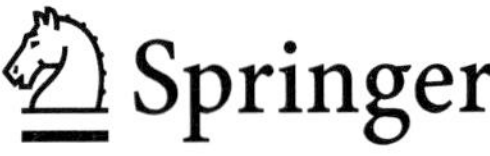
Springer

Alfredo Guglielmi
Andrea Ruzzenente
Calogero Iacono
General Surgery A, Department of Surgery and Gastroenterology
University Hospital G.B. Rossi
Verona, Italy

in cooperation with
Luigi Marchiori, Silvia Pachera, Luca Bortolasi
General Surgery A, Department of Surgery and Gastroenterology
University Hospital G.B. Rossi
Verona, Italy

Riccardo Manfredi
Department of Radiology
University Hospital G.B. Rossi
Verona, Italy

Paola Capelli
Department of Pathology
University Hospital G.B. Rossi
Verona, Italy

The publication and the distribution of this volume have been supported by the Italian Society of Surgery

Library of Congress Control Number: 2007931745

ISBN 978-88-470-0728-4 Milan Heidelberg New York
e-ISBN 978-88-470-0729-1

Springer is a part of Springer Science+Business Media
springer.com
© Springer-Verlag Italia 2008

Cover design: Simona Colombo, Milan, Italy
Typesetting: Graphostudio, Milan, Italy
Printing and binding: Arti Grafiche Nidasio, Assago, Italy

Printed in Italy
Springer-Verlag Italia S.r.l. – Via Decembrio 28 – I-20137 Milan

Updates in Surgery

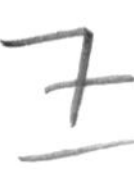

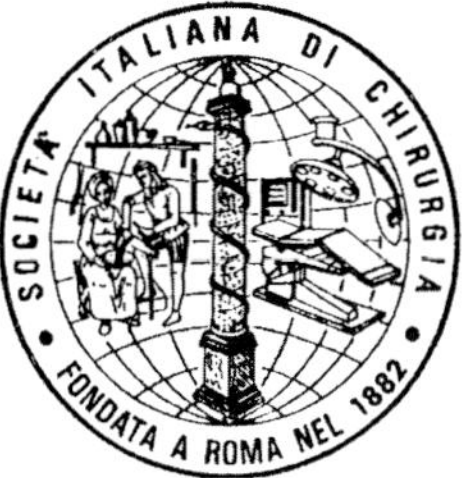

Foreword

In the 10 years since the presentation of Gazzaniga's excellent monograph on extrahepatic biliary tumours at the SIC Congress in 1997, interesting developments in the field have pressed upon us an undoubted need to reassess the complex topic of hepatobiliary surgery. It is therefore with great pleasure that, at the proposal of the Steering Committee of the Italian Society of Surgery (SIC), we present to Italian surgeons this monograph on the treatment of hilar and intrahepatic cholangiocarcinoma, prepared by Alfredo Guglielmi, professor and chairman of Surgical Department A at the University School of Medicine of Verona, and his colleagues.

The volume is divided into two parts. The first relates to hilar cholangiocarcinomas, about which there are a number of complex and still controversial issues; the second relates to intrahepatic cholangiocarcinomas, which are frequently treated like other primary tumours of the liver. The monograph includes preliminary information about molecular biology, and diagnostic and treatment methods are extensively examined in relation to type of neoplastic spread. In our opinion the most interesting part of the book concerns the treatment of these tumours with both interventional radiology and surgery, which can range from simple hepatectomies to liver transplantation. We would like to point out that Professor Guglielmi carried out the first liver transplantation in the University of Verona surgical department.

The monograph is aimed at those in clinical practice, and is written by a colleague for whom the most important objective of his work is to perform the best surgery in the light of the most recent developments and to achieve results in the interests of his patients. Just as usually happens in clinical practice, pathologists and radiologists have participated in the making of this book. This type of "disease management team" improves the quality and results of surgery.

Over the last 20 years, Alfredo Guglielmi has followed with enthusiasm and intelligence the progress made in hepatobiliary surgery. He has connections with European, American and Japanese surgical institutes; he performed an in-depth study of the surgical treatment of cholangiocarcinoma at the University of Nagoya under the guidance of Yuji Nimura, a pioneer in this field. The mutuality of this professional relationship and sincere friendship is attested to by several visits of Yuji Nimura to the surgical department of the University School of Medicine of Verona.

It is for all these reasons that we are proud to present to Italian surgeons this monograph, which conveys the most recent orientations of the SIC. For the first time it is being published in English by a publishing house with an international presence. We think that this is the best way to share our experiences with colleagues from other countries. We also feel that this volume will be an excellent instrument for the achievement of the aims of the SIC Steering Committee. We hope it will achieve wide circulation and great success.

Verona, October 2007   *Claudio Cordiano*
Past President, Italian Society of Surgery

Rome, October 2007   *Roberto Tersigni*
President, Italian Society of Surgery

Preface

I would like to thank the Steering Committee of the Italian Society of Surgery (SIC) for giving me the opportunity of writing this book. I accepted the task enthusiastically, because the surgery of cholangiocarcinoma is a fascinating and complex part of hepatobiliary surgery that has undergone numerous changes over recent decades. My aim has been to provide an update on the diagnosis, staging, preoperative management and treatment of hilar and intrahepatic cholangiocarcinoma, and to provide a critical review of diagnostic and therapeutic tools in the light of the published literature and personal experience.

Cholangiocarcinoma is a rare neoplasm, but its incidence is increasing in Western and Eastern countries. It was described in rare reports before the 1950s, and only in 1965 did Klatskin collect 13 cases and describe the clinical and pathological characteristics of the disease. Classically, cholangiocarcinoma is categorised into intrahepatic and extrahepatic types according to the location of the tumour along the biliary tract. However, the frequently mixed type of growth of these tumours often makes this type of classification difficult to apply. This monograph has therefore been divided into two parts to analyse the differences between the two types of cholangiocarcinoma, emphasising that the treatment of these two neoplasms often requires combined hepatic and bile duct resection.

The modern era of surgery of hilar cholangiocarcinoma began in 1954 when Brown performed the first bile duct resection for hilar cholangiocarcinoma. The first experiences of bile duct resection associated with liver resection were published during the 1960s. From the 1970s onwards, Longmire, Fortner and Launois reported the first surgical series with good survival results but with a high rate of mortality and complications. After the 1980s, the clinico-anatomical study of the hepatic hilum and the segmental biliary drainage proposed by Nimura led to further progress in precise preoperative diagnosis of tumour extent and surgical planning.

More recently, progress in non-invasive diagnostic tools has further improved the preoperative evaluation, with a reduction in invasive diagnostic techniques. During the past decade, improvements in surgical techniques and preoperative optimisation of liver function (preoperative biliary drainage and portal vein embolisation) have made it possible to perform extended liver resection combined with vascular resection and reconstruction with low mortality and morbidity. The higher curative resection rate of this type of surgical approach has also improved long-term results.

The surgery of cholangiocarcinoma is still changing today, and several controversies in preoperative and surgical management remain. These open issues provide stimulus for further research and new ideas on the treatment of this tumour.

I am extremely grateful to Professor Claudio Cordiano, who in his surgical department stimulated and supported me in the development of hepatobiliary surgery. I owe a debt of thanks to my "maestro". I also thank Professor Yuji Nimura for all the teachings he gave me, with great willingness and undisputed expertise, over the last 15 years. His thoughts are present in many places in the pages of this book.

Thanks also go to all the colleagues who helped me during the writing of the book, of whom I asked dedication and diligence, and into whom I hope I have instilled my passion for this challenging branch of surgery.

Finally, thank you to Giovanni Paolo Pianegonda for his wonderful drawings.

Alfredo Guglielmi

Contents

Part 1: Hilar Cholangiocarcinoma

Reporting Cholangiocarcinoma: Pathological Aspects 3

  Definitions 3

  Clinical Information 4

  Intraoperative Consultation 5

  Macroscopic Examination 6

  Pathology Findings in Non-Neoplastic Liver 9

  Lymph Nodes (Location, Number) 10

  Frozen Tissue (Molecular Studies) 10

  Microscopic Examination 10

  Additional Pathology Findings 12

  Immunohistochemistry 13

Diagnosis 17

  Ultrasound (Endoscopic, Intraductal, Transabdominal) 17

  Computed Tomography 20

  Magnetic Resonance Imaging 21

  Positron Emission Tomography 23

  Direct Cholangiography (ERCP and PTC) 23

  Cholangioscopy (Peroral, Percutaneous) 24

  Angiography 25

Preoperative Staging 29

  Evaluation of the Biliary Involvement (Longitudinal Extent) 30

  Evaluation of Radial Extent: Vascular Involvement,
Parenchymal Involvement and Hepatic Lobar Atrophy 33

  Preoperative Assessment of Tumour Resectability (T) 35

  Evaluation of Lymph Node Status (N) 36

  Evaluation of Metastases (M) 37

  Conclusions 37

The Role of Laparoscopy in Preoperative Staging 43

    Technique 43

    Results 44

    Laparoscopic Ultrasound 45

    Conclusions 46

Preoperative Assessment of Liver Function 49

Preoperative Biliary Drainage 57

    Drainage: Pros 58

    Drainage: Cons 59

    Conclusions 62

Preoperative Portal Vein Embolization 67

    Physiopathology of PVE 67

    Indications 69

    Contraindications 69

    Technique 69

    Results 71

    Post-PVE Course and Timing of Resection 72

    Conclusions 72

Prognostic Factors 75

    Gross Type 75

    Microscopic Pattern 76

    Biological and Molecular Prognostic Factors 76

    T Category 77

    N Category 81

    M Category 82

    Prognostic Significance of TNM UICC/AJCC Classification 82

Staging Systems 87

    Bismuth-Corlette Classification 87

    TNM Staging System According to UICC/AJCC 6th Edition 88

    Comparison between 5th and 6th Edition of TNM UICC/AJCC 91

    Staging System According to JSBS 91

    Early Cancer 96

    Gazzaniga Staging System 96

    Memorial Sloan-Kettering Cancer Center Staging 98

    Conclusions 99

Surgical Anatomy of the Hepatic Hilus 101

Anatomy of the Bile Duct Branches 102

Anatomy of the Portal Vein Branches 105

Anatomy of the Hepatic Artery Branches 107

Surgical Anatomy of the Caudate Lobe 108

Surgical Treatment 113

General Principles 113

Assessment of Resectability 115

Indication for Surgical Resection 120

Isolated Extrahepatic Bile Duct Resection 121

Independent Caudate Lobectomy (S1) 122

Central Hepatic Resections 123

Extended Right Resections 124

Extended Left Resections 125

Surgical Technique 129

Position of the Patient 129

Incision 129

Intraoperative Exploration 130

Hepatic Pedicle Dissection and Lymphadenectomy 130

Bile Duct Resection Alone 131

Independent Caudate Lobectomy (S1) 132

Right Hepatectomy with Caudate Lobectomy (S4a, S5, S6, S7, S8 + S1) 133

Right Trisectionectomy with Caudate Lobectomy (S4, S5, S6, S7, S8 + S1) 135

Left Hepatectomy with Caudate Lobectomy (S2, S3, S4 + S1) 138

Left Trisectionectomy with Caudate Lobectomy (S2, S3, S4, S5, S8 + S1) 139

Central (Preserving) Hepatectomy 141

Hepatectomy with Portal Resection and Reconstruction 143

Hepatectomy with Arterial Resection and Reconstruction 148

Hepatopancreatoduodenectomy (HPD) 149

Biliary Anastomosis 150

Results of Surgery 153

Morbidity and Mortality 153

Long-term Results 157

Recurrence 159

The Role of Liver Transplantation 163

Indications and Results 163

Combined Transplantation 165

Transplantation with Adjuvant and Neoadjuvant Treatments 166
Conclusions 167

Adjuvant and Neoadjuvant Treatments 169
Chemotherapy 169
Radiotherapy 170
Chemoradiation Therapy 170
Neoadjuvant Therapy 171
Conclusions 172

Palliative Treatments 175
Palliation of Jaundice 175
Chemotherapy, Radiotherapy and Photodynamic Therapy 179

Part 2: Intrahepatic Cholangiocarcinoma

Diagnosis 187
Ultrasound 187
Computed Tomography 188
Magnetic Resonance Imaging 190
Angiography 192

Prognostic Factors 193
Gross Type 193
T Category 195
N Category 196
Microscopic Pattern 199

Staging Systems 203
TNM Staging System According to UICC/AJCC 203
TNM Classification According to the LCSGJ 206
Conclusions 210

Surgical Treatment 213
Intraoperative Assessment of Resectability 213
Indications for Surgical Resection 214
Type of Surgical Resection 214
Indications for Lymphadenectomy 217
Extrahepatic Metastases 219

Results of Surgery 221
    Morbidity and Mortality 221
    Long-Term Survival 222
    Recurrence 226

The Role of Liver Transplantation 229

Adjuvant and Palliative Treatments 233
    Adjuvant Therapy 233
    Palliative Therapy 235

Subject Index 239

Part 1
Hilar Cholangiocarcinoma

Reporting Cholangiocarcinoma: Pathological Aspects

Definitions

Cholangiocarcinoma is a malignant tumour composed of cells resembling those of the bile ducts. According to WHO classification [1] the term cholangiocarcinoma is reserved for carcinomas arising in the intrahepatic bile ducts. For this reason, tumours arising from extrahepatic bile ducts should be designated as extrahepatic bile duct carcinomas. However clinical and pathological differentiation of intrahepatic from extrahepatic bile duct cancers can be difficult. Cancers arising from the bile duct epithelium of the right and left hepatic ducts and at the bifurcation are also considered cholangiocarcinomas and are called "hilar cholangiocarcinomas". Intrahepatic (or peripheral) cholangiocarcinoma is a primary liver cancer and can arise from any portion of the intrahepatic bile duct epithelium [2].

The TNM staging system of the American Joint Committee on Cancer (AJCC) and the International Union Against Cancer (UICC) applies to all primary carcinomas of the liver, including hepatocellular carcinomas, intrahepatic bile duct carcinomas and mixed tumours [3]. General Rules for the Clinical and Pathological Study of Primary Liver Cancer of the Liver Cancer Study Group of Japan also applies to all primary carcinomas of the liver [4]. Hilar cholangiocarcinoma arises from the extrahepatic bile ducts (right and left hepatic ducts at or near their junction) and is considered an extrahepatic carcinoma [5]. The TNM staging system for malignant tumours of the extrahepatic bile ducts of the American Joint Committee on Cancer (AJCC) and the International Union against Cancer (UICC) is recommended [3]. Classification of Biliary Tract Carcinoma of the Japanese Society of Biliary Surgery (JSBS) is also applied [6].

In most peripheral cholangiocarcinomas, hard, compact, and grayish-white massive or nodular lesions are found in the liver. They may grow inside the dilated bile duct lumen or show an infiltrative growth along the portal pedicle. Usually the tumours are not big compared to the whole liver. Haemorrhage and necrosis are infrequent, and the association with cirrhosis is only occasional. Tumour located just beneath the capsule of the liver shows umbilication, as in metastatic liver cancer.

A. Guglielmi, A. Ruzzenente, C. Iacono (eds.) *Surgical Treatment of Hilar and ICC.*
© Springer 2008

In most hilar cholangiocarcinomas, the tumour infiltrates and proliferates along the extrahepatic bile duct, which is thickened in most cases. Mass formation may be minimal and there could be thickening and enlargement of the portal region. The infiltration in the liver has an arborescent appearance. Extensive parenchymal infiltration in also observed in most cases.

In the peripheral type, there is no dilatation of intrahepatic bile ducts in non-cancerous areas; in the hilar type this dilatation is often prominent. Moreover, in hilar cholangiocarcinoma there is frequently cholestasis, biliary fibrosis and cholangitis with abscess formation. These findings may also be present in peripheral cholangiocarcinoma, which involves the hepatic hilum.

Differentiation of intrahepatic from extrahepatic bile duct cancer may be difficult in cases with massive tumour at the hilum of the liver. In surgical cases, cancers occurring in the hilum are often small and can be identified relatively easily as being intra- or extrahepatic of origin.

Maybe the pathological differentiation of intra- and extrahepatic bile duct carcinoma will become easier thanks to morphological, immunohistochemical and molecular studies.

Clinical outcome of intra- and extrahepatic cholangiocarcinoma will become more evident after studying a larger number of surgically resected cases.

However it is difficult to compare the benefits of different surgical approaches described in many studies since there are several discrepancies. First of all, different stage classification systems are applied (Japanese vs. UICC), resulting in different tumour stages. Second, there is no consensus on the extent of the pathomorphological examination of the resection specimens; consequently results can vary considerably.

In this study we used a checklist based on a standardized pathological staging of specimens and resection margins for cholangiocarcinoma that closely follows the surgical procedure and also includes the pathological details necessary for comparison with other series, both Japanese and American.

Clinical Information

- *Relevant history*. Family history of liver tumours; prior surgery for cancer; ulcerative colitis; viral hepatitis (HBV, HCV); haemochromatosis; cirrhosis; bile duct disease (e.g. sclerosing cholangitis); inflammatory bowel disease.
- *Relevant findings*. Tumoural markers, jaundice.
- *Relevant imaging studies*. CT, MRI, US, ECPR. They should be sent to the Pathologist, especially when there is a hilar cholangiocarcinoma, in order to correlate radiological and pathological findings.
- *Prior diagnostic procedure*. Fine needle aspiration (FNA), brushing, needle biopsy.
- *Clinical diagnosis description*.
- *Procedure description*. lobectomy, partial hepatectomy, total hepatectomy,

non-neoplastic liver biopsy, needle biopsy, wedge biopsy, segmental bile duct resection.

Intraoperative Consultation

Resection margin assessment includes bile ducts at the cut margin and the hepatic section surface (Fig. 1). Intraoperative examination of the bile ducts at the cut margin is recommended in order to evaluate the lining epithelium for invasive carcinoma or in situ carcinoma or dysplasia (intraepithelial neoplasia). It is important to evaluate carefully all surgical margins on frozen section (en face) (Figs. 2,3), with the option of re-resection, including an assessment of vascular (lymphatic and blood vessel) and perineural invasion. Local recurrence is often related to residual tumour located in the proximal or distal surgical margins of the bile duct or to tumour located along the dissected soft tissue margin in the portal areas (circumferential or radial margin).

Local recurrence (usually at the surgical margins) is most common with carcinoma arising in the extrahepatic bile duct.

In some cases it may be difficult to evaluate margins on frozen section preparations because of inflammation and reactive atypia of the surface epithelium or within intramural mucous glands. If surgical margins are free of carcinoma, the distance between the closest margin and the tumour edge should be measured.

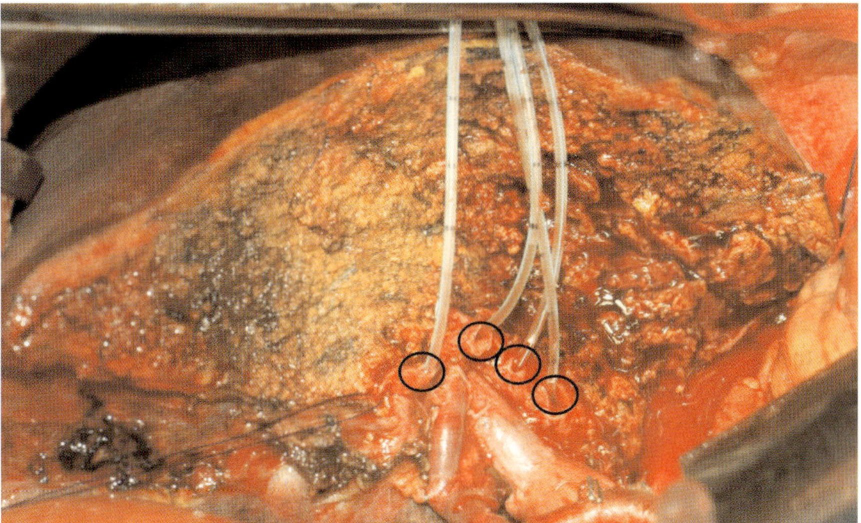

Fig. 1 Operative field after left hepatectomy, intraoperative histological evaluation of the bile duct resection margins

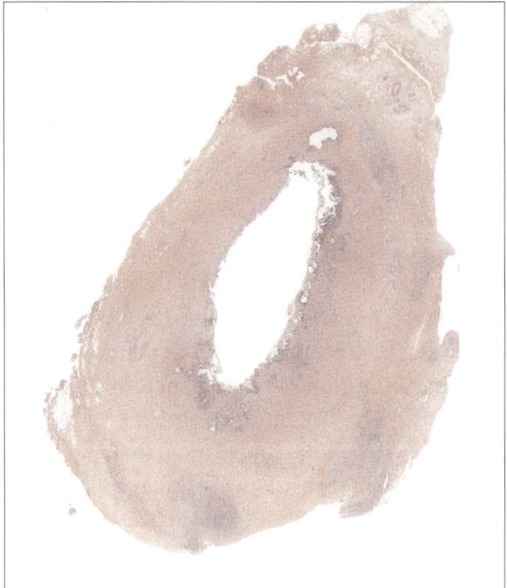

Fig. 2 Bile duct cross section for evaluation of surgical resection margin

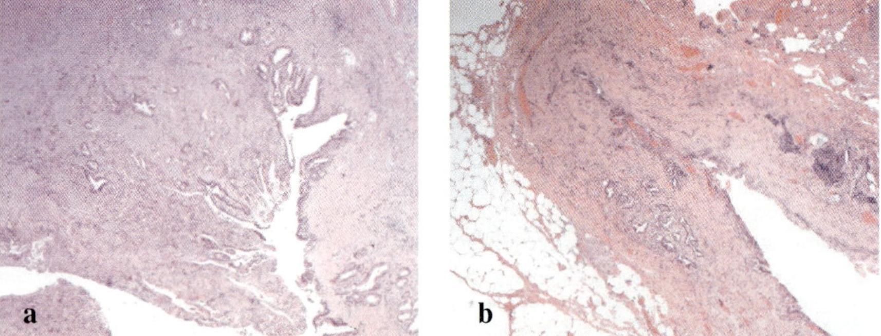

Fig. 3a,b a Presence of adenocarcinoma at surgical margin of the bile duct. **b** Negative bile duct margin

Macroscopic Examination

It is mandatory to examine the specimen in a fresh, unfixed state, in the operating theatre in close cooperation with the surgeons. The bile ducts should be probed and the site of origin of the carcinoma must be identified exactly. This is more important for carcinoma arising in the extra hepatic bile duct, in relation to the longitudinal extension of the neoplasia (Bismuth-Corlette Classification) [7]. The tumour should then be recorded in relation to the main branches/trunk of the portal vein or hepatic artery, also using radiological data.

In case of suspected tumour adherence to the portal vein requiring vessel resection, the segment should be separated from the specimen, serially sectioned and submitted "in toto" so that tumour invasion can be checked histologically. Both ends and perivascular tissue have to be considered as additional resection margins.

Local tumour extension and invasion of adjacent structures should also be reported.

Specimen

– *Liver.* Size (3 dimensions); Weight; Descriptive features (external/cut surfaces); Bile duct / vessels on cut surface
– *Extrahepatic Bile Duct.* Dimension of bile ducts (length and thickness of wall); External surface; Obstruction (partial / complete)
– *Margins.* Transection margin, Bile duct margin

The intraoperative examination of the bile ducts at the cut margin is recommended in order to evaluate the lining epithelium for carcinoma in situ or dysplasia.

The raw surface of a hepatectomy may be large, rendering it impractical for complete examination. The surgeon should be consulted to determine the critical foci that may require microscopic evaluation. Grossly positive margins should be microscopically confirmed and documented. If the margins are grossly free of tumour, judicious sampling of the cut surface in the region closest to the nearest identified tumour nodule is indicated.

If the neoplasm is found near the surgical margin, the distance from the margin should be reported.

The adipose tissue is very important for carcinoma arising in the extrahepatic bile: it is difficult to investigate and represents the periductal soft tissue dissected in the portal area. The outer surface should be marked with India ink and the tissue, with the bile duct inside, should be sectioned perpendicularly in subsequent, numbered specimens that should be submitted for histological examination.

The hepatic section margin should also be marked with India ink, and the whole specimen should be cut with sections made perpendicularly to the capsule (pay attention to the hepatic hilum).

Tumour(s)

– *Location.* With reference to the bile ducts: intrahepatic or hilar (Fig. 4)
– *Extent of Biliary Involvement.* For hilar cholangiocarcinoma: involvement of right hepatic duct - left hepatic bile duct - junction of right and left hepatic ducts - common bile duct (Bismuth classification). If more than one anatomical portion is involved, all involved portions should be recorded in the order of involvement, first indicating the portion in which the bulk of the tumour is located.

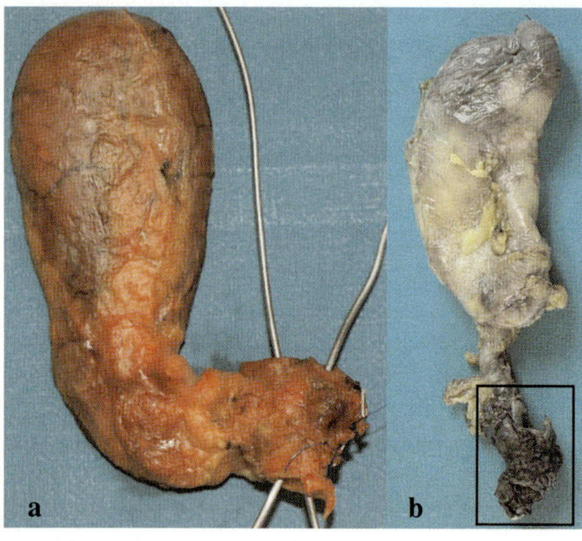

Fig. 4a,b Hilar cholangio-carcinoma. **a** Neoplasm of the bile duct without liver parenchyma involvement. **b** Fatty tissue margin (radial margin) marked with India ink

If possible specify the growth pattern in the bile duct wall (papillary, nodular, flat type)

– *Size*
– *Tumour Margins*
– *Gross Type*
  Mass forming. The nodular type of cholangiocarcinoma is relatively well demarcated but it is not encapsulated. In the vast majority of cases there is a single nodule. Often there are small metastatic nodules around the principal tumour (Fig. 5)
  Infiltrating (periductal). Tumour infiltrates and proliferates along the bile duct, which is usually thickened. There is minimal mass formation and thickening and enlargement of the portal region. The infiltration in the liver has an arborescent appearance. In most cases there is also extensive parenchymal infiltration (Fig. 6)
  Intraductal polypoid growth
– *Nodule/Number of Nodules*. In the diffuse involvement of the liver, there are small (usually <1 cm) tumour nodules distributed uniformly over the entire liver. Nodules are not sharply demarcated from the non-neoplastic parenchyma
– *Tumour appearance*. E.g., number of nodules, color, consistency, haemorrhage, necrosis, bile, stones
– *Extension* to adjacent organs/tissues (e.g., gallbladder, pancreas, etc.)
– *Vessel invasion* (portal vein, hepatic artery)

Samples from different areas of the tumour and from the tumour-free parenchyma should be submitted for histological evaluation.

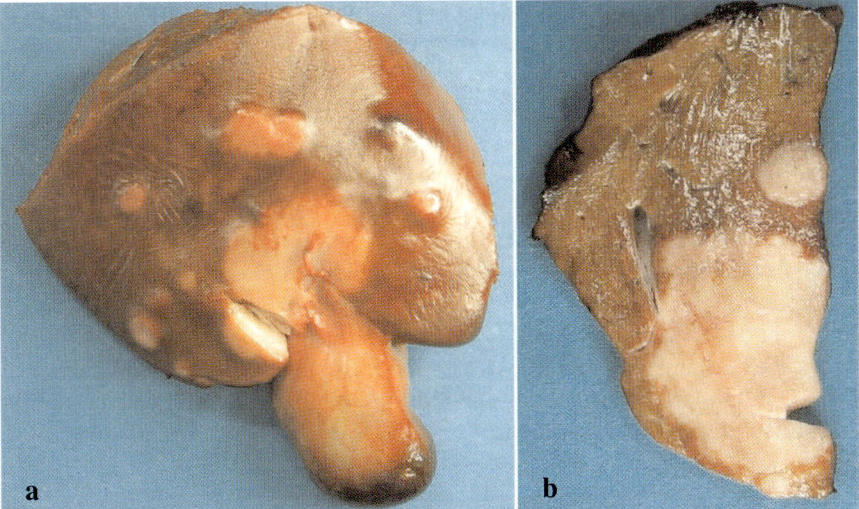

Fig. 5a,b Intrahepatic cholangiocarcinoma: mass forming type. **a** Surgical specimen with multiple nodules on surface. **b** The section of the liver discloses large tumour mass with satellite lesions

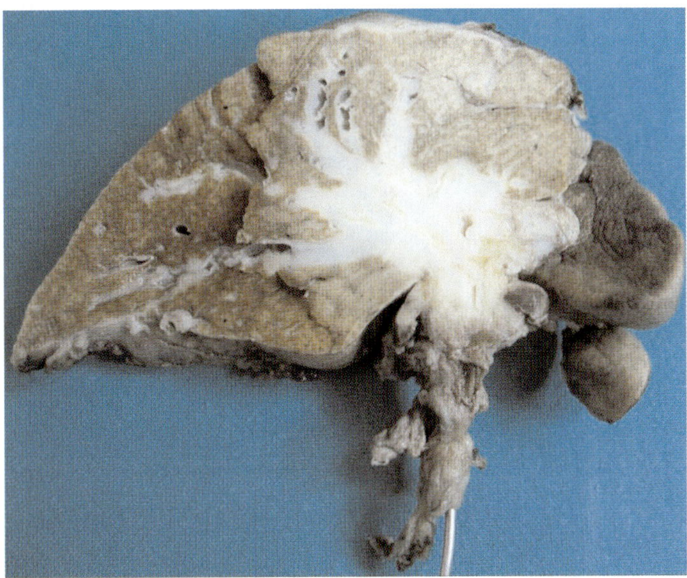

Fig. 6 Intrahepatic cholangiocarcinoma periductal infiltrating: tumour proliferate along the bile duct in an infiltrative pattern

Pathology Findings in Non-Neoplastic Liver

Cirrhosis, atrophy, duct obstructions/dilatation, calcifications, cysts, abscess, other.

Lymph Nodes (Location, Number)

The removed lymph nodes should be classified and numbered according to the Japanese classification. Although this classification is a complex system, it should be applied to be sure that the individual nodes are precisely defined.

According to UICC criteria the regional lymph nodes must be separated from non-regional lymph nodes; the involvement of non-regional lymph nodes is defined as distant metastases. The last classification reflects the anatomical site of larger node groups in relation to the liver and also closely follows the surgical procedure, since most nodes are already dissected and submitted separately.

All nodes should be submitted separately for histological examination and nodes with a diameter >1 cm should be half-sectioned. If lymph nodes cannot be identified on macroscopy the fibrofatty tissue should be investigated in order to detect neural tissue and lymphatics (Fig. 7).

Frozen Tissue (Molecular Studies)

-   Neoplastic liver / Non-neoplastic liver

Microscopic Examination

Tumour(s)

–   *Histological type.* Histological tumour classification should be performed according to the generally accepted principles of the WHO. Although most carcinomas are adenocarcinomas, other histological types must be considered.

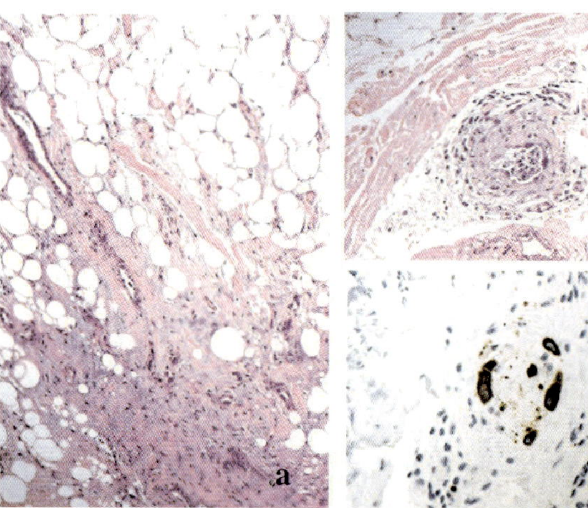

Fig. 7a–c Fibrofatty tissue of hepatoduodenal ligament infiltrated by adenocarcinoma. a Macroscopically evident infiltration. b,c Microscopic infiltration: presence of isolated adenocarcinoma glands (**b**), evidenced by keratin positivity (**c**)

- *Histological grade*. Well differentiated; Moderately differentiated; Poorly differentiated (Fig 8). The grade should be recorded according to the criteria of the WHO, based on architectural and cytological features. Well-differentiated cholangiocarcinomas form relatively uniform tubular or papillary structures; moderately-differentiated cholangiocarcinomas have moderately distorted tubular patterns with cribriform formations and/or a cord-like pattern; poorly-differentiated cholangiocarcinomas show severely distorted tubular structures with marked cellular pleomorphism.
- *Pattern of growth*
  Intrahepatic Cholangiocarcinoma: nodular (mass forming); number and location of nodules; infiltrating (periductal infiltrating); involvement of bile ducts.
  Hilar Cholangiocarcinoma: extension of biliary involvement. Involvement of right hepatic duct - left hepatic bile duct - junction of right and left hepatic ducts - common bile duct (Bismuth-Corlette classification). Involvement of bile duct wall (confined to or beyond the wall). Involvement of bile duct wall should be evaluated on cross-sectional circumference of the duct wall.

If confined to the wall, if possible specify the deepest involved layer (mucosa, fibromuscular layer, subserosa, serosa surface).

Involvement of intrahepatic ducts or hepatic parenchyma: if there is involvement of hepatic parenchyma, if possible specify the depth of invasion (<5 mm, ≥5 mm, <20 mm, ≥20 mm)

Extent of Invasion

- *Vessel invasion*. If possible, specify the depth of invasion: adventitia, media, intima
- *Adjacent tissue/organs*. If possible, specify the depth of invasion: in mm if parenchyma or layer of wall or organ. Involvement of: liver capsule, hepatic falciform ligament, adipose tissue of porta hepatis
- *Blood / lymphatic invasion* (Fig. 9)
- *Peri-endoneural invasion* (Fig. 10)

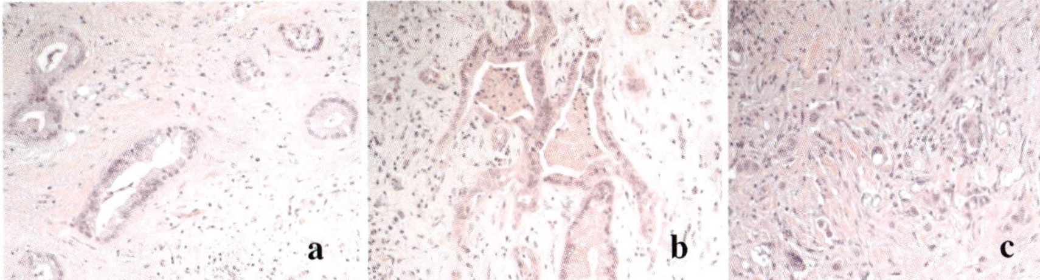

Fig. 8a–c Grading: well (**a**), moderated (**b**), and poorly (**c**) differentiated adenocarcinoma

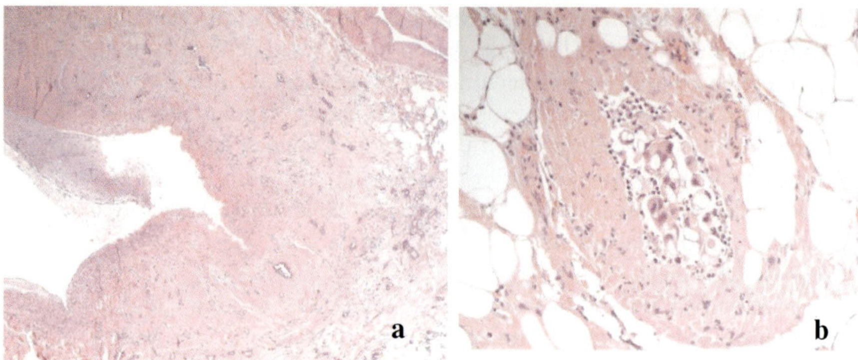

Fig. 9a,b a Macroscopic vessel invasion: adenocarcinoma infiltrating tonaca media of portal vein. **b** Miscoscopic vascular invasion

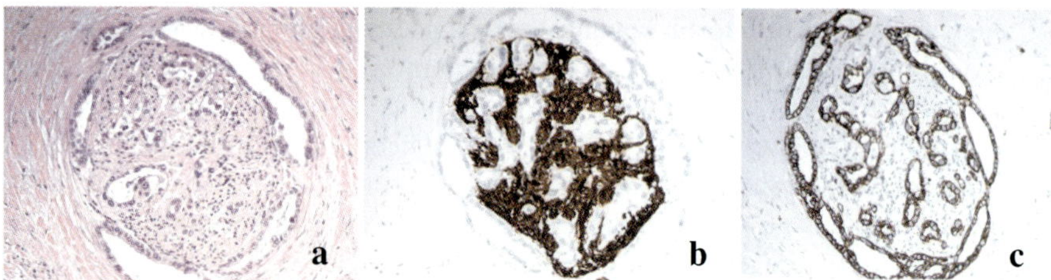

Fig. 10a–c Periendoneural-invasion. **a** Ematossilin-eosin. **b** S100 protein: nerve positivity. **c** Cytokeratin: neoplastic glands positivity

Peri-endoneural and lymphatic invasion are common in the extrahepatic bile duct carcinomas. They should be specifically evaluated since they are associated with adverse outcome.

Additional Pathology Findings (if Present)

– *Bile Duct Dysplasia*. Biliary intraepithelial neoplasia (dysplasia) is characterized by abnormal epithelial cells with multilayering of nuclei and micropapillary projections into the duct lumen. Abnormal cells have an increased nuclear-cytoplasmic ratio, a partial loss of nuclear polarity and nuclear hyperchromasia. These lesions are divided into low-grade and high-grade lesions. Some data suggest a hyperplasia-dysplasia-carcinoma sequence in the biliary tree.
– *Papillomatosis*. This lesion consists of dilated intrahepatic and extrahepatic bile ducts filled with papillary or villous excrescences. Microscopically, these excrescences are papillary or villous adenomas with a fibrovascular stalk covered with a columnar or glandular epithelium. Biliary papillomatosis is soft and white, red or tan. Sometimes there is some atypia and multi-

layering of nuclei. Occasionally, foci of in situ or invasive carcinoma are observed.
- *Benign tumour(s)*
- *Cirrhosis/fibrosis*
- *Haemosiderosis*
- *Portal vein thrombosis*
- *Hepatitis*
- *Other*

Margins

- *Parenchymal margin*
  Cannot be assessed
  Uninvolved by invasive carcinoma
  Distance of invasive carcinoma from closest margin
  Involved by invasive carcinoma
- *Bile duct margin (proximal-hepatic; distal-duodenal)*
  Cannot be assessed
  Uninvolved by invasive carcinoma
  Presence of in situ carcinoma or dysplasia (specify margin)
  Involved by invasive carcinoma (specify margin)

Specify extent / type of invasion (lymphatic and /or blood vessel invasion, dissemination of tumour cells). If the margins are free of cancer, the distance in millimeters between the tumour edge and the surgical cut end should be recorded.

Lymph Nodes

- *Number*
- *Number with metastasis* (specify location of nodes with metastases if possible)

The total number of nodes should be counted during the histological examination, as well as the number of metastatic nodes and any perinodal invasion, in particular lymphatic and perineural invasion should be noted.

Immunohistochemistry

Cholangiocarcinoma cells express cytokeratins 7 and 19, carcinoembryonic antigen—CEA, epithelial membrane antigen—EMA, BER-EP4 and blood group antigens. Hepatocyte antigen is not usually expressed by cholangiocarcinoma. Mucus core (MUC) proteins 1, 2, 3 are also detectable in carcinoma cells.

Immunohistochemistry can be useful in distinguishing cholangiocarcinoma from metastatic carcinoma, especially in bioptic specimens. Occasionally, dysplastic changes in neighboring bile ducts suggest biliary origin. In addition, diffuse expression of cytokeratin 20 favors metastatic adenocarcinoma, particularly from the colon (also CDX2 positive) (Figs. 11,12).

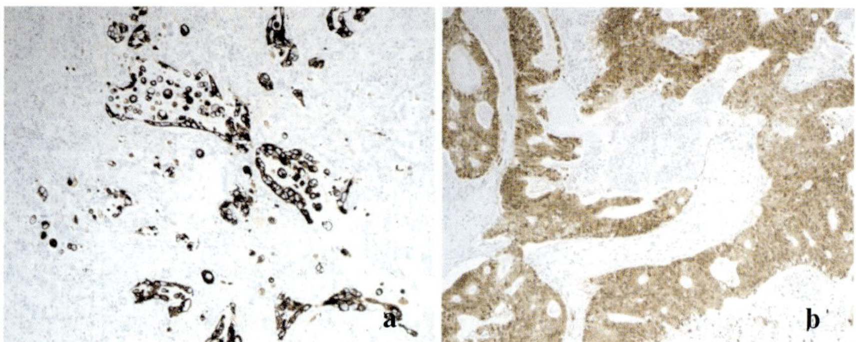

Fig. 11a,b Immunohistochemistry. **a** Cholangiocarcinoma: CK 7 positivity. **b** Liver metastasis of colonic adenocarcinoma CDX2 positivity

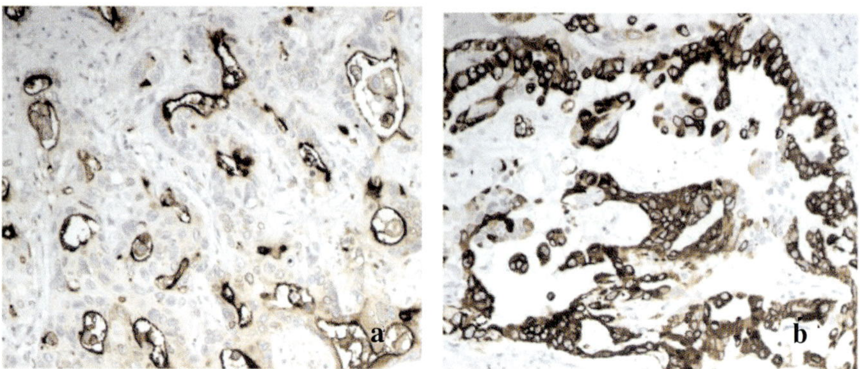

Fig. 12a,b Cholangiocarcinoma: positive immunostaining for MUC1 (**a**) and MUC 2 (**b**)

References

1. Hamilton SR, Aaltonen LA (2000) Pathology and genetics of tumours of the digestive system:WHO classification of tumours. IARC Press, Lyon
2. Ishak KG, Goodman ZD, Stocker JT (2001) Tumours of the liver and intrahepatic bile ducts. Atlas of tumour pathology, 3rd Series, Fascicle 31. Armed Forces Institute of Pathology, Washington DC
3. Greene FL, Page DL, Fleming ID et al (eds) (2003) AJCC Cancer staging manual, 6th edition. Springer, New York
4. Liver Cancer Study Group of Japan (2003) General rules for clinical and pathological study of primary liver cancer, 2nd English edition. Kanehara, Tokyo.
5. Albores-Saavedra J, Henson DE, Klimstra DS (2000) Tumours of the gallbladder, extrahepatic bile ducts, and ampulla of vater. Atlas of tumour pathology, 3rd Series, Fascicle 27. Armed Forces Institute of Pathology, Washington DC
6. Japanese Society of Biliary Surgery (2004) Classification of biliary tract carcinoma, 2nd English edition. Kanehara, Tokyo
7. Bismuth H, Corlette MB (1975) Intrahepatic cholangioenteric anastomosis in carcinoma of the hilus of the liver. Surg Gynecol Obstet 140(2):170–178

Diagnosis

Diagnosis of cholangiocarcinoma is usually suspected in presence of obstructive jaundice or high cholestasis in blood test values. Currently, many preoperative studies can be used to achieve a correct diagnosis; they can be direct or indirect, invasive or non-invasive (Table 1).

In absence of previous operations a stenosis of the biliary tree associated with the aforesaid symptoms arouses suspicions of a probable hilar cholangiocarcinoma. However, it must be emphasisized that not all stenoses are neoplastic; in fact until now from 5 to 15% [1–3] of patients resected due to suspected cholangiocarcinoma turn out to be non-neoplastic or suffering from other neoplasms at the definitive pathology examination [4]. Since treatment of these lesions is surgical in any case, in patients with a resectable hilar lesion a pathological diagnosis prior to surgical exploration is not mandatory [4].

Ultrasound (Endoscopic, Intraductal, Transabdominal)

Ultrasound represents the technique of choice for confirming obstructive jaundice. In fact it allows easy detection of the dilatation of the intra- and extrahepatic biliary systems. However, although it shows high diagnostic reliability (80–94%) in detecting biliary dilatation and the level of obstruction, its reliability in diagnosing the cause of obstruction decreases.

Hilar cholangiocarcinoma may be presumed at ultrasound in presence of a hilar hypoechoic mass that has spread along the biliary tract, determining dilatation of the upstream biliary system. Sometimes the lesion may be surrounded by hyperechoic tissue resulting from fibrosis [5]; other indirect signs suggestive of a correct diagnosis are the ductal abnormalities, ductal obstruction, or vascular involvement of hilar structures that this technique can reveal (Fig. 1).

A. Guglielmi, A. Ruzzenente, C. Iacono (eds.) *Surgical Treatment of Hilar and ICC*.
© Springer 2008

Table 1 Sensitivity of different diagnostic tools for preoperative staging of hilar cholangiocarcinoma

	US/Doppler US	CT	MRI/MRCP	EUS/FNA	ERCP	PTC	Cholangioscopy	PET
Tumour diagnosis	±	+++	+++	+++	+++	+++	+++	+
Staging according to Bismuth-Corlette	±	++	+++	+	++	+++	+++	-
Portal vein involvement	+++	+++	+++	-	-	-	-	-
Hepatic artery involvement	++	++	++	-	-	-	-	-
Lobar atrophy	++	+++	+++	-	+	+	-	-
I level lymph nodes	+	++	++	+++	-	-	-	++
II level lymph nodes	+	++	++	+	-	-	-	++
Liver metastasis	++	++	++	-	-	-	-	++
Extrahepatic metastasis	-	++	+	-	-	-	-	++
Peritoneal carcinomatosis	-	+	+	-	-	-	-	++

US, Ultrasonography; *CT*, computed tomography; *MRI*, magnetic resonance imaging; *MRCP*, magnetic resonance cholangiopancreatography; *EUS*, endoscopic ultrasonography; *FNA*, fine-needle aspiration; *ERCP*, endoscopic retrograde cholangiopancreatography; *PTC*, percutaneous transhepatic cholangiography; *PET*, positron emission tomography; ±, useless; +++, very useful; ++, useful +, few useful

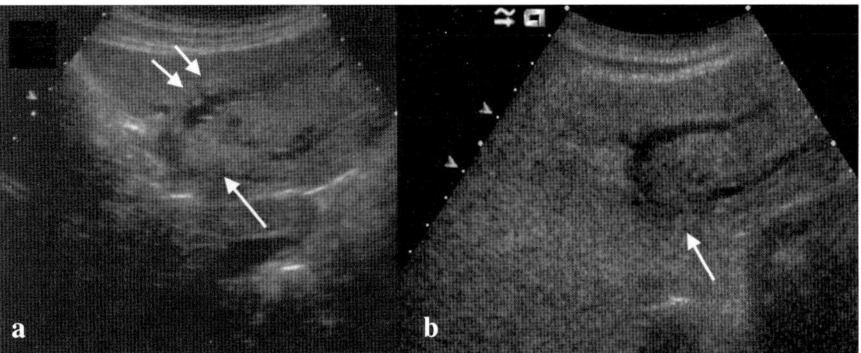

Fig. 1a,b Ultrasound images of hilar cholangiocarcinoma. **a** Hilar hypoechoic mass is visible (*white arrow*) with dilatated bile duct for hepatic segment 2 and segment 3 (*double white arrow*); **b** contrast enhanced US showing hypovascular mass with dilatated bile ducts in the left lobe

The introduction of sonographic contrast agents has enhanced the diagnostic accuracy of this technique, as the hilar lesion can be better typified during the different phases of vascular uptake; however this method is not useful for evaluating intraductal spreading [6].

Endoscopic ultrasound can aid in approaching hilar cholangiocarcinoma although it has been shown to be more useful in the study of pancreatic and peri-ampullary neoplasms. Echoendoscopy may show the neoplasm as a round or fusiform hypoechoic mass involving the wall of the duct and/or surrounding tissue.

Echoendoscopy presents sensitivity similar to endoscopic retrograde cholangiopancreatography (ERCP) and greater than transabdominal ultrasound and CT in the identification of small tumours [7,8]. In a recent study De Witt [9] reports a detection rate of 96% (23 of 24 cases) for proximal biliary mass, and in 16 of these patients the other procedures failed to show the lesion. The main advantage of echoendoscopy consists in guiding fine needle aspiration for cytology in patients with a doubtful stenosis or negative cytology after ERCP. Two recent studies [9,10] show high sensitivity, specificity and diagnostic accuracy rates: 89, 100 and 91% [10] and 77, 100 and 79% [9], respectively. The limit of this latter study is that pathological correlation has been carried out in only 8 of 24 resected patients (33%). Echoendoscopy associated with FNA seems a sensitive method for diagnosing hilar lesions; it has a low negative predictive value (29%) but in the case of negative examination, neoplastic disease cannot be excluded.

A more advanced use of ultrasonography comes with intraductal ultrasound which can be performed through percutaneous or endoscopic routes. This method is not widespread in clinical practice and it is mainly used in a few Asian centers. Compared to echoendoscopy it offers more advantages for exploration of the proximal biliary tract with better results in diagnosis and staging. Analogously for the pancreas the main limit of intraductal ultrasound is the low penetration of the transducer. Nevertheless, in the future it may provide good results that need to be evaluated with prospective studies.

In 2005 Stavropoulos et al. [11] reported the results in 61 patients with jaundice without mass at preoperative workup, with a biliary tract stenosis documented by ERCP (malignant obstruction in 43 cases and benign in 18); subjects underwent ultrasound with a high frequency probe (20 MHz). While ERCP showed 25 false negative cases, 22 of whom had malignant stenosis, intraductal ultrasound showed only 7 false-negative cases and 3 false-positive. The percentage of patients with positive diagnosis for malignant disease was 2.06 times higher for intraductal echography than ERCP. The diagnostic accuracy has changed from 58% in ERCP alone, to 90% in ERCP combined with intraductal ultrasound. Recently Japanese authors [12] introduced intraductal tridimensional ultrasonography, that would have a role of great magnitude compared to the standard technique of evaluating the extent of the neoplasm and its relationship to the portal axis. In addition, this novel technique would allow performing the volumetric assessment of the tumour, which appear to have significant prognostic value, and allow evaluation of the efficacy of palliative therapy such as laser and photodynamic therapy.

Computed Tomography

As to pathological findings, hilar cholangiocarcinoma shows three different aspects at CT scan [13,14]:
1. Infiltrative: determines a focal stenosis of biliary ducts and comprises more than 70% of cases;
2. Nodular: shows a hilar mass resembling peripheral cholangiocarcinoma and therefore it is difficult to differentiate a main duct neoplasm from advanced peripheral neoplasm invading the biliary ducts at the confluence;
3. Papillary: rare, appears as an intraductal polypoid lesion.

The infiltrative pattern on enhanced CT scan with contrast agents is demonstrated as a focal area of ductal involvement with lumen occlusion; the neoplastic area shows high attenuation compared to normal parenchyma in 80% of cases. The nodular pattern on CT appears as a large area of low attenuation with a hypervascular peripheral rim as intrahepatic cholangiocarcinoma [13]. The nodular variant presents as an intraductal lesion with low attenuation of the intensity compared with surrounding parenchyma and biliary dilatation. Those rare forms are often multiple and disseminated to the entire biliary tree.

Multislice spiral CT allows diagnostic accuracy of 86% [15] which in the experience of Tillich et al. reaches 100% [16]. Arterial contrast phase has allowed a diagnostic rate of 100% for both infiltrating and nodular types. Multislice technique allows better acquisition of information and a complete visualization of the biliary tree during the different phases of contrast injection. The infiltrating type lesion is showed as a nodular or round mass with high attenuation during arterial contrast phase and subsequently it presents attenuation features similar to hepatic parenchyma in the dominant portal phase. These characteristics allow differentiating infiltrative cholangiocarcinoma from other benign lesions or lymph nodes that do not usually form a mass or result hypodense. The nodular variant is hypodense compared to normal liver during both the dominant arterial and portal phases, as in intrahepatic cholangiocarcinoma (Fig. 2).

A recent study considered the hypothesis of differentiating cholangiocarcinoma from periductal fibrosis in patients with hepatolithiasis through CT scan; the parameters considered are density of periductal tissue, presence of ascites, portal vein occlusion, lymph node enlargement and biliary stones.

Magnetic Resonance Imaging

The use of T2-weighted sequences permits acquisition of images that present a low signal in solid tissue and circulating blood and a high signal in static fluids such as bile or pancreatic juice. This provides a MR-cholangiopancreatography without using specific contrast, an invasive maneuver that can cause complications. Another advantage is that it permits cholangiographic study even in patients who had previously undergone upper digestive tract surgery.

Data from the literature show that there are no differences between imaging obtained from MR-cholangiography vs. ERCP; comparative and prospective studies have shown that MR-cholangiography is better than ERCP for recognizing the proximal extent of the tumour since it allows one to detect dilatation above the stenosis, not communicating and therefore untraceable by direct cholangiography. The accuracy of MR-cholangiography to assess the level and biliary extent is similar to that obtained with direct cholangiographic techniques (ERCP, PTC) [17–20]. It is the best technique for studying the biliary tract since it allows evaluation above and below the lesion (Fig. 3).

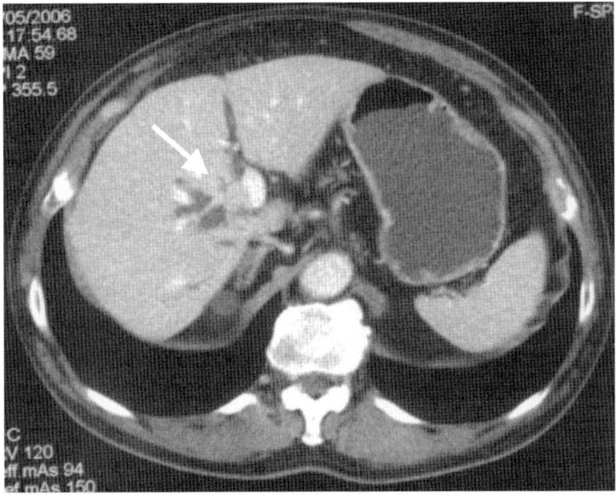

Fig. 2 Axial CT image shows an hyperattenuating mass at the biliary confluence (*white arrow*)

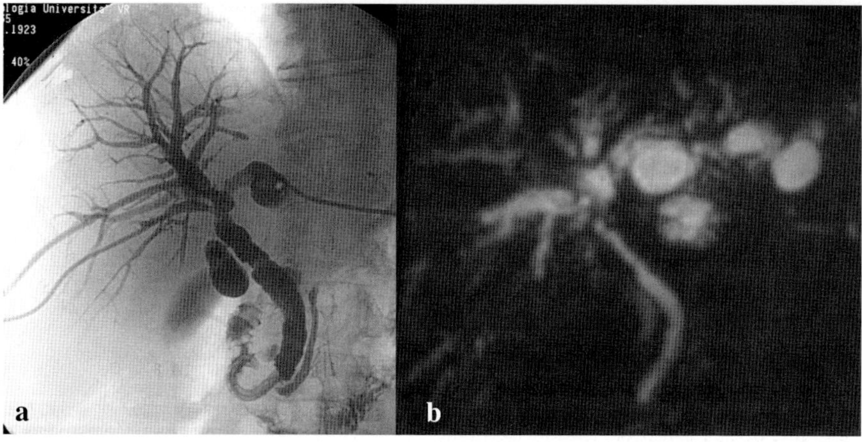

Fig. 3a,b Hilar cholangiocarcinoma. **a** Transhepatic cholangiogram showing hilar cholangio-carcinoma with the involvement of bile duct confluence and of the left hepatic bile duct. **b** MRCP confirms infiltration of the left hepatic duct with upstream dilation

Hilar cholangiocarcinoma has an intensity of signal similar to that of the intrahepatic on MRI in both T1- and T2-weighted images (Fig. 4). The majority of these tumours are hypovascular compared to adjacent parenchyma, showing a progressively increasing heterogeneous uptake that reaches the highest peak in late sequences [21].

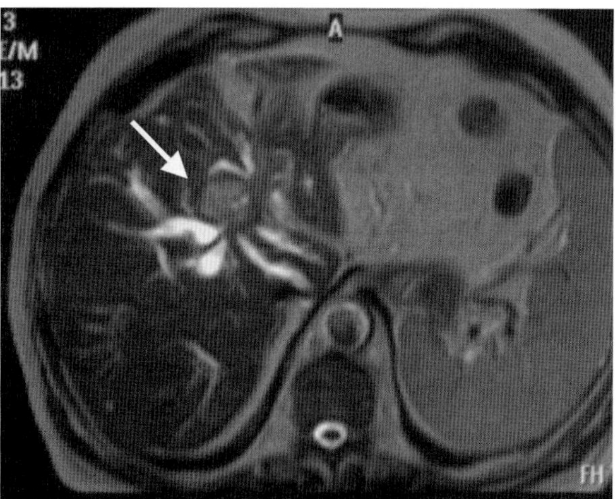

Fig. 4 Axial T2-weighted image shows a hyperintense mass in the hepatic hilum (*white arrow*)

Positron Emission Tomography

At the end of the 1990s Delbeke [22] foresaw a potential role for this technique in the diagnosis of these neoplasms; nevertheless today this diagnostic technique seems more useful in preoperative staging than in the diagnosis of hilar cholangiocarcinoma. In the identification of peripheral cholangiocarcinoma it shows an accuracy of 95 vs 69% of the extrahepatic one. This difference is due to the different size of the presenting tumours, the former being larger. In hilar cholangiocarcinoma it is useful to recognize the nodular type even in lesions larger than 1 cm (sensitivity 85%) while its utility is low for the infiltrative type that is more frequent (sensitivity 18%) [23]. It could have a role in the diagnosis of cholangiocarcinoma presenting with atypical radiological aspects or in absence of histologic malignant diagnosis [23]. Conversely, in the experience of Kluge et al. [24] in 2001, PET presented a high sensitivity (92.3%) and specificity (92.9%) in diagnosing and localizing cholangiocarcinoma while it only played a minor role in staging, particularly lymph node staging; in fact it has identified metastatic lymph nodes in only 2 of 15 cases while for distant metastases it has an accuracy of 70% (7 of 10 cases).

In a comparative study between CT vs. PET FDG, in 30 cases with extrahepatic cholangiocarcinoma CT resulted reliable in 80% of the cases while PET was reliable in 60% of cases [25].

Direct Cholangiography (ERCP and PTC)

Direct visualization of the biliary tree is achieved by means of endoscopic retrograde cholangiography and percutaneous transhepatic cholangiography that provide a precise and complete opacification with contrast material.

Since the introduction of ultrasound (CT and especially MRCP) in clinical practice, indication of these techniques for diagnosis has decreased and they are mainly applied for operative purposes. The application of these direct and invasive techniques has to be proposed by the hepatobiliary team since the choice of method, either ERCP or PTC, is fundamental. If the latter is chosen, it is necessary to specify the right or left approach; in fact the choice of the exact method must be tailored to the needs of the patient, considering the diagnostic purpose as well as the therapeutic possibility (surgical resection, surgical palliation, nonsurgical palliation).

The techniques show noticeable complication rates; PTC has a morbidity rate of 3–5% and the main complications are cholangitis, biliary leakage with potential bile peritonitis or perihepatic biliary collection (biloma), haemobilia, bilhemia, and subcapsular or intrahepatic haematoma. The complications of ERCP are cholangitis whose risk is enhanced by severe stenosis, since the introduction of the contrast that is not drained increases infective risk; to prevent infection, biliary decompression after the diagnostic procedure of the stenosis is mandatory.

Success rates of PTC range from 95 to 100% of jaundiced patients with biliary obstruction, while for ERCP with a recognized papilla, the rate is about 90%.

Of the two procedures PTC allows a better evaluation of cholangiocarcinoma, especially hilar compared to ERCP since it can better visualize the proximal biliary tract above the stenosis. The advantage of ERCP compared to PTC and MRCP is the possibility of performing brushing cytology or intraductal biopsy for pathological evaluation; however the success rate of these technique is low, about 50–60% [26].

On direct cholangiography, cholangiocarcinoma shows as an annular stricture since most of the tumour is infiltrative. Polypoid type is rare and some forms producing mucin present intraluminal defects.

PTC performed by experienced personnel [27] and in large series correctly shows the site of stenosis in a range between 96 and 99% and reveals the nature of the lesion at a rate of between 93 to 99%, respectively.

Cholangioscopy (Peroral, Percutaneous)

Cholangioscopy associated with biopsy has an important role in the differential diagnosis of biliary stenosis [28–32]. It can be performed through a peroral endoscopic or a percutaneous approach [30–33]; the former is the less invasive route and does not necessarily require sphincterectomy, with the advantage that it can be performed at the same time as ERCP, reducing the time of diagnosis and preoperative hospitalization. Conversely percutaneous transhepatic cholangioscopy requires a gradual dilatation of the PTBD path.

Although both techniques are useful diagnostic tools, peroral cholangioscopy is less efficacious compared to percutaneous transhepatic for evaluating the longitudinal extent of the tumour due to the technical and mechanical limitations of this approach [32,33].

As mentioned above, the cytological and histological results obtained through endoscopic trans-papillary approach or percutaneously under fluoroscopy are not good: Ponchon reports a sensitivity rate in malignant lesions of 36% with cytology and 43.5% with pinch biopsy (47% in cholangiocarcinoma) [31]. On the other hand, when cyto-histological samples are taken under cholangioscopy results improve as the sample is taken on direct vision of the suspect area; this improvement is reflected in a sensitivity rate arriving at 78% for diagnosis of malignancy and 82.4% for cholangiocarcinoma [31]. In Nimura's experience with 257 cholangioscopies the sensitivity rate was 81% in malignant stenosis and 96% in cholangiocarcinoma [34]. Neuhaus reports sensitivity values above 75%, as well [35].

Fokuda [32] reports similar results in the peroral approach: he identifies with ERCP/tissue sampling 22/38 cases of malignant stenosis and 35/38 benign lesions (in three cases the samples were inadequate) with an accuracy of 78%, a sensitivity of 57.9% and a specificity of 100%; the results change significantly after the application of peroral cholangioscopy, which allows identifying 38 of 38 malignant lesions and 33 of the 38 benign lesions with an accuracy of 93.4%, sensitivity of 100% and specificity of 86.8%.

The recent introduction of the Narrow Band Imaging technique increases reliability compared to White Light Imaging. The Nagoya group, which is one of the supporters of percutaneous cholangioscopy, has introduced this technique into the workup of cholangiocarcinoma [36].

Angiography

In the last 20 years the role of angiography has diminished after the introduction of new imaging techniques. Once believed fundamental for assessing loco regional diffusion in hilar neoplasms, especially when evaluating portal and arterial involvement, today these evaluations are carried out by spiral CT, MRI and color-Doppler sonography. Angiography is no longer performed and now belongs to the history of these tumours.

References

1. Gerhards MF, Vos P, van Gulik TM et al (2001) Incidence of benign lesions in patients resected for suspicious hilar obstruction. Br J Surg 88(1):48–51
2. Knoefel WT, Prenzel KL, Peiper M et al (2003) Klatskin tumours and Klatskin mimicking lesions of the biliary tree. Eur J Surg Oncol 29(8):658–661
3. Nakayama A, Imamura H, Shimada R et al(1999) Proximal bile duct stricture disguised as malignant neoplasm. Surgery 125(5):514–521
4. Jarnagin WR, D'Angelica M, Blumgart LH (2006) Intrahepatic and extrahepatic biliary cancer. In: Blumgart LH (ed) Surgery of the liver, biliary tract, and pancreas. 4th edn. Saunders Elsevier, Philadelphia
5. Dancygier H, Nattermann C (1994) The role of endoscopic ultrasonography in biliary tract disease: obstructive jaundice. Endoscopy 26(9):800–802
6. Schuessler G, Ignee A, Hirche T, Dietrich CF (2003) [Improved detection and characterisation of liver tumours with echo-enhanced ultrasound]. Gastroenterol Z 41(12):1167-1176 (German)
7. Sugiyama M, Atomi Y, Wada N et al (1996) Endoscopic transpapillary bile duct biopsy without sphincterotomy for diagnosing biliary strictures: a prospective comparative study with bile and brush cytology. Am J Gastroenterol 91(3):465–467
8. Tio TL, Reeders JW, Sie LH et al(1993) Endosonography in the clinical staging of Klatskin tumour. Endoscopy 25(1):81–85
9. DeWitt J, Misra VL, Leblanc JK et al (2006) EUS-guided FNA of proximal biliary strictures after negative ERCP brush cytology results. Gastrointest Endosc 64(3):325–333

10. Fritscher-Ravens A, Broering DC, Knoefel WT et al (2004) EUS-guided fine-needle aspiration of suspected hilar cholangiocarcinoma in potentially operable patients with negative brush cytology. Am J Gastroentero 99(1):45–51

11. Stavropoulos S, Larghi A, Verna E (2005) Intraductal ultrasound for the evaluation of patients with biliary strictures and no abdominal mass on computed tomography. Endoscopy 37(8):715–721

12. Inui K, Miyoshi H (2005) Cholangiocarcinoma and intraductal sonography. Gastrointest Endosc Clin N Am 15(1):143–155

13. Han JK, Choi BI, Kim AY et al (2002) Cholangiocarcinoma: pictorial essay of CT and cholangiographic findings. Radiographics 22(1):173–187

14. Lim JH (2003) Cholangiocarcinoma: morphologic classification according to growth pattern and imaging findings. AJR Am J Roentgenol 181(3):819–827

15. Zandrino F, Benzi L, Ferretti ML et al (2002) Multislice CT cholangiography without biliary contrast agent: technique and initial clinical results in the assessment of patients with biliary obstruction. Eur Radiol 12(5):1155-1161

16. Tillich M, Mischinger HJ, Preisegger KH et al (1998) Multiphasic helical CT in diagnosis and staging of hilar cholangiocarcinoma. AJR Am J Roentgenol 171:651–658

17. Manfredi R, Masselli G, Maresca G et al (2003) MR imaging and MRCP of hilar cholangiocarcinoma. Abdom Imaging 28:319–325

18. Manfredi R, Barbaro B, Masselli G et al (2004) Magnetic resonance imaging of cholangiocarcinoma. Semin Liver Dis 24(2):155–164

19. Lee WJ, Lim HK, Jang KM et al (2001) Radiologic spectrum of cholangiocarcinoma: emphasis on unusual manifestations and differential diagnoses. Radiographics 21: S97-S116

20. Lopera JE, Soto JA, Munera F (2001) Malignant hilar and perihilar biliary obstruction: use of MR cholangiography to define the extent of biliary ductal involvement and plan percutaneous interventions. Radiology 220:90–96

21. Slattery JM, Sahani DV (2006) What is the current state-of-the-art imaging for detection and staging of cholangiocarcinoma? Oncologist 11(8):913–922

22. Delbeke D, Martin WH, Sandler MP et al (1998) Evaluation of benign vs. malignant hepatic lesions with positron emission tomography. Arch Surg 133(5):510–515; discussion 515–516

23. Anderson CD, Rice MH, Pinson CW et al (2004) Fluorodeoxyglucose PET imaging in the evaluation of gallbladder carcinoma and cholangiocarcinoma. J Gastrointest Surg 8(1):90–97

24. Kluge R, Schimdt F, Caca K et al (2001) Positron emission tomography with (18F)fluoro-2-deoxy-D-glucose for diagnosis and staging of bile duct cancer. Hepatology 33:1029–1035

25. Kato T, Tsukamoto E, Kuge Y et al (2002) Clinical role of (18)F-FDG PET for initial staging of patients with extrahepatic bile duct cancer. Eur J Nucl Med Mol Imaging 29(8):1047–1054

26. Rustgi AK (1989) Malignant tumours of the bile ducts: diagnosis by biopsy during endoscopic cannulation. Gastroinst Endosc 35:248–251

27. Gazzaniga GM, Faggioni A, Bondanza G et al (1990) Percutaneous transhepatic biliary drainage twelve years' experience. Hepatogastroenterology 37(5):517–523

28. Kim DI, Kim MH, Lee SK et al (2001) Risk factors for recurrence of primary bile duct stones after endoscopic biliary sphincterotomy. Gastrointest Endosc 54(1):42–48

29. Lee SS, Kim MH, Lee SK et al (2002) MR cholangiography versus cholangioscopy for evaluation of longitudinal extension of hilar cholangiocarcinoma. Gastrointest Endosc 56(1):25–32

30. Nimura Y, Kamiya J, Hayakawa N, Shionoya S (1989) Cholangioscopic differentiation of biliary strictures and polyps. Endoscopy 21(Suppl 1):351–356

31. Ponchon T, Genin G, Mitchell R et al (1996) Methods, indications, and results of percutaneous choledochoscopy. A series of 161 procedures. Ann Surg 223(1):26–36

32. Fukuda Y, Tsuyuguchi T, Sakai Y et al (2005) Diagnostic utility of peroral cholangioscopy for various bile-duct lesions. Gastrointest Endosc 62(3):374–382

33. Nagino M, Nimura Y (2006) Perihilar cholangiocarcinoma with emphasis on presurgical management. In: Blumgart LH (ed) Surgery of the liver, biliary tract, and pancreas. 4th edn. Saunders Elsevier, Philadelphia, pp 804–814
34. Nimura Y, Kamiya J (1998) Cholangioscopy. Endoscopy 30(2):182–188
35. Neuhaus H (1994) Cholangioscopy. Endoscopy 26(1):120–125
36. Nimura Y (2007) Cholangiocarcinoma- Diagnostic Work up. 7th Congress of EHPBA, Verona, Italy, June 6–9 2007

Preoperative Staging

The only successful treatment of cholangiocarcinoma is curative resection; evaluation of biliary involvement, either longitudinal or radial, loco-regional diffusion and presence of distant metastases are important for planning the therapeutic strategy.

The introduction of imaging techniques, especially spiral CT and MRI associated with MRCP, have changed evaluation of preoperative staging of cholangiocarcinoma; these procedures allow to obtain high definition images, and make possible to elaborate and perform tridimensional reconstructions in order to obtain a better definition of the tumour.

The required parameters for the two most widespread classifications of hilar cholangiocarcinoma [1,2] are obtained nowadays with non-invasive imaging techniques. Nevertheless the majority of series report underestimation rates of preoperative staging due to undiagnosed hepatic and peritoneal metastases, lymph-node metastases, major involvement of vascular structures and greater diffusion of the disease along the biliary ducts [2]. On the other hand, only a German study [3] reports errors of overstatement that risk excluding patients from the only treatment that can ensure a good outcome.

The questions that a hepatobiliary surgeon asks to the imaging in order to determine the correct therapeutic approach concern: definition of hilar anatomy; extent of the tumour along the biliary ducts, especially towards second order confluences; vascular relationship of the tumour with hepatic artery, portal vein and their left and right branches; presence or absence of parenchymal atrophy secondary to long-term portal branch involvement; volume and pattern of residual liver in order to plan surgical resection, preoperative biliary decompression and/or vascular embolisation.

A. Guglielmi, A. Ruzzenente, C. Iacono (eds.) *Surgical Treatment of Hilar and ICC.*
© Springer 2008

Evaluation of the Biliary Involvement (Longitudinal Extent)

Ultrasound

Transabdominal ultrasound does not contribute any information to the evaluation of this parameter. However echoendoscopy appears to be useful in staging cholangiocarcinoma; the lesion is detected as a hypoechoic mass within the lumen of the duct, frequently with infiltration of surrounding tissue. Sometimes the lesion is encased by hyperechoic tissue that is the expression of peritumoral fibrosis [4]. Tio et al. [5] reported a correct evaluation of T-stage in 85% of 43 cases with carcinoma of hilar and of the common hepatic duct. The limit of echoendoscopy is that exploration of the hilum is not always possible; in fact some authors report fewer data in proximal cholangiocarcinoma compared to distal cholangiocarcinoma [4].

MRCP

MRCP has an accuracy similar to direct cholangiography and is more powerful than CT in evaluating ductal involvement; it also allows detection of isolated obstructed ducts that are not communicating and thus are not identified by ERCP and/or PTC. In a comparative study between ERCP and MRCP in 40 patients, both techniques permitted diagnosis of biliary obstruction in 100% of cases, but MRCP was superior to ERCP in evaluating the extent of the tumour [6]. In another study comparing the two techniques, MRCP permitted correct Bismuth-Corlette classification of 78% of the patients and underestimated 22%. The authors noted that if management of the patients had relied only on MRCP, the definitive treatment would have been modified in 28% of the cases (five of 18 patients); this is mainly due to a mistaken assessment of second order ductal involvement. As a matter of fact, in Bismuth-Corlette stages I and II MRCP showed an accuracy of 90%, whereas in stage III and IV it presented errors of underestimation in three of seven cases. The authors concluded that MRCP must be considered a useful technique in the therapeutic planning for malignant hilar neoplasms: "accurate depiction of high grade strictures for which endoscopic drainage is not the option of choice can preclude unnecessary invasive imaging" [7]. Manfredi has shown that MRCP gives similar results of direct cholangiographic techniques although it is less effective in identifying the extent of small hilar lesions [8]; evaluating biliary involvement according to Bismuth-Corlette, he obtained accuracy in 84% of the cases (10 of 12).

Spiral CT

The diagnostic accuracy of CT in evaluating longitudinal diffusion is not particularly satisfying; in fact it ranges between 54 and 64% [13,14]. These low percentages are related to the type of diffusion of cholangiocarcinoma. It occurs under the epithelium along the wall of the biliary duct, and in the periductal tissue without affecting the epithelium, and therefore are difficult to assess on CT [15,16]. The use of biliary contrast materials administered orally or intravenously, which could have provided advantages, present some limitations since they are not correctly excreted in the patients with an obstructed biliary tract [17]. To increase diagnostic accuracy in evaluating longitudinal diffusion, Kim et al. [18] have proposed the use of spiral CT associated with direct cholangiography obtained by injection of contrast material in the nasobiliary or in the percutaneous transhepatic drainage with this technique Kim et al. have correctly assessed the involvement of primary confluence in 11 of 11 patients, and of second level confluence in 18 of 19 (95%). The correct extent of the neoplasm was achieved in 10 of 11 patients; the procedure showed a false positive case in the evaluation of second order confluence involvement [18]. Sensitivity, specificity, positive predictive value and negative predictive value rates were 100, 90, 90 and 100%, respectively.

In Lee's study [19], the association of CT and direct cholangiography allowed identifying the correct extent of the disease along the ducts in 46 of 55 patients (accuracy 84%), underestimation in seven of 55 patients, and overestimation in only two patients.

ERCP/PTC

If the majority of authors report underestimation errors in the evaluation of longitudinal diffusion, others [3] report a high rate of overestimation due to peritumoral fibrosis. Comparing the data of ERCP, PTC, and MRCP with surgical specimens the German authors report a correct evaluation with ERCP in 29% of the cases, with MRCP in 36%, and with PTC in 53%, an overestimation rate of 42, 41 and 31%, and underestimation rate of 31, 23 and 16%, respectively. In the experience of these authors the most reliable technique for studying hilar cholangiocarcinoma is PTC: significantly better than ERCP ($p<0.008$), slightly superior to MRCP ($p=0.06$), while ERCP and MRCP have similar results. The limit of ERCP is the evaluation of proximal extension of the tumour, determined by the absent or incomplete opacification of the intrahepatic biliary tree. MRCP, conversely, allows a correct image of both the hepatic lobes in about 90% of cases, while it has a lower ability than PTC ($p<0.019$) to evaluate the edges of the neoplasm. The main diagnostic problems concern stages III and IV of Bismuth-Corlette, which are better studied with PTC than ERCP or MRCP.

Rotational Cine-cholangiography

To overcome the limits of direct cholangiography a rotational cholangiographic technique has been proposed that allows correct evaluation of ductal anatomy and a better evaluation of intraductal diffusion of the tumour [9–11]. Miura [10] performed rotational cine-cholangiography in 60 patients with obstructive jaundice; he evaluated the biliary anatomy and the ability to visualise the main confluence as well as second order ductal confluences, and he compared the radiological findings with the pathological reports in 26 resected patients.

The percentage of primary confluence visualization was 97.6% with rotational cine-cholangiography, while it was 87% for right anterior-posterior confluence and 93.1% for medial left duct confluent. The diagnostic accuracy of neoplastic diffusion was 91.7% for common hepatic duct, 100% for right hepatic duct, 91.7% for left hepatic duct, 100% for right anterior duct, 83.3% for right posterior duct, and 100% for left medial duct. Nevertheless, the author concluded that rotational cine-cholangiography is a useful method for evaluating the anatomy of first and second order confluences and also for identifying the intraductal spread of the carcinoma [10].

Recently a new technique of rotational three-dimensional cholangiography was suggested [12] that is obtained by injecting contrast material through percutaneous transhepatic drainage and using the technique of digital angiography subtraction of images and 3-D reconstruction; this method would allow an accurate anatomical study of the biliary tree.

Cholangioscopy

Different authors, especially Japanese, believe that percutaneous transhepatic cholangioscopy is unrivalled for identifying superficial diffusion of cholangiocarcinoma [20–24].

Lee compared MRCP with percutaneous transhepatic cholangioscopy in the evaluation of longitudinal extent of cholangiocarcinoma and reported in the infiltrative form an optimal correlation between the two techniques: in 16/18 cases for type I of Bismuth-Corlette (88.9%), in 14/16 for type II (87.5%), in 19/23 for type IIIa (82.6%), in 14/14 for type IIIb (100%), and in 24/28 for type IV (85.7%), so that it is believed that MRCP must replace cholangioscopy; on the other hand cholangioscopy was more reliable for assessing polypoid and diffuse sclerosing types [25].

Nimura [24] confirmed these results and suggested that cholangioscopy aimed at preoperative diagnosis of cancer extent is indicated in patients with papillary type or nodular type cholangiocarcinoma since the mucosal extension of the tumour is easily observable. The evaluation of tumoral extension must be performed not only in the intrahepatic portion but also in the distal bile duct in order to tailor the resection (hepatobiliary or hepatopancreatoduodenectomy).

Evaluation of Radial Extent: Vascular Involvement, Parenchymal Involvement and Hepatic Lobar Atrophy

Echo-Doppler, echoendoscopy, CT and MRI contribute to evaluating the radial extension of cholangiocarcinoma.

Ultrasound

The involvement of vascular structures can be assessed by conventional ultrasound (US). Ultrasound presents a good evaluation of the vascular relationship also when it is performed endoscopically (EUS); a prospective study of Japanese authors [26] compared EUS with US, CT and angiography in a group of patients with hilar neoplasm who underwent hepatic resection with or without vascular resection: EUS has shown higher diagnostic accuracy (93%) compared to 74% of US, 84% of CT and 89% of angiography.

When transabdominal US is associated with Doppler US it allows correct evaluation of vascular correlation, particularly with respect to the main portal vein (Fig. 1). In the MSKCC study, this technique presented a sensitivity rate of 93% and a specificity of 99%, with a positive predictive value of 97% [27,28]; when compared to angio-CT, it presented similar or even better results (sensitivity 90%, specificity 99%, positive predictive value 95% for angio-CT).

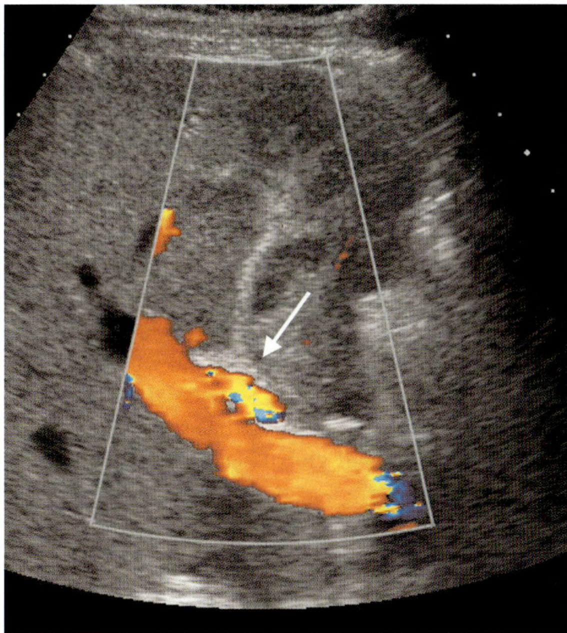

Fig. 1 Hilar cholangiocarcinoma. Doppler US showing involvement of left hepatic artery (*white arrow*)

MRI

MRI with angio-MR technique has results similar to those of angiography in evaluating vascular involvement in patients with hilar cholangiocarcinoma, showing an accuracy rate of 67%, overestimation of 8% and underestimation of 25% [29]. Lee et al. [30] compared angio-MR with angiography for image subtraction in 36 patients with hilar cholangiocarcinoma to evaluate the relationship of the tumour with hepatic artery, portal vein and their right and left branches. The percentage of visualisation of hepatic artery and portal vein was obtained in 78 and 94% of cases, respectively, with a sensitivity, specificity, and accuracy in detecting arterial infiltration of 58, 93 and 89% vs. 75, 99 and 96% for angiography. In evaluation of portal infiltration the percentages were comparable in the two techniques (sensitivity, specificity, and diagnostic accuracy of 78, 91, 89% for angio-MR, vs. 78, 92 and 90% for angiography). No statistical differences were shown between the two techniques; angiography was more specific only in the evaluation of arterial infiltration. These data confirm that angio-MR must replace angiography in the diagnosis and evaluation of vascular involvement in patients with suspected hilar cholangiocarcinoma.

CT

To assess the radial diffusion dynamic CT seems to have a high diagnostic reliability even superior to MRI [31]. It allows a vascular study with arterial and portal phases, analogous or superior to angiography (Fig. 2). In Lee's experience [19] CT showed an arterial involvement in 20 of 55 cases, and surgery confirmed this datum in 19 patients; only one case resulted false positive. Only three cases of the 35 patients in whom vascular involvement was excluded were underestimated with sensitivity of 86.4%, specificity of 97%, positive predictive value of 95%, negative predictive value of 91.4% and a global accuracy of 92.7%.

In this study, the authors utilised a single detector CT in the first phase of the study and subsequently a multi-detector CT. Comparing the results of the two different types of CT the authors showed that the former presented a greater number of false positive and false negative results with sensitivity, specificity, positive and negative predictive values and global accuracy of 72.8, 94, 87.5, 88.9, 88.5%, respectively, while on multi-detector CT the percentages were higher, 92.3, 100, 100, 94, and 96.6%, respectively. The data show better results with multi-detector CT but the difference are not statistically significant (p=0.406) [19]. In the evaluation of portal involvement CT has sensitivity, specificity, positive and negative predictive value and global accuracy of 76.9, 93.1, 81.8 and 85.5%.

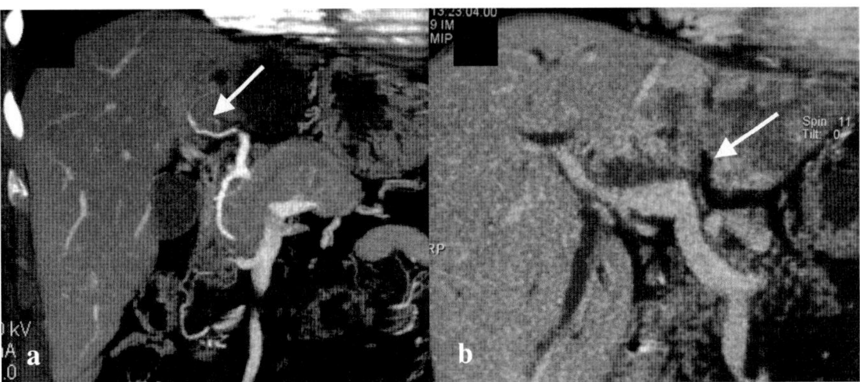

Fig. 2a,b CT image shows a hyperattenuating mass centered on the biliary confluence. Coronal reformatted image (**a**) shows infiltration of the left hepatic artery (*white arrow*). **b** Reformatted coronal CT-angiography shows infiltration of the left portal branch (*white arrow*)

Evaluation of Lobar Atrophy and Parenchymal Involvement

An important factor in Jarnagin and Blumgart staging is the parenchymal atrophy.

Lobar atrophy can be identified by abdominal ultrasound but is better evaluated by CT and MRI; it is characterised by a small hypovascular lobe with dilated ducts (Fig. 3).

In evaluating hepatic parenchymal involvement, which is present in about 60% of cases of hilar cholangiocarcinoma [32], CT and MRI prove useful. The diagnostic sensitivity of assessing this factor was 87% in Hanninen's study [32] and 75% in Manfredi's study, with an underestimation in 25% of the cases [29].

Preoperative Assessment of Tumour Resectability (T)

The diagnostic accuracy of CT in the evaluation of resectability varies from 60 to 74.5% [14,30,33]. Tillich believes that since spiral CT is unable to assess correctly the proximal extension of the tumour, it cannot be considered a definitive investigation for evaluating resectability. To achieve better results, Lee [19] associated it with direct cholangiography to increase reliability from 60 to 75%; 30 of 42 patients were correctly considered resectable while 12 patients were underestimated: six for longitudinal diffusion, three for diffusion of the tumour along the hepatoduodenal ligament, and three for vascular underestimation of the vascular involvement [19], with a positive predictive value of 71.4%. Of the

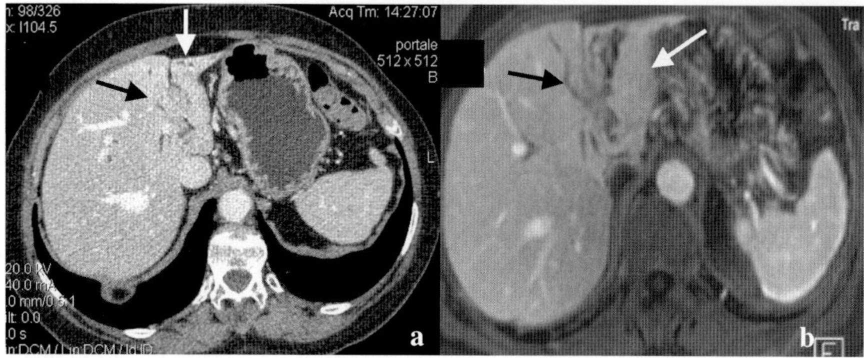

Fig. 3a,b CT image (**a**) shows hilar cholangiocarcinoma with involvement of left portal vein (*black arrow*) and left lobar atrophy (*white arrow*). **b** MRI portal phase confirms CT findings

13 cases considered unresectable, 11 were correctly assessed (negative predictive value 84.6%) while in two cases vascular involvement was overestimated. As previously mentioned, Otto [3] reported higher overestimation than underestimation rates in the valuation of Bismuth-Corlette staging; the same group reported that CT and MRI assessment of vascular involvement was only 50%, while in 24% of the patients who were shown to be without vascular involvement on preoperative studies, such involvement was confirmed on the operating table [3]. Evaluating Bismuth-Corlette classification, Otto [3] was able to stratify the surgical strategy preoperatively in a prospective study. In 48 of 59 cases, the surgical operation was the same as that estimated; in four cases the diffusion in the considerably involved biliary hemisystem was ignored, and in five and two patients respectively, resection was more or less extended than planned.

Evaluation of Lymph Node Status (N)

This parameter has been Achilles' heel of preoperative staging of all neoplasms; all investigations have failed to accurately identify this parameter, which is important not only for surgery but also for prognosis. Lymph-node involvement is present in 36–50% of patients with cholangiocarcinoma at diagnosis [32].

Transabdominal ultrasound does not provide sufficient information, while EUS has a diagnostic accuracy of 53–64% [5], with a sensitivity of 93% and a specificity of 18%. When echoendoscopy is associated with FNA, the accuracy is >90% [34].

Also CT accuracy is not high, especially in the evaluation of second level lymph nodes with a rate of 50% [19] (eight patients of 15 with N2 positive nodes); of the 40 patients with negative CT, two had lymph-node metastases.

Correct lymph node staging was obtained in 46/55 cases (83.6%).

MRI presents a value of reliability comparable to EUS. Hanninen [32] reported an accuracy of 60%. The limit is that size is not a reliable parameter; in fact lymph nodes of normal size may be metastatic; instead enlarged nodes may be inflammatory and non-metastatic [32].

A recent study [35] showed the utility of a lymph node-specific contrast agent (ultrasmall particles of iron oxide) used in the detection of lymph nodes in patients with prostate cancer. The results regarding the accuracy of this study are excellent but this agent has not yet been introduced in clinical practice.

PET results are discordant: some authors report a low rate of lymph-node metastasis detection (two of 15 cases in Kluge's experience [36]), while others [37] report an 86% accuracy rate; sensitivity is similar to CT, but specificity of PET is 100% vs. 59% of CT ($p<0.01$).

Evaluation of Metastases (M)

Abdominal ultrasound enhanced with contrast agent can better identify and typify hepatic lesions than conventional US; CT and MRI are also useful to focalise this parameter. PET is effective for staging due to its ability to detect distant metastases. Anderson [38] reported that 30% of the patients with distant metastases were not diagnosed with other radiological tests, while Kim [39] identified distant metastases in four of 21 patients with peripheral cholangiocarcinoma, not detected by other diagnostic techniques. In Kluge's study, the reliability rate in diagnosing distant metastases was 70% (peritoneum, lung) [36].

Preoperative workup often fails to ascertain the presence of peritoneal and hepatic metastases that are shown only by preliminary laparoscopy or laparotomy, since the small size of these lesions cannot be assessed by preoperative imaging.

Conclusions

In our opinion, the diagnostic flow chart reported in Figure 4 allows a correct evaluation of resectability without performing direct cholangiography.

Further diagnostic investigation, such as the probable use of invasive technique, biliary drainage, or restoring hepatic function, should be decided by the hepatobiliary team based on the performance status of the patient (presence/absence of sepsis, alteration of hepatic function, malnutrition) and the feasible therapeutic approach.

Optimising management allows to avoid invasive, risky and useless manoeuvres, long hospitalisation and delay of definitive treatment, and can facilitate selection of the patients for different therapeutic options.

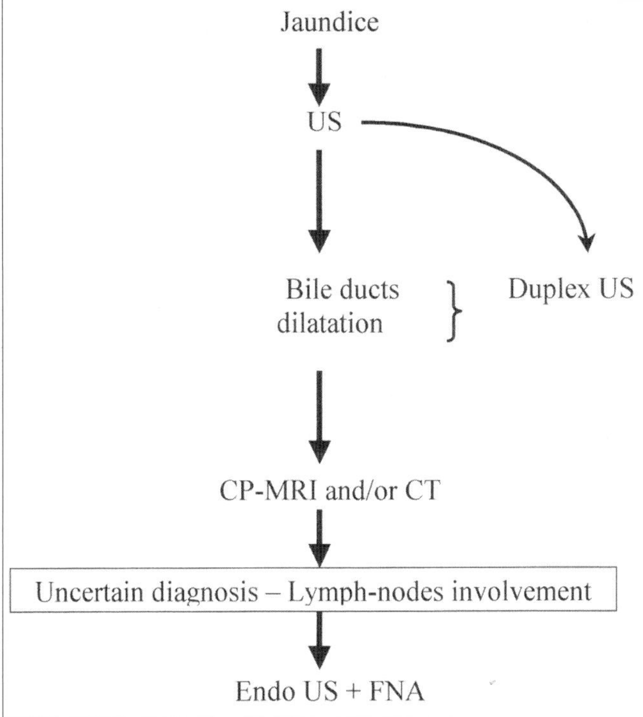

Fig. 4 Proposed non-invasive diagnostic flow chart for hilar cholangiocarcinoma

Study with MRI and MRCP, associated or not with CT and/or EUS, shows whether a cholangiocarcinoma is resectable or not. In presence of resectable tumour at preoperative non-invasive studies, a decision must be made considering jaundice, the concomitant presence of infection, the extent of the tumour along the biliary tract (Bismuth-Corlette staging), and the evaluation of remnant liver.

In presence of jaundice without signs of infection and in absence of lobar atrophy, one can proceed directly to surgery. In presence of cholangitis, preoperative biliary drainage is mandatory, preferably unilateral on the future remnant liver, bilateral or multiple if bilirubin level does not decrease or cholangitis persists. In presence of homolateral lobar atrophy, the atrophic lobe does not need draining, unless the patient presents signs of sepsis sustained by the undrained lobe when the volume of the future remnant liver is less than 30–40% of the total liver volume, it can prove useful to adopt the technique of portal vein embolisation, with preventive biliary drainage (Fig. 5).

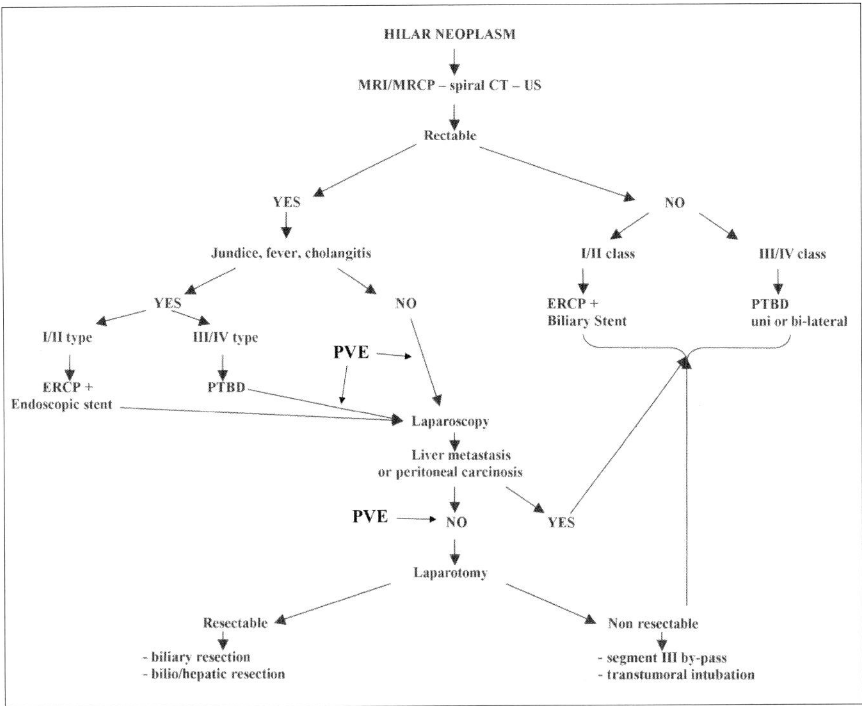

Fig. 5 Proposed diagnostic and therapeutic workup for hilar cholangiocarcinoma

References

1. Bismuth H, Corlette MB (1975) Intrahepatic cholangioenteric anastomosis in carcinoma of the hilus of the liver. Surg Gynecol Obstet 140(2):170–178
2. Jarnagin WR, Fong Y, DeMatteo RP et al (2001) Staging, resectability, and outcome in 225 patients with hilar cholangiocarcinoma. Ann Surg 234(4):507–517; discussion 517–519
3. Otto G, Romaneehsen B, Hoppe-Lotichius M, Bittinger F (2004) Hilar cholangiocarcinoma: resectability and radicality after routine diagnostic imaging. J Hepatobiliary Pancreat Surg 11(5):310–318
4. Dancygier H, Nattermann C (1994) The role of endoscopic ultrasonography in biliary tract disease: obstructive jaundice. Endoscopy 26(9):800–802
5. Tio TL, Reeders JW, Sie LH et al (1993) Endosonography in the clinical staging of Klatskin tumour. Endoscopy 25(1):81–85
6. Yeh TS, Tseng JH, Chiu CT et al (2006) Cholangiographic spectrum of intraductal papillary mucinous neoplasm of the bile ducts. Ann Surg 244(2):248–253
7. Zidi SH, Prat F, Le Guen L et al (2000) Performance characteristics of magnetic resonance cholangiography in the staging of malignant hilar strictures. Gut 46:103–106

8. Manfredi R, Brizi MG, Masselli G et al (2001) Malignant biliary hilar stenosis: MR cholangiopancreatography compared with direct cholangiography. Radiol Med 102:48–54

9. Furukawa H, Sano K, Kosuge T et al (1997) Analysis of biliary drainage in the caudate lobe of the liver: comparison of three-dimensional CT cholangiography and rotating cine cholangiography. Radiology 204(1):113–117

10. Miura F, Asano T, Okazumi S et al (1999) Rotational cine cholangiography: evaluation for use in diagnosing bile duct carcinoma. AJR Am J Roentgenol 173(4):1043–1048

11. Furukawa H, Sano K, Kosuge T et al (2000) Hilar cholangiocarcinoma evaluated by three-dimensional CT cholangiography and rotating cine cholangiography. Hepatogastroenterology 47(33):615–620

12. Uchida M, Abe T, Nishimura K et al (2002) Rotational three-dimensional cholangiography: initial clinical experience. Radiat Med 20(4):213–215

13. Nesbit GM, Johnson CD, James EM et al (1988) Cholangiocarcinoma: diagnosis and evaluation of resectability by CT and sonography as procedures complementary to cholangiography. AJR Am J Roentgenol 151(5):933–938

14. Tillich M, Mischinger HJ, Preisegger KH et al (1998) Multiphasic Helical CT in diagnosis and staging of hilar cholangiocarcinoma. AJR Am J Roentgenol 171:651–658

15. Wiston C, Teitcher J (2006) Computer tomography of the liver, biliary tract, and pancreas. Blumgarth H (ed) Surgery of the liver, biliary tract, and pancreas, 4th edn. Saunders Elsevier, Philadelphia, pp 266–305

16. Feydy A, Vilgrain V, Denys A et al (1999) Helical CT assessment in hilar cholangiocarcinoma: correlation with surgical and pathologic findings. AJR Am J Roentgenol 172(1):73–77

17. Fleischmann D, Ringl H, Schofl R et al (1996) Three-dimensional spiral CT cholangiography in patients with suspected obstructive biliary disease: comparison with endoscopic retrograde cholangiography. Radiology 198(3):861–868

18. Kim JH, Kim TK, Eun HW et al (2006) CT findings of cholangiocarcinoma associated with recurrent pyogenic cholangitis. AJR Am J Roentgenol 187(6):1571–1577

19. Lee HY, Kim SH, Lee JM et al (2006) Preoperative assessment of resectability of hepatic hilar cholangiocarcinoma: combined CT and cholangiography with revised criteria. Radiology 239(1):113–121

20. Iwahashi N, Hayakawa N, Yamamoto H et al (1998) Mucosal bile duct carcinoma with superficial spread. J Hepatobiliary Pancreat Surg 5(2):221–225

21. Kim DI, Kim MH, Lee SK et al (2001) Risk factors for recurrence of primary bile duct stones after endoscopic biliary sphincterotomy. Gastrointest Endosc 54(1):42–48

22. Sano T, Nimura Y, Hayakawa N et al (1997) Clinical utility of percutaneous transhepatic cholangioscopy in defining tumour extent: a case of mucin-producing bile duct carcinoma originating in the left caudate lobe. Gastrointest Endosc 46(5):455–458

23. Ponchon T, Genin G, Mitchell R et al (1996) Methods, indications, and results of percutaneous choledochoscopy. A series of 161 procedures. Ann Surg 223(1):26–36

24. Nagino M, Nimura Y (2006) Perihilar cholangiocarcinoma with emphasis on presurgical management. In: Blumgart H (ed) Surgery of the liver, biliary tract, and pancreas. 4th edn. Saunders Elsevier, Philadelphia, pp 804–814

25. Lee SS, Kim MH, Lee SK et al (2002) MR cholangiography versus cholangioscopy for evaluation of longitudinal extension of hilar cholangiocarcinoma. Gastrointest Endosc 56(1):25–32

26. Sugiyama M, Hagi H, Atomi Y, Saito M (1997) Diagnosis of portal venous invasion by pancreatobiliary carcinoma: value of endoscopic ultrasonography. Abdom Imaging 22(4):434–438

27. Hann LE, Greatrex KV, Bach AM et al (1997) Cholangiocarcinoma at the hepatic hilus: sonographic findings. AJR Am J Roentgenol 168(4):985–989

28. Jarnagin WR, D'Angelica M, Blumgart LH (2006) Intrahepatic and extrahepatic biliary cancer. In: Blumgart H (ed) Surgery of the liver, biliary tract, and pancreas, 4th edn. Saunders Elsevier, Philadelphia

29. Manfredi R, Barbaro B, Masselli G et al (2004) Magnetic resonance imaging of cholangio-carcinoma. Semin Liver Dis 24(2):155–164

30. Lee MG, Park KB, Shin YM et al (2003) Preoperative evaluation of hilar cholangiocarcino-ma with contrast-enhanced three-dimensional fast imaging with steady-state precession magnetic resonance angiography: comparison with intraarterial digital subtraction angiography. World J Surg 27(3):278–83

31. Zhang Y, Uchida M, Abe T et al (1999) Intrahepatic peripheral cholangiocarcinoma: comparison of dynamic CT and dynamic MRI. J Comput Assist Tomogr 23(5):670–677

32. Hanninen EL, Pech M, Jonas S et al (2005) Magnetic resonance imaging including magnetic resonance cholangiopancreatography for tumour localization and therapy planning in malignant hilar obstructions. Acta Radiol 46(5):462–470

33. Cha JH, Han JK, Kim TK et al (2000) Preoperative evaluation of Klatskin tumour: accuracy of spiral CT in determining vascular invasion as a sign of unresectability. Abdom Imaging 25(5):500–507

34. Hoffman BJ, Hawes RH (1995) Endoscopic ultrasonography-guided puncture of the lymph nodes: first experience and clinical consequences. Gastrointest Endosc Clin N Am 5(3):587–593

35. Harisinghani MG, Barentsz J, Hahn PF et al (2003) Noninvasive detection of clinically occult lymph-node metastases in prostate cancer. N Engl J Med 348(25):24912499

36. Kluge R, Schimdt F, Caca K et al (2001) Positron emission tomography with (18F)fluoro-2-deoxy-D-glucose for diagnosis and staging of bile duct concer. Hepatology 33:1029–1035

37. Kato T, Tsukamoto E, Kuge Y et al (2002) Clinical role of (18)F-FDG PET for initial staging of patients with extrahepatic bile duct cancer. Eur J Nucl Med Mol Imaging 29(8):1047–1054

38. Anderson CD, Rice MH, Pinson CW et al (2004) Fluorodeoxyglucose PET imaging in the evaluation of gallbladder carcinoma and cholangiocarcinoma. J Gastrointest Surg 8(1):90–97

39. Kim YJ, Yun M, Lee WJ et al (2003) Usefulness of 18F-FDG PET in intrahepatic cholangiocarcinoma. Eur J Nucl Med Mol Imaging 30(11):1467–1472

The Role of Laparoscopy in Preoperative Staging

Hilar cholangiocarcinoma often presents in an advanced stage when the disease is not resectable. Despite the evolution of imaging techniques such as CT, MRI, ultrasonography and PET scan, it is often difficult to identify small liver and peritoneal metastases at preoperative staging, and the precise extent of the disease along the hepato-duodenal ligament is difficult to determine. In about 25–46% of patients the condition of non-resectability is confirmed only at laparotomy [1,2].

Diagnostic laparoscopy has been proposed as a staging tool in hepatobiliary neoplasms [3]; its main aim is to identify the patients with disseminated disease not diagnosed at preoperative workup, in whom the disadvantages of an unnecessary laparotomy can be avoided. In non-resectable patients the laparoscopic approach significantly reduces the length of stay, cost and the time of initiation of palliative therapies [4].

In the literature, reports on the use of laparoscopy in cholangiocarcinoma staging are limited. Some authors suggest carrying out laparoscopic exploration immediately before laparotomy; others use it as a staging method preliminary to invasive procedures such as portal vein embolisation and/or biliary drainage [5].

Technique

Laparoscopic examination is generally performed under general anaesthesia. The laparoscopic access is done in the line of the planned laparotomy incision [6]. Usually two or more port sites are used in order to more easily manipulate the structures and obtain biopsy samples of suspect lesions. A 30-degree scope is usually used to provide an optimal view from the periumbilical or right upper quadrant access. Laparoscopic examination entails careful inspection of the entire abdominal cavity, with particular attention to the parietal peritoneum which is often the site of carcinomatosis. The next exploration evaluates the superior and inferior surfaces of right and left lobes, hepatoduodenal ligament

A. Guglielmi, A. Ruzzenente, C. Iacono (eds.) *Surgical Treatment of Hilar and ICC.*
© Springer 2008

and porta hepatis; examination allows a direct view of the aspect of hepatic parenchyma, and the possible presence of cirrhosis or lobar atrophy not seen at preoperative studies. The occurrence of evident parietal and visceral peritoneal localisations must be confirmed by frozen-section histology, which is not indicated, due to the risk of neoplastic seeding for lesions that will not change the criteria of resectability (i.e. regional lymph-node metastases) [7]. The dissection of hilar structures is not indicated due to the highly demanding laparoscopic manoeuvre and its limited utility in evaluating the local extent of the disease.

Results

Diagnostic laparoscopy has a low morbidity and almost no mortality. In the literature, the complication rate of laparoscopy for hepatobiliary neoplasms varies from 0 to 4% [5,7–10]. Major and more frequently observed complications are postoperative bleeding, intestinal perforation and intra-abdominal infection. Minor complications are wound infection, abdominal pain and pulmonary complications.

Neoplastic seeding in the port sites is described in the laparoscopy studies for hepatobiliary neoplasms. Nieveen reported an incidence of 2% in his study of 420 diagnostic laparoscopies for upper gastrointestinal neoplasms [7]. Other reports confirmed the occurrence of port site metastases (Shoup observed an incidence of 0.8% in a series of 1,650 diagnostic laparoscopies [11]).

In the literature, the yield of laparoscopy is variable and the frequency of identification of preoperative misdiagnosed lesions ranges from 20 to 40% [5,6,9,12]. Many factors contribute to this variability: limited series, different type of cholangiocarcinoma (i.e. hilar cholangiocarcinoma and gallbladder neoplasm), long observation time during which the new preoperative imaging techniques are not employed.

The most frequent causes of unresectability are peritoneal carcinomatosis, vascular invasion, hepatic metastases, and involvement of non-regional lymph nodes. The accuracy of laparoscopy in detecting the causes of non-resectability is highly variable; while it is very useful for identifying hepatic and peritoneal metastases, it is of little value in evaluating vascular invasion and lymph-node metastases. Laparoscopic sensitivity in defining peritoneal carcinomatosis is over 80% in some series; it permits identification of more than 60% of patients with hepatic metastases, while detection of metastatic lymph nodes is lower than 30% and it rarely allows identification of patients who are non-resectable due to local advanced disease [5,6]. The usefulness of laparoscopy is also determined by the stage of the disease; in a series of 84 patients Connor observed that the accuracy of laparoscopy for T3 lesions according to the MSKCC preoperative staging system was significantly higher compared to stage T1-2 patients. The cause of non-resectability was metastatic disease, which was 68% in T3, 37% in T2, and 26% in T1 ($p<0.05$) [12].

Other authors have proposed the use of peritoneal lavage with instillation of 100–200 cc saline solution to enhance the accuracy of laparoscopy; however, in the literature the only experience with hilar cholangiocarcinoma shows a low accuracy. In a series of 26 patients Martin [13] reported a positive peritoneal cytology in only 2 of 6 cases with peritoneal carcinomatosis.

Laparoscopic Ultrasound

Laparoscopic ultrasound can be useful for increasing the sensitivity and accuracy of laparoscopic staging. Laparoscopic ultrasound probe is linear at high frequency (8–10 MHz) and gives high-resolution images; besides Doppler ultrasound evaluation it permits identification of vascular structure infiltration. An ultrasound probe is inserted through the 10-mm umbilical or right upper quadrant port and a complete examination of hepatic parenchyma is performed, since it can detect hepatic lesions smaller than a few millimeters. The initial ultrasound examination evaluates the left and right lobes; subsequently positioning the probe transversely to the hepato-duodenal ligament, the common hepatic duct, hepatic artery and portal vein are inspected, as are the main lymph node stations. Laparoscopic ultrasound can guide biopsy of suspect lesions.

In the literature, many experiences have been reported on the use of laparoscopic ultrasound, but are limited to small series of patients [7,12,14–16]. Although laparoscopic ultrasound allows precise visualisation of the hepatic parenchyma and hilar structures its utility in the definition of resectability of hilar cholangiocarcinoma is not supported by the literature.

Van Delden was the first to propose the technique; in his series of 31 patients with unresectable hilar cholangiocarcinoma, only 10 patients (28%) were identified by traditional laparoscopy and the diagnosis was obtained by ultrasound in only one patient [16]. This fact was confirmed by more recent observations which reported that the procedure was useful in less than 20% of cases [6,8,9]. Only one author showed a significant increase in laparoscopic examination through ultrasound; in his experience, in 84 patients the yield of laparoscopy alone was 24%, while it was 41% in the case of laparoscopy associated with ultrasound [12]. The causes of the limited usefulness of laparoscopic ultrasound are correlated with the difficulties in correctly defining the local neoplastic extent at the hepatic hilum, due to inflammatory alterations and the presence of biliary stents [6]. Sensitivity of ultrasound in diagnosing hepatic metastases is very high; however, these patients often have hepatic lesions that emerge from the hepatic surface and are easily detected by direct vision. Ultrasound evaluation of regional and non-regional lymph nodes does not distinguish between metastatic and inflammatory lymph nodes; moreover lymph node biopsy under ultrasound control is very demanding. Tillman underlined the fact that very often the ultrasound suspicion of unresectability is not confirmed at subsequent laparotomy; in his study of 110 patients, ultrasound revealed a non-resectable disease in 19 cases, but at subsequent laparotomy the diagnosis was confirmed in only one patient.

Despite a better sensitivity in diagnosing hepatic metastases, ultrasound evaluation does not offer any useful elements for evaluating lymph-node involvement at the hepatic hilum.

Conclusions

Diagnostic laparoscopy in hilar cholangiocarcinoma has a low yield since the neoplasm is often unresectable because locally advanced. The accuracy of the procedure is high in the identification of peritoneal and hepatic metastases but its sensibility is low even with ultrasound support, as it does not allow identification of patients with local advanced disease or metastatic lymph nodes. In advanced disease, when the percentage of metastatic disease is high, the methodical use of laparoscopy could be helpful.

References

1. Hemming AW, Reed AI, Fujita S et al (2005) Surgical management of hilar cholangiocarcinoma. Ann Surg 241(5):693–699; discussion 699–702
2. Lang H, Sotiropoulos GC, Fruhauf NR et al (2005) Extended hepatectomy for intrahepatic cholangiocellular carcinoma (ICC): when is it worthwhile? Single center experience with 27 resections in 50 patients over a 5-year period. Ann Surg 241(1):134–143
3. D'Angelica M, Jarnagin W, Dematteo R et al (2002) Staging laparoscopy for potentially resectable noncolorectal, non-neuroendocrine liver metastases. Ann Surg Oncol 9(2):204–209
4. Cuschieri A (2001) Role of video-laparoscopy in the staging of intra-abdominal lymphomas and gastrointestinal cancer. Semin Surg Oncol 20(2):167–172
5. Goere D, Wagholikar GD, Pessaux P et al (2006) Utility of staging laparoscopy in subsets of biliary cancers: laparoscopy is a powerful diagnostic tool in patients with intrahepatic and gallbladder carcinoma. Surg Endosc 20(5):721–725
6. Weber SM, DeMatteo RP, Fong Y et al (2002) Staging laparoscopy in patients with extrahepatic biliary carcinoma. Analysis of 100 patients. Ann Surg 235(3):392–399
7. Nieveen van Dijkum EJ, de Wit LT (1999) Staging laparoscopy and laparoscopic ultrasonography in more than 400 patients with upper gastrointestinal carcinoma. J Am Coll Surg 189(5):459–465
8. Vollmer CM, Drebin JA, Middleton WD et al (2002) Utility of staging laparoscopy in subsets of peripancreatic and biliary malignancies. Ann Surg 235(1):1–7
9. Tilleman EH, de Castro SM, Busch OR et al (2002) Diagnostic laparoscopy and laparoscopic ultrasound for staging of patients with malignant proximal bile duct obstruction. J Gastrointest Surg 6(3):426–430; discussion 430–431
10. Jarnagin WR, Bodniewicz J, Dougherty E et al (2000) A prospective analysis of staging laparoscopy in patients with primary and secondary hepatobiliary malignancies. J Gastrointest Surg 4(1):34–43
11. Shoup M, Brennan MF, Karpeh MS et al (2002) Port site metastasis after diagnostic

laparoscopy for upper gastrointestinal tract malignancies: an uncommon entity. Ann Surg Oncol 9(7):632–636

12. Connor S, Barron E, Wigmore SJ et al (2005) The utility of laparoscopic assessment in the preoperative staging of suspected hilar cholangiocarcinoma. J Gastrointest Surg 9(4):476–480

13. Martin RC 2nd, Fong Y, DeMatteo RP et al (2001) Peritoneal washings are not predictive of occult peritoneal disease in patients with hilar cholangiocarcinoma. J Am Coll Surg 193(6):620–625

14. Callery MP, Strasberg SM, Doherty GM et al (1997) Staging laparoscopy with laparoscopic ultrasonography: optimizing resectability in hepatobiliary and pancreatic malignancy. J Am Coll Surg 185(1):33–39

15. Lo CM, Lai EC, Liu CL et al (1998) Laparoscopy and laparoscopic ultrasonography avoid exploratory laparotomy in patients with hepatocellular carcinoma. Ann Surg 227(4):527–532

16. van Delden OM, de Wit LT, Nieveen van Dijkum EJ et al (1997) Value of laparoscopic ultrasonography in staging of proximal bile duct tumours. J Ultrasound Med 16(1):7–12

Preoperative Assessment of Liver Function

Many elements contribute to the optimal selection of patients who will undergo surgery for hilar cholangiocarcinoma, including:
- Improvement of the preoperative diagnosis in the definition of size, site and tumour extent related to intrahepatic vascularisation
- Findings of the intraoperative workup
- Knowledge of the biological behavior of the tumour
- Effects of biliary obstruction and jaundice
- Effects of parenchymal inflammatory process and of cholangitis on clinical course and prognosis
- Nutritional state
- Adjuvant therapy

The choice of resection must take into consideration the need to remove the tumour completely as well as the need to maintain residual volume of parenchyma to carry on hepatic function.

In surgery of hilar cholangiocarcinoma, which also requires extended resection, attention must be focused not only on the amount of hepatic parenchyma removed but mainly to the residual quantity and its ability to guarantee acceptable postoperative residual liver function. Depending on the type of growth, cholangiocarcinoma can bring about complete or selective obstruction of one or more segments of the intrahepatic biliary tree. The obstacle to bile flow is responsible for worsened global hepatic function with a major risk of septic phenomena and relevant systemic effects. In presence of biliary obstruction, biliary pressure increases from 5–10 to 30 cm of H_2O with destruction of the junctions between hepatocytes and biliary cells. The results are: (1) compression by dilated biliary tract on capacity portal vessels with reduction of portal flow; (2) negative influence on humoral factors involved in initiating and maintaining the regeneration with a decrease in growth-related factors; (3) activation of hepatocellular apoptosis process by accumulation of toxic bile salts; (4) increased cholangiole permeability with direct bile reflux in sinusoids and beginning of inflammatory response; (5) decreased bile excretion by hepatocytes; (6)

A. Guglielmi, A. Ruzzenente, C. Iacono (eds.) *Surgical Treatment of Hilar and ICC.*
© Springer 2008

decreased excretory activity of hepatocytes with a direct reflux of metabolites in circulatory system and consequent systemic toxicity; (7) alteration of micro- and macro-vascular perfusion.

Protide synthesis is altered with albumin level reduction, alteration of coagulation factors and a fall in immunoglobulins. The effects of obstruction extend to detoxification activity of the liver with decreased excretion of the substances metabolised in the liver. The systemic effects of biliary obstruction are evident with regard to cardiovascular activity, renal function, and the coagulation process. Jaundiced patients are more susceptible to developing postoperative shock consequent to depression of left ventricular activity and decreased peripheral vascular resistance as well as plasmatic volume. Renal function is impaired by hyperbilirubinemia, due to the reduction of renal perfusion related to cardiac pump impairment and to renal causes themselves, as natriuretic effects of bile salts and direct parenchymal toxicity of endotoxaemia; renal failure in jaundice patients has a mortality that can reach 70% [1]. Deprivation of bile at the intestinal level interferes with vitamin K absorption, with prolongation of prothrombin time. The effects of bile deprivation on the intestine and the interruption of enterohepatic circulation determine the loss of emulsive and antitoxic activity of bile salts, permitting the abundant amount of endotoxins present in the intestinal lumen to be absorbed by the portal circulation [2]. With a normal biliary pressure (7–14 cm of H_2O) bacteremia in portal circulation is cleared by Kuppfer cells; in presence of biliary obstruction their activity is impaired with decreased bacterial and endotoxin clearance and antigen presentation. High concentration of bacteria in the bile and biliary hypertension are the causes of cholangitis and biliary sepsis. Decompression of the biliary system, with a normalisation of bilirubinemia values, produces such improvement of biochemical circulating parameters and hepatic function that it allows performance of extended hepatectomies with 70% hepatic volume resection without or with very low postoperative hepatic insufficiency [3–6]. Jaundice resolution is considered able to restore a hepatic reserve similar to that of patients with normal hepatic function [4]. However, external drainage does not restore enterohepatic circulation and does not affect bacterial translocation. Bile replacement has been proposed in jaundiced patients to repair intestinal mucosa integrity and reduce septic complications [7]. The need for preoperative drainage in patients with hilar cholangiocarcinoma is debated; in patients with cholangitis, long-term jaundice, severe malnutrition, and bilirubinemia >5 mg/ml, who require major hepatectomy (more than 60%), preoperative drainage is considered efficacious [8–11]. In the same way, biliary drainage of the future remnant liver is considered mandatory prior to performing PVE since expected hypertrophy requires normal values of bilirubinemia [12,13]. In all other cases of biliary obstruction there are two different schools of thought: Western thinking supports early resection in jaundiced patients with hilar cholangiocarcinoma, considering that biliary drainage presents the risk of complications (peritonitis, cholangitis, bleeding) from 3 to 5% [14,15]; also, the potential risk of neoplastic seeding, although rare, is considered able to jeopardise the radicality of surgery [16]. On the other hand, Asian authors support the use of biliary drainage [17,18] that is addressed to normalising liver function with an improvement of cholestatic liver tolerance to ischemia, to decrease transfusion therapy and to improve regeneration capacity. Clinical randomised trials have not shown until now that biliary drainage, internal or external, is of benefit prior to resection. Even the modalities of drainage (endoscopic/percutaneous, segmental/lobar, single/multiple, trans-stenotic or not) are under discussion and require further study. Unilateral biliary drainage should be used on the side of the future remnant liver. Drainage of atrophic liver is contraindicated due to unlikelihood of reversing hepatic volume and function loss from atrophy. Prior evaluation of resection of hepatic function and investigation of predictive factors to assess hepatic volume and the reserve of residual function are taken into consideration in order to reduce operative risk [19].

Tests that measure the serum value of hepatic enzymes are commonly defined standard liver function tests and reflect the hepatocytes' integrity or the presence of cholestasis. Albuminemia and prothrombin time are related to the functioning hepatic mass, but are not specific to hepatopathy [20]; although not unanimously recognised, a predictive value to the standard liver function test is not given until nowadays [21]. Child score, an indicator of excretion and synthesis function and portal hypertension utilised in the surgery of the cirrhotic liver, is not useful in cholangiocarcinoma in the non-cirrhotic liver. Many qualitative tests have been proposed using different substrates (Table 1); in spite of being precise, they are impractical in a clinical setting for various reasons such as excessive cost, need for multiple samples and prolonged catheterisation, and risk of allergic reaction.

Table 1 Quantitative tests. Adapted from [19]

Quantitative Tests	Function Tested
Aminopyridine breath test	Microsomial function
Antipyridine clearance	Microsomial function
Caffeine clearance	Microsomial function
Lidocaine clearance (MEGX)	Microsomial function
Methacetin breath test	Microsomial function
Galactose elimination capacity (GEC)	Cytosolic function
Low-dose galactose clearance	Hepatic perfusion (liver blood flow)
Sorbitol clearance	Hepatic perfusion (liver blood flow)
Indocyanine green disappearance	Hepatic perfusion, anion excretion
Albumine synthesis	Synthetic function
Urea synthesis	Synthetic function

The maximal enzymatic liver function capacity has been re-proposed based on the C-methacetin breath test (LiMAx test) [22]; it shows a significant correlation with remnant liver volume, but its recent introduction requires further validation. Of the proposed tests for anticipating the postoperative residual liver function, ICG clearance is considered the most powerful predictive test of operative mortality after hepatectomy if compared to other tests such as the aminoacid clearance test or aminopyrine breath test [23,24]. The model of retention rate (ICG-15) is the one most frequently used. The percentage of retention can be measured by pulsed spectrophotometry using an optical sensor [25]. There is no unanimous consensus on the cut-off value of IGC retention with a predictive value of postoperative hepatic failure, but it is believed that IGC-15 equal to or greater than 15% is indicative of inadequate clearance with limited hepatic reserve; therefore major hepatectomy is unwise. ICG and bilirubin bind to the same carrier in the transport phase in hepatocytes, determining a competitive inhibition. In patients with obstructive jaundice hyperbilirubinemia is independent of the reserve of hepatic function and ICG retention is therefore not valid. In these cases 99-m TC-GSA scintigraphy is proposed, which assumes the role of a quantitative test of hepatic function [19]. Scintigraphy with 99-m TC-GSA (diethylenetriamine-pentaacetic acid with galactosyl human serum albumin) is a dynamic technique that provides information on the density of specific receptors on the plasma membrane of hepatocytes, whose density directly reflects the functioning hepatic mass. The liver can tolerate considerable reduction of its volume since mechanisms of compensatory hypertrophy are activated, but inadequate hepatic volume after resection (small remnant liver volume) can have a negative influence on the postoperative course with the risk of hepatic failure. Two events can occur: (1) the residual volume of a normo-functioning liver can be insufficient for providing an adequate hepatic reserve; (2) the hepatic reserve can be reduced due to a concomitant pre-existing hepatocellular impairment (in the case of hilar cholangiocarcinoma, obstructed biliary tract with jaundice, steatosis, fibrosis, cirrhosis) even in presence of an apparently sufficient volume. Techniques of preoperative measurement of hepatic volume on CT scans have been introduced [26]. The volumetric findings of hepatic resection and transplantation have shown a close correlation between actual and CT-calculated volumes allowing a precise evaluation of each hepatic segment [27–29]. The minimal volume of residual liver after resection that can guarantee a normal function is at least 25–30% of the initial functioning liver. This percentage must be increased to 40% and more, in patients with chronic hepatic disease or who have undergone previous chemotherapy [28,30,31]. The acquisition of hepatic volumetry allows evaluation of the efficacy of the procedure as PVE addressed to initiate preoperatively the compensatory hypertrophy of the future remnant liver.

The presence of cirrhosis greatly affects hepatic regeneration, and as an indication for hepatic resection in the cirrhotic patient, is subject to debate.

Particular attention must be paid to steatosis; diabetic, obese and patients who have undergone previous chemotherapy are likely to develop steatosis. Insulin is considered a promoting factor of hepatic regeneration; diabetic and obese patients present insulin resistance with a risk of developing postoperative failure related to the degree of steatosis [32]. In presence of steatosis PVE is indicated, to optimise the hepatic reserve [33]. None of the tests used alone can recognise the individuals who can tolerate hepatic resection, or determine the amount of resection. Laboratory data, diagnostic and quantitative tests are integrated and contribute, together with the surgeon's opinion, to formulating the correct surgical indication [21]. Two elements, biliary drainage and portal vein embolisation, combined on the basis of bilirubinemia values and future remnant liver characteristics, in our opinion acquire a prominent value in the preoperative assessment (Fig. 1); they are also important for recovering sufficient hepatic function in the patient candidate for biliary-hepatic resection due to hilar cholangiocarcinoma.

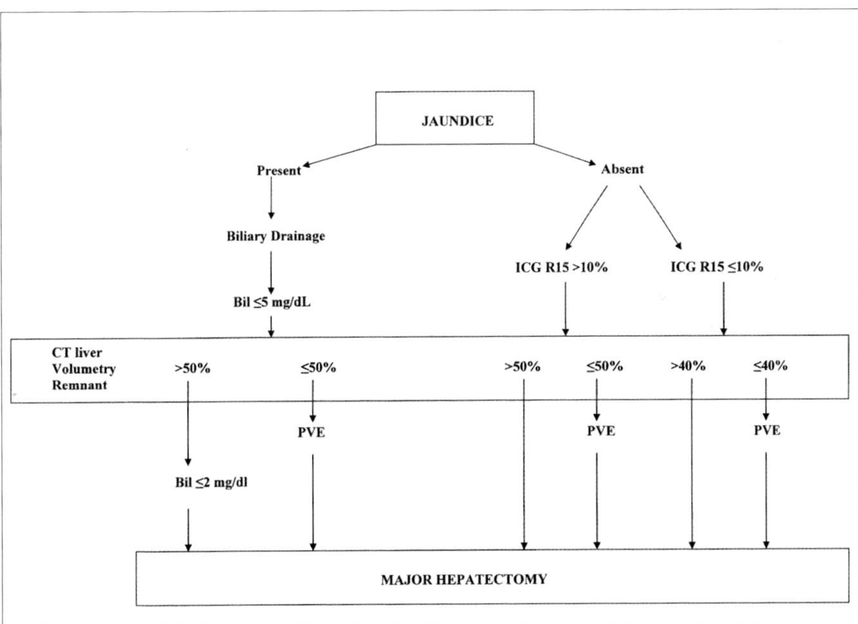

Fig. 1 Flowchart of preoperative preparation of hepatic resection for hilar cholangiocarcinoma. In presence of normal bilirubinemia, after ICG clearance, indication for PVE is taken on the assessment of volumetry of future remnant liver. In jaundiced patients biliary drainage allows normalisation of bilirubinemia with the possibility of performing PVE if future remnant liver is not sufficient. Modified from [3]

References

1. Fogarty BJ, Parks RW, Rowlands BJ, Diamond T (1995) Renal dysfunction in obstructive jaundice. Br J Surg 82(7):877–884
2. Yokoyama Y, Nagino M, Nimura Y (2007) Mechanism of impaired hepatic regeneration in cholestatic liver. J Hepatobiliary Pancreat Surg 14(2):159–166
3. Seyama Y, Makuuchi M (2007) Current surgical treatment for bile duct cancer. World J. Gastroenterol 13(10):1505–1515
4. Takahashi T, Togo S, Tanaka K et al (2004) Safe and permissible limits of hepatectomy in obstructive jaundice patients. World J Surg 28(5):475–481
5. Nimura Y, Kamiya J, Kondo S et al (1995) Technique of inserting multiple biliary drains and management. Hepatogastroenterology 42(4):323–331
6. Kawasaki S, Imamura H, Kobayashi A et al (2003) Results of surgical resection for patients with hilar bile duct cancer: application of extended hepatectomy after biliary drainage and hemihepatic portal vein embolization. Ann Surg 238(1):84–92
7. Kamiya S, Nagino M, Kanazawa H et al (2004) The value of bile replacement during external biliary drainage: an analysis of intestinal permeability, integrity, and microflora. Ann Surg 239(4):510–517
8. Bismuth H, Nakache R, Diamond T (1992) Management strategies in resection for hilar cholangiocarcinoma. Ann Surg 215(1):31–38
9. Vauthey JN, Blumgart LH (1994) Recent advances in the management of cholangiocarcinomas. Semin Liver Dis 14(2):109–114
10. Nakeeb A, Pitt HA, Sohn TA et al (1996) Cholangiocarcinoma. A spectrum of intrahepatic, perihilar, and distal tumours. Ann Surg 224(4):463–473; discussion 473–475
11. Cherqui D, Benoist S, Malassagne B et al (2000) Major liver resection for carcinoma in jaundiced patients without preoperative biliary drainage. Arch Surg 135(3):302–308
12. Makuuchi M, Thai BL, Takayasu K et al (1990) Preoperative portal embolization to increase safety of major hepatectomy for hilar bile duct carcinoma: a preliminary report. Surgery 107(5):521–527
13. Nagino M, Nimura Y, Hayakawa N et al (1993) Logistic regression and discriminant analyses of hepatic failure after liver resection for carcinoma of the biliary tract. World J Surg 17(2):250–255
14. Lai EC, Mok FP, Fan ST et al (1994) Preoperative endoscopic drainage for malignant obstructive jaundice. Br J Surg 81(8):1195–1198
15. Liu CL, Lo CM, Lai EC, Fan ST (1998) Endoscopic retrograde cholangiopancreatography and endoscopic endoprosthesis insertion in patients with Klatskin tumours. Arch Surg 133(3):293–296
16. Chapman WC, Sharp KW, Weaver F, Sawyers JL (1989) Tumour seeding from percutaneous biliary catheters. Ann Surg 209(6):708–713; discussion 713–715
17. Nimura Y, Hayakawa N, Kamiya J et al (1990) Hepatic segmentectomy with caudate lobe resection for bile duct carcinoma of the hepatic hilus. World J Surg 14(4):535–543; discussion 544
18. Miyagawa S, Makuuchi M, Kawasaki S (1995) Outcome of extended right hepatectomy after biliary drainage in hilar bile duct cancer. Arch Surg 130(7):759–763
19. Imamura H, Sano K, Sugawara Y et al (2005) Assessment of hepatic reserve for indication of hepatic resection: decision tree incorporating indocyanine green test. J Hepatobiliary Pancreat Surg 12(1):16–22
20. Giannini EG, Testa R, Savarino V (2005) Liver enzyme alteration: a guide for clinicians. CMAJ. Feb 1;172(3):367–379
21. Mullin EJ, Metcalfe MS, Maddern GJ (2005) How much liver resection is too much? Am J Surg 190(1):87–97
22. Stockmann M, Schwabauer E, Videv N et al (2006) The new intravenous LiMax test (maximal enzymatic liver function capacity based on 13-c-methacetin kinetics) for mentoring of

liver function after liver transplantation.Am J Transplant 6(Suppl 2):725
23. Nonami T, Nakao A, Kurokawa T et al (1999) Blood loss and ICG clearance as best prognostic markers of post-hepatectomy liver failure. Hepatogastroenterology 46(27):1669–1672
24. Hemming AW, Scudamore CH, Shackleton CR et al (1992) Indocyanine green clearance as a predictor of successful hepatic resection in cirrhotic patients. Am J Surg 163(5):515–518
25. Okochi O, Kaneko T, Sugimoto H et al (2002) ICG pulse spectrophotometry for perioperative liver function in hepatectomy. J Surg Res 103(1):109–113
26. Vauthey JN, Abdalla EK, Doherty DA et al (2002) Body surface area and body weight predict total liver volume in Western adults. Liver Transpl 8(3):233–240
27. Heymsfield SB, Fulenwider T, Nordlinger B et al (1979) Accurate measurement of liver, kidney, and spleen volume and mass by computerized axial tomography. Ann Intern Med 90(2):185–187
28. Kubota K, Makuuchi M, Kusaka K et al (1997) Measurement of liver volume and hepatic functional reserve as a guide to decision-making in resectional surgery for hepatic tumours. Hepatology 26(5):1176–1181
29. Madoff DC, Abdalla EK, Vauthey JN (2005) Portal vein embolization in preparation for major hepatic resection: evolution of a new standard of care. J Vasc Interv Radiol 16(6):779–790
30. Abdalla EK, Hicks ME, Vauthey JN (2001) Portal vein embolization: rationale, technique and future prospects. Br J Surg 88(2):165–175
31. de Baere T, Roche A, Elias D et al (1996) Preoperative portal vein embolization for extension of hepatectomy indications. Hepatology 24(6):1386–1391
32. Behrns KE, Tsiotos GG, DeSouza NF et al (1998) Hepatic steatosis as a potential risk factor for major hepatic resection. J Gastrointest Surg 2(3):292–298
33. Bennett JJ, Blumgart LH (2005) Assessment of hepatic reserve prior to hepatic resection. J Hepatobiliary Pancreat Surg 12(1):10–15

Preoperative Biliary Drainage

One of the most important factors of morbidity in hilar cholangiocarcinoma is the presence of jaundice as a consequence of physiopathologic changes following cholestasis, described in Chap. "Preoperative Assessment of Liver Function". The close association of this complex disease with high operative risk, determined by increased postoperative mortality and morbidity, has led to the belief that preoperative drainage of jaundice would have decreased the risk of a major resection (i.e. pancreaticoduodenectomy or hepatic resection).

In fact, the first retrospective [1–3] and randomized studies [4] after percutaneous drainage and endoscopic stent [5] showed decreased mortality and in some cases morbidity in jaundiced patients who had been drained. Nevertheless, controlled randomized studies [6–8] and more recent studies [9–11] showed not only a lack of significant advantages but even an increased mortality in drained patients [12]. However, it is important to underline that in all these studies patients who underwent hepatic resection were few since most underwent pancreaticoduodenectomy for pancreatic or periampullary disease.

Recent prospective studies with larger series [12–16] offer variable results regarding the comparison drained/not drained: from the absence of significant differences in mortality and morbidity [15] to an increased rate of wound infection with unchanged mortality [13,14,16] to a significant increase in complications (specifically, infective and abscess) and fourfold increased mortality in drained patients [12]. Even a recent published meta-analysis on the worth of preoperative biliary drainage shows that percutaneous transhepatic biliary drainage (PTBD) for neoplastic jaundice would not provide clear benefits and should not be carried out routinely [17]. The probable advantages of PTBD regarding percentage of mortality and morbidity do not appear to balance the procedure's disadvantages. The metanalysis concludes that controlled randomized studies and a better drain technique are necessary in order to correctly define the problem; another point is that jaundice in patients with hilar cholangiocarcinoma who are candidates for major liver resection presents different problems than jaundice in patients who are candidates for pancreaticoduodenectomy; for this reason specific randomized studies are required.

A. Guglielmi, A. Ruzzenente, C. Iacono (eds.) *Surgical Treatment of Hilar and ICC.*
© Springer 2008

In the cited meta-analysis the number of patients with hilar cholangiocarcinoma were 34 of 312 patients (11%) in randomized studies, while the number was 113 of 372 patients (30%) in non-randomized studies [17]. Only one randomized study [10] and two non-randomized studies [18,19] consider the role of PTBD in patients with proximal cholangiocarcinoma. All three studies do not show advantages of PTBD; however the authors of the meta-analysis underline that the data reported are not sufficient for a correct analysis [17]. Figueras [19] reports a morbidity rate of 100% in the 11 drained patients vs. 66% in the 9 non-drained patients (p=0.8) and a postoperative hospitalization time that is longer in drained patients (25 vs. 13 days, p=0.009).

Drainage: Pros

Considerations derived from these studies lead to the hypothesis of a change in trend that will determine a radical reduction in preoperative drainage [12] or at least a restriction based on the following precise indications [13–17,20,21]:
- Need to resolve cholangitis
- Need to avoid exacerbation of severe jaundice while awaiting completion of the workup
- To correct severe malnutrition
- To improve jaundice-related renal or hepatic insufficiency
- To plan neoadjuvant treatment
- To improve hypertrophy of the remnant liver after PVE

Mean duration of preoperative biliary drainage is 2 weeks and in the literature it varies from 12 to 26 days in randomized studies and from 10 to 32 days in non-randomized studies [17]; at the end of this period the values of bilirubinemia are reduced on average to one-fourth of the initial value. An absent or slow decrease in bilirubinemia suggests a malfunction of the drainage or impaired liver function. The abovementioned timing and bilirubinemia values in patient candidates for pancreaticoduodenectomy can be considered adequate; however, in patients who are destined for hepatobiliary resection it is mandatory to re-establish bilirubinemia levels under 2 mg/dL as well as hepatic function, which requires 4–6 weeks as previously shown.

In literature many studies show that hepatic resection in jaundiced patients is associated with significant morbidity and mortality rates consequent to haemorrhage, subphrenic abscesses secondary to biliary leak, sepsis and hepatic insufficiency [22–25]. For these reasons and to increase resectability and feasibility of major hepatectomy many authors (mainly Asian) prefer to perform PTBD routinely [26–29]. Even Belghiti [30], following Japanese indications, has observed that preoperative PTBD increases resectability rate; in fact dividing his series in two different time periods he noticed that in the first period (1992–1995) 39% of 31 patients underwent PTBD and resectability rate was 32% (10 of 31 patients), vascular resection/reconstruction was performed in only 2 of the 10 resected patients (20%) while in the second time period (1995–2001) 70% of 37 patients with hilar cholangiocarcinoma underwent PTBD with a resectability rate of 59% (2 cases) and vascular resection/reconstruction in 8 of 22 resected patients (36%) [30]. Extensive use of this procedure has determined a smaller rate of septic complications in the French study that the author also ascribes to improved skill (60% in the first period vs. 20% in the second) [30].

Drainage: Cons

A critical evaluation of the indiscriminate use of preoperative biliary drainage has revealed functional limits and undeniable side effects:

– After biliary drainage bilirubinemia normalizes in only two-thirds of the treated cases [5,31] and 4–8 weeks are required for complete disappearance of jaundice [32]. Watanapa [33] has shown in preoperative and postoperative functional studies that the liver rcsumes its normal functions 6 weeks after surgical operation entailing jaundice drainage with decompression of both hepatic lobes. It has been shown experimentally that normalization of impaired mitochondrial function caused by jaundice requires at least 6 weeks after biliary decompression [34] and pathological alterations become completely reversible 8 weeks after restoration of normal bile drainage [35].
– Retrograde endoscopic drainage and most frequently percutaneous drains are the causes of biliary tract, peritoneal and parietal infection with increased operative mortality [11,12,18,36].
– Periductal and hepatoduodenal fibrosis caused by stents or drains increase operative difficulties during dissection; moreover, reduction of duct size following biliary decompression can be the reason for a demanding bilio-digestive anastomosis.
– Seeding along the site of percutaneous drainage [19,29,37–39].

Conversely, Cherqui [25] plans a non-invasive work-up to stage the disease and perform an early operation, believing that the utility of preoperative drainage has not been proved. Two groups of neoplastic patients similar for age, size of tumour, type of resection and vascular occlusion were compared; 20 jaundiced patients who underwent a major hepatic resection and 27 non-jaundiced patients were selected from the institutional database of 261 patients. Haemotransfusion was performed in 85% of patients in the jaundiced group vs. 48% in the non-jaundiced group, morbidity rate, which was determined mainly by subphrenic abscess ($p=0.02$) and biliary leak ($p=0.04$) observed only in the jaundiced group, was 50 vs. 15% ($p=0.006$). Mortality rate (5 vs. 0%), hepatic insufficiency rate (5 vs. 0%) and postoperative alteration of hepatic function were similar in the two groups. Eventually the authors concluded that: (1) even major hepatic resection can be performed safely in jaundiced patients without preventive biliary drainage; however the increased rate of complications and blood transfusion is similar to that observed in patients who underwent PTBD; (2) no evidence supports the concept that preoperative PTBD can decrease these complications.

An experimental study on rats [40] shows that cholestatic liver is largely exposed to complications related to post-ischemic reperfusion, probably due to decreased antioxidant activity and increased inflammatory response; on the other hand these alterations are lessened after biliary decompression. The results of the study support a high risk of inflammatory events after the Pringle maneuver during hepatic resection in presence of cholestasis.

Endoscopic or Percutaneous Drainage

The endoscopic route is currently the procedure of choice for treating obstruction of middle and distal biliary tract [41,42] with a 90–95% success rate; however this percentage is lower in proximal obstruction when the procedure is compared to percutaneous drainage [43] although one study reports a higher success rate for endoscopic route (81–87%) vs. PTBD (57–83%) [44]. Considering the major risks of transhepatic biliary drainage and longer preoperative hospitalization required, endoscopic drainage can be indicated in stage I and possibly stage II of Bismuth-Corlette classification, planning a fortnightly replacement to prevent occlusion [45]. PTBD is instead the treatment of choice in stages III e IV [42,44,46] as the endoscopic route has a success rate of only 15% in these patients; only one study in the literature [47] reports a success rate of 100% in this group of patients after placement of an endoscopic plastic stent. In the future the high quality of MRCP imaging and the use of better endoscopic stents will increase the endoscopic approach even for proximal obstruction [30].

Percutaneous Drainage Technique

Transhepatic percutaneous drainage can be performed either under fluoroscopy [26,48,49] or sonographic guidance [50,51], external or internal, unilateral, bilateral or multiple. Success rate for experienced personnel is high at first attempt: 99.2% of 501 patients in the Nagoya group, arriving at 100% when a further pass was performed, with no mortality and 9.2% morbidity rate [49]. Takada [51] reports a complication rate of 6% in 603 cases of PTBD under fluoroscopy and 0.7% in 409 cases of PTBD under sonography. To prevent cholangitis in case of obstructed confluence cholangiogram does not need to be performed, but according to Makuuchi would be carried out only to place the drain or the evening prior to surgery [20].

Uni- vs. Bilateral PTBD

The initial approach must be unilateral on the future hepatic remnant lobe [26,29,30,32] but if the decision is not made about which hepatic lobe will be resected Nimura suggests draining the left hepatic duct [26]. In case the intrahepatic biliary ducts are separated because involved by the neoplasm (as in Bismuth-Corlette stages II, III, and IV) the indication changes according to the institution: if the contralateral ductal system is not contrast-injected it is enough to drain a single hepatic system [43], while other authors [30] believe that bilateral drainage is required only in presence of cholangitis not resolved by monolateral PTBD. In the Nimura group's experience bilateral drainage can be obtained by means of a single percutaneous catheter [26] and when this is not feasible, a second PTBD is always required; in advanced cases when second order confluences are involved, the placement of multiple drains is needed, as well [52]; conversely the Watanapa study [53] does not report any significant differences in hepatic function after complete vs. monolateral hepatic drainage 6 weeks after biliary decompression; the only difference is that monolateral drainage cannot prevent cholangitis in the non-drained lobe. The choice of multiple drains is determined by segmental cholangitis [26], which represents the major prognostic factor for outcome in major hepatic resection for hilar cholangiocarcinoma [49,53]. In contrast, Kawasaki [52] does not consider useful the meticulous evaluation of intrahepatic diffusion of the tumour through direct cholangiography due to the limits of the procedure; moreover, as the infection rate increases the number of required drains, he supports monolateral drainage of the hepatic remnant even in the patient candidate for preliminary PVE. The same opinion is corroborated by the Makuuchi group that in recent reports [20,21] sustains the superiority of selective drainage of the future hepatic remnant since it does not increase cholangitis compared with complete liver drainage and associated with PVE, and eases residual hepatic hypertrophy, assuring a good hepatic function.

Internal vs. External Drainage

Another unresolved and much-debated problem is that of deciding between an internal or external drainage; when the biliary tract is drained through the endoscopic route the drainage is always internal and it is aggravated by a noticeable rate of biliary tract infection (up to 50% and more of the cases [54]), whereas transhepatic percutaneous drainage is either internal or external: internal drainage re-institutes bile flow in the duodenum and presents some advantages in comparison with an external drain, above all in stimulating hepatic regeneration [55,56], and maintaining the intestinal barrier [57,58]. External drainage, preferred by the Nimura group, permits decompression of the biliary system proximally to the stenosis reducing the risk of ascending contamination as occurs in internal drainage placed in the duodenum; although other authors [59] utilize PTBD or trans-tumoral stents, they prefer to place the tip of the catheter in the common hepatic duct to preserve sphincter function. In presence of external drainage the Nagoya group [26], and the Makuuchi as well [20,21], consider it important to reintroduce the drained bile per os through a nasogastric tube or jejunostomy before and after hepatic resection to increase hepatic regeneration [53,56,60,61] and to maintain the barrier function of the small bowel. However other studies are needed to evaluate if intestinal bile restoration prevents bacterial translocation and therefore the incidence of postoperative septic complications [58].

Conclusions

Currently there are two schools of thought, the Western and the Eastern points of view, concerning preoperative biliary drainage in jaundiced patients who are candidates for major hepatectomy. The Asian school [9,25,62,63] believes that the theoretical advantages of preoperative drainage are annulled by the high percentages of procedural complications, and the risk of recurrence along the path of the drain that can compromise the results of curative resection. For these reasons the procedure is not applied systematically prior to hepatic resection but only in a subgroup of malnourished patients with hypoalbuminemia, cholangitis or long-lasting jaundice. The Asian school [20,21,26], also followed by some European groups [30], regularly utilize single or multiple PTBD. However these differences reveal a diverse philosophy regarding the surgical approach to this type of disease: the Euro-American being less aggressive and the Asian more aggressive. This idea is supported by the evaluation of the series of patients and resectability rate, hepatobiliary resection associated with vascular resection and reconstruction, percentage of trisegmentectomies and of patients who underwent PVE to determine hypertrophy of the residual hepatic segments.

Makuuchi [21] suggests the following guidelines in managing patients with cholangiocarcinoma:
– In patient candidates for hepatobiliary resection, biliary drainage is required
– Cholangiogram must be performed only when the drain is introduced on the evening prior to surgery
– Selective and external PTBD of the remnant liver is the treatment of choice
– Drained bile must be reintroduced per os
– Bile cultures with antibiogram need to be performed routinely
– In stage II–IV the endoscopic route must not be used for biliary drainage
– Whenever a stent is positioned endoscopically it must be substituted every 15 days
– Hepatic resection must be carried out only when hepatic function is restored

References

1. Denning DA, Ellison EC, Carey LC (1981) Preoperative percutaneous transhepatic biliary decompression lowers operative morbidity in patients with obstructive jaundice. Am J Surg 141(1):61–65
2. Norlander A, Kalin B, Sundblad R (1982) Effect of percutaneous transhepatic drainage upon liver function and postoperative mortality. Surg Gynecol Obstet 155(2):161–166
3. Gundry SR, Strodel WE, Knol JA et al (1984) Efficacy of preoperative biliary tract decompression in patients with obstructive jaundice. Arch Surg 119(6):703–708
4. Smith RC, Pooley M, George CR, Faithful GR (1985) Preoperative percutaneous transhepatic internal drainage in obstructive jaundice: a randomized, controlled trial examining renal function. Surgery 97(6):641–648
5. Neff R, Fantochen E, Cooperman AM et al (1987) The radiologic management of malignant biliary obstruction. Clin Radiol 34:143–146
6. Hatfield AR, Tobias R, Terblanche J et al (1982) Preoperative external biliary drainage in obstructive jaundice. A prospective controlled clinical trial. Lancet 2(8304):896–899
7. McPherson GA, Benjamin IS, Hodgson HJ (1984) Pre-operative percutaneous transhepatic biliary drainage: the results of a controlled trial. Br J Surg 71(5):371–375
8. Pitt HA, Gomes AS, Lois JF et al (1985) Does preoperative percutaneous biliary drainage reduce operative risk or increase hospital cost? Ann Surg 201(5):545–553
9. Nakeeb A, Pitt HA (1995) The role of preoperative biliary decompression in obstructive jaundice. Hepatogastroenterology 42(4):332–337
10. Lai EC, Mok FP, Fan ST et al (1994) Preoperative endoscopic drainage for malignant obstructive jaundice. Br J Surg 81(8):1195–1198
11. Heslin MJ, Brooks AD, Hochwald SN et al (1998) A preoperative biliary stent is associated with increased complications after pancreatoduodenectomy. Arch Surg 133(2):149–154
12. Povoski SP, Karpeh MS Jr, Conlon KC et al (1999) Association of preoperative biliary drainage with postoperative outcome following pancreaticoduodenectomy. Ann Surg 230(2):131–142
13. Sohn TA, Yeo CJ, Cameron J et al (2000) Do preoperative biliary stents increase postpancreaticoduodenectomy complications? J Gastrointest Surg 4(3):258–267; discussion 267–268
14. Pisters PW, Hudec WA, Hess KR et al (2001) Effect of preoperative biliary decompression on pancreaticoduodenectomy-associated morbidity in 300 consecutive patients. Ann Surg 234(1):47–55
15. Martignoni ME, Wagner M, Krahenbuhl L et al (2001) Effect of preoperative biliary drainage on surgical outcome after pancreatoduodenectomy. Am J Surg 181(1):52–59; discussion 87
16. Srivastava S, Sikora SS, Kumar A et al (2001) Outcome following pancreaticoduodenectomy in patients undergoing preoperative biliary drainage. Dig Surg 18(5):381–387
17. Sewnath ME, Karsten TM, Prins MH et al (2002) A meta-analysis on the efficacy of preoperative biliary drainage for tumours causing obstructive jaundice. Ann Surg 236(1):17–27
18. Hochwald SN, Burke EC, Jarnagin W al (1999) Association of preoperative biliary stenting with increased postoperative infectious complications in proximal cholangiocarcinoma. Arch Surg 134(3):261–266
19. Figueras J, Llado L, Valls C et al (2000) Changing strategies in diagnosis and management of hilar cholangiocarcinoma. Liver Transpl 6(6):786–794
20. Ishizawa T, Hasegawa K, Sano K et al (2007) Selective vs. total biliary drainage for obstructive jaundice caused by a hepatobiliary malignancy. Am J Surg 193(2):149–154
21. Seyama Y, Makuuchi M (2007) Current surgical treatment for bile duct cancer. World J Gastroenterol 13(10):1505–1515
22. Su CH, P'eng FK, Lui WY (1992) Factors affecting morbidity and mortality in biliary tract surgery. World J Surg 16(3):536–540

23. Clements WD, Diamond T, McCrory DC, Rowlands BJ (1993) Biliary drainage in obstructive jaundice: experimental and clinical aspects. Br J Surg 80(7):834–842

24. Su CH, Tsay SH, Wu CC et al (1996) Factors influencing postoperative morbidity, mortality, and survival after resection for hilar cholangiocarcinoma. Ann Surg 223(4):384–394

25. Cherqui D, Benoist S, Malassagne B et al (2000) Major liver resection for carcinoma in jaundiced patients without preoperative biliary drainage. Arch Surg 135(3):302–308

26. Nagino M, Nimura Y (2006) Perihilar cholangiocarcinoma with emphasis on presurgical management. In: Blumgart LH (ed) Surgery of the liver, biliary tract, and pancreas. 4th edn. Saunders Elsevier, Philadelphia, pp 804–814

27. Miyagawa S, Makuuchi M, Kawasaki S (1995) Outcome of extended right hepatectomy after biliary drainage in hilar bile duct cancer. Arch Surg 130(7):759–763

28. Ebata T, Nagino M, Kamiya J (2003) Hepatectomy with portal vein resection for hilar cholangiocarcinoma: audit of 52 consecutive cases. Ann Surg 238(5):720–727

29. Seyama Y, Kubota K, Sano K et al (2003) Long-term outcome of extended hemihepatectomy for hilar bile duct cancer with no mortality and high survival rate. Ann Surg 238(1):73–83

30. Belghiti J, Ogata S (2005) Preoperative optimization of the liver for resection in patients with hilar cholangiocarcinoma. HPB Surg 7:252–253

31. Pellegrini CA, Thomas MJ, Way LW (1982) Bilirubin and alkaline phosphatase values before and after surgery for biliary obstruction. Am J Surg 143(1):67–73

32. Howard JH, Jordan GL, Reber HA(1987) Surgical disease of the pancreas. Lea&Febriger, Philadelphia

33. Watanapa P (1996) Recovery patterns of liver function after complete and partial surgical biliary decompression. Am J Surg 171(2):230–234

34. Koyama K, Takagi Y, Ito K, Sato T (1981) Experimental and clinical studies on the effect of biliary drainage in obstructive jaundice. Am J Surg 142(2):293–299

35. Aronson DC, Chamuleau RA, Frederiks WM (1993) Reversibility of cholestatic changes following experimental common bile duct obstruction: fact or fantasy? J Hepatol 18(1):85–95

36. Temudom T, Sarr MG, Douglas MG, Farnell MB (1995) An argument against routine percutaneous biopsy, ERCP, or biliary stent placement in patients with clinically resectable periampullary masses: a surgical perspective. Pancreas 11(3):283–288

37. Jarnagin WR, Burke E, Powers C et al (1998) Intrahepatic biliary enteric bypass provides effective palliation in selected patients with malignant obstruction at the hepatic duct confluence. Am J Surg 175(6):453–460

38. Soyer P, Pelage JP, Dufresne AC et al (1998) CT of abdominal wall implantation metastases after abdominal percutaneous procedures. J Comput Assist Tomogr 22(6):889–893

39. Sakata J, Shirai Y, Wakai T et al (2005) Catheter tract implantation metastases associated with percutaneous biliary drainage for extrahepatic cholangiocarcinoma. World J Gastroenterol 11(44):7024–7027

40. Kloek JJ, Marsman HA, van Vliet AK et al (2007) Biliary drainage attenuates post-ischemic reperfusion injury in the cholestatic rat liver. J Hepatobiliary Pancreat Surg 9(Suppl 2):11, abs 34

41. Sherman S (2001) Current status of endoscopic pancreaticobiliary interventions. J Vasc Interv Radiol 12:120–155

42. England RE, Martin DF (1996) Endoscopic and percutaneous intervention in malignant obstructive jaundice. Cardiovasc Intervent Radiol 19(6):381–387

43. Hatzidakis A, Adam A (2003) The interventional radiological management of cholangiocarcinoma. Clin Radiol 58(2):91–96

44. Nelsen KM, Kastan DJ, Shetty PC et al (1996) Utilization pattern and efficacy of nonsurgical techniques to establish drainage for high biliary obstruction. J Vasc Interv Radiol 7(5):751–756

45. Jagannath P, Dhir V, Shrikhande S et al (2005) Effect of preoperative biliary stenting on immediate outcome after pancreaticoduodenectomy. Br J Surg 92(3):356–361

46. Cowling MG, Adam A (2001) Internal stenting in malignant biliary obstruction. World J Surg 25:355–361

47. Gerhards MF, den Hartog D, Rauws EA et al (2001) Palliative treatment in patients with unresectable hilar cholangiocarcinoma: results of endoscopic drainage in patients with type III and IV hilar cholangiocarcinoma. Eur J Surg 167(4):274–280

48. Takada T, Hanyu F, Kobayashi S, Uchida Y (1976) Percutaneous transhepatic cholangial drainage: direct approach under fluoroscopic control. J Surg Oncol 8(1):83–97

50. Kanai M, Nimura Y, Kamiya J et al (1996) Preoperative intrahepatic segmental cholangitis in patients with advanced carcinoma involving the hepatic hilus. Surgery 119(5):498–504

50. Singhal D, van Gulik TM, Gouma DJ (2005) Palliative management of hilar cholangiocarcinoma. Surg Oncol 14(2):59–74

51. Takada T, Yasuda H, Hanyu F (1995) Technique and management of percutaneous transhepatic cholangial drainage for treating an obstructive jaundice. Hepatogastroenterology 42(4):317–322

52. Kawasaki S, Imamura H, Kobayashi A (2003) Results of surgical resection for patients with hilar bile duct cancer: application of extended hepatectomy after biliary drainage and hemihepatic portal vein embolization. Ann Surg 238(1):84–92

53. Nimura Y, Kamiya J, Kondo S (2000) Aggressive preoperative management and extended surgery for hilar cholangiocarcinoma: Nagoya experience. J Hepatobiliary Pancreat Surg 7(2):155–162

54. Rerknimitr R, Attasaranya S, Kladchareon N et al (2002) Feasibility and complications of endoscopic biliary drainage in patients with malignant biliary obstruction at King Chulalongkorn Memorial Hospital. J Med Assoc Thai 85(Suppl 1):S48-S53

55. Saiki S, Chijiiwa K, Komura M et al (1999) Preoperative internal biliary drainage is superior to external biliary drainage in liver regeneration and function after hepatectomy in obstructive jaundiced rats. Ann Surg 230(5):655–662

56. Suzuki H, Iyomasa S, Nimura Y, Yoshida S (1994) Internal biliary drainage, unlike external drainage, does not suppress the regeneration of cholestatic rat liver after partial hepatectomy. Hepatology 20(5):1318–1322

57. Ogata Y, Nishi M, Nakayama H et al (2003) Role of bile in intestinal barrier function and its inhibitory effect on bacterial translocation in obstructive jaundice in rats. J Surg Res 115(1):18–23

58. Kamiya S, Nagino M, Kanazawa H et al (2004) The value of bile replacement during external biliary drainage: an analysis of intestinal permeability, integrity, and microflora. Ann Surg 239(4):510–517

59. Brown KT (2006) Interventional radiologic techniques in hilar and intrahepatic biliary tumours. In: Blumgart LH (ed) Surgery of the liver, biliary tract, and pancreas. 4 edn. Saunders Elsevier, Philadelphia, pp 814–822

60. Iyomasa S, Terasaki M, Kuriki H et al (1992) Decrease in regeneration capacity of rat liver after external biliary drainage. Eur Surg Res 24(5):265–272

61. Takeuchi E, Nimura Y, Nagino M et al (1997) Human hepatocyte growth factor in bile: an indicator of posthepatectomy liver function in patients with biliary tract carcinoma. Hepatology 26(5):1092–1099

62. Bismuth H, Nakache R, Diamond T (1992) Management strategies in resection for hilar cholangiocarcinoma. Ann Surg 215(1):31–38

63. Parc Y, Frileux P, Vaillant JC et al (1999) Postoperative peritonitis originating from the duodenum: operative management by intubation and continuous intraluminal irrigation. Br J Surg 86(9):1207–1212

Preoperative Portal Vein Embolization

Curative treatment of hilar cholangiocarcinoma leads to a major reduction of hepatic function due to the need for extended hepatectomy with biliary tract resection; therefore, it is exposed to the risk of postoperative hepatic failure [1,2]. Makuuchi [3] can take the credit for introducing preoperative embolic occlusion of portal branches (PVE) in patients with hilar cholangiocarcinoma to stimulate compensatory hypertrophy of the future remnant liver (FRL) and prevent the sudden increase of portal pressure after hepatectomy. Diversion of portal flow following PVE entails an improvement of the functional reserve of residual liver and allows extending the indications for surgical therapy even in patients with a marginal hepatic function.

Physiopathology of PVE

Despite the intense metabolic commitment, normally only a small part of hepatocytes (0.0012–0.01%) is involved in mitotic activity [4]. The liver does not show a lively replication attitude until it is involved by toxic insult or hepatic resection. In the case of hepatic resection an impressive hepatic cellular proliferation occurs, that in 2 weeks restores two-thirds of the functional mass. The mechanisms that direct and regulate this proliferation process are humoral and haemodynamic, and present analogously after hepatic resection and PVE, even though they are more rapid after hepatectomy (Fig. 1) [5,6].

At laparotomy the embolized lobe appears smaller than normal and with a softer texture, while no inflammatory processes are described on the hepatoduodenal ligament or gallbladder [3]. The entity of regeneration is 12–21 cm^3/day at 2 weeks, 11 cm^3/day at 4 weeks and 6 cm^3/day at 32 days after PVE [7]. Regeneration power is directly in proportion to the grade of stimulation and this fact explains why cellular replication after PVE is less prompt than the one after resection. A suppression effect on hepatic regeneration by obstructive jaundice, diabetes, alcohol abuse, nutritional status, male gender, advanced age and con-

A. Guglielmi, A. Ruzzenente, C. Iacono (eds.) *Surgical Treatment of Hilar and ICC.*
© Springer 2008

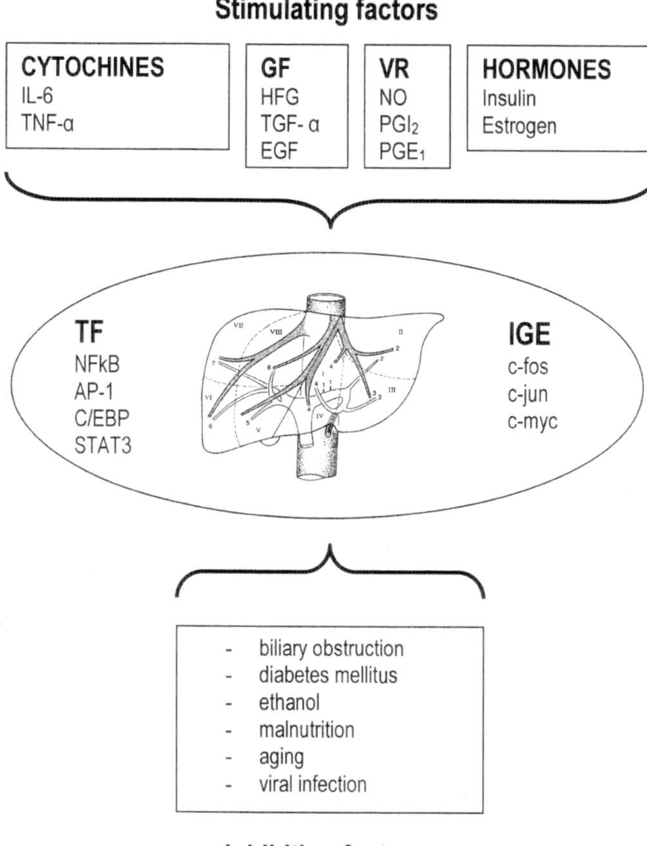

Fig. 1 Mechanism of hepatic regeneration after PVE, with stimulating factors and inhibiting factors that can modulate cellular proliferation. *IL-6*, Interleukin-6; *TNF-α*, tumour necrosis factor; *GF*, growth factors; *HGF*, hepatocyte growth factor; *TGF-α*, transforming growth factor; *EGF*, epidermal growth factor; *VR*, vasoregulators; *NO*, nitric oxide; *PGI₂*, prostaglandine I₂; *PGE₁*, prostaglandine E₁; *TF*, transcriptional factors; *NFκB*, nuclear factor κB; *AP-1*, activator protein 1; *C/EBPβ*, CCAAT enhancer-binding protein β; *Stat3*, signal transducers and activators of transcription 3; *IEG*, immediate early genes (c-fos; c-jun; c-myc). Modified from [6]

comitant infection is recognized. Regeneration rate in presence of diabetes or cirrhosis is 9 cm³/day at 2 weeks [8].

Portal flow in the non-embolized liver increases significantly and decreases thereafter until basal value after 11 days. It is interesting to notice as portal flow is correlated to parenchymal hypertrophy [9,10].

Indications

PVE is indicated in extended in liver tumour. There is a general consensus in retaining that in a normal liver the minimum essential volume of the FRL is between 25 and 30% [2,11–13]. A major percentage of FRL is required in patients with compromised hepatic function or in whom the planned procedure is difficult, e.g. in cholangiocarcinoma, to reduce the postoperative risks. Future remnant liver can be at least 40% in patients with cholestasis or chronic hepatic disease (steatosis, cirrhosis) or previous systemic chemotherapy [14,15]. The absence of lobar hypertrophy of the non-embolized lobe after PVE is considered an indicator of the failure of the liver to regenerate and represents a contraindication to major resection [16,17].

Jaundice and PVE

The majority of patients with hilar cholangiocarcinoma have cholestatic liver injury. High values of total bilirubinemia when PVE is performed decreases the hypertrophy amplitude of the non-embolized lobe [18], but only an elevated concentration of bile salts can induce hepatocellular apoptosis. The reason for the negative effect of jaundice on hepatic regeneration is determined by haemodynamic causes (portal flow is correlated to parenchymal hypertrophy) and humoral regulation [5]. Hence the need for biliary drainage of FRL before PVE is unanimously recognized as indispensable [3,19,20]. In Nagino's experience, in 193 jaundiced patients with biliary neoplasm PVE was performed after biliary drainage with a drop of bilirubinemia under 5 mg/dl [21].

Contraindications

The contraindications to PVE are: (1) dilated biliary ducts in the FRL, (2) presence of untreatable coagulopathy, (3) moderate portal hypertension, and (4) renal insufficiency in dialyzed patients. In presence of portal neoplastic invasion the portal flow is already diverted, therefore there are no indications for PVE. The presence of neoplastic extent to FRL or extrahepatic metastases is itself a contraindication to resection, as is the occurrence of evident portal hypertension. PVE is not needed when documented lobar atrophy or clear neoplastic portal stenosis are shown.

Technique

The approach to the portal system depends on the technical preferences of the operator, on the types of planned hepatic resection, on embolization extent and the embolizing agent. Independently of the chosen route, the aim is to occlude completely the portal branches of the portion of hepatic parenchyma that is going to be resected; this prevents the development of porto-portal collaterals that can negatively condition the volumetric increase of the residual part of the liver [22]. The type of planned resection regulates the choice of the segments to be embolized. If right hepatectomy is planned, segments V–VIII are embolized, with extension to IVa and IVb if right extended hepatectomy is required to allow surgical radicality and amplify hypertrophy of the FRL. The extension of embolization to segment IV (PVE "trisegment") in patients with hilar cholangio-carcinoma has been shown to decrease the technical difficulties of trisectionec-tomy and to increase hypertrophy of segments II and III. On percentage, the use of left extended hepatectomy (4 of 240 extended hepatectomies for biliary neo-plasm in Nagino's experience [21]) with preventive embolization of left and right anterior portal branches results lower. The technique requires antibiotic prophylaxis and even if general anesthesia may be needed, PVE can be per-formed under local anesthesia with intravenous sedative. Under ultrasound con-trol the most suitable access to the portal system is identified. Access to the por-tal system is achieved under ultrasound or fluoroscopic guidance in a prepared antiseptic field. Transparenchymal portal puncture is carried out by Chiba nee-dle and the porta vein is cannulated by means of the Seldinger technique. The angiographic study with right and left selective injections in different projec-tions allow definition of the portal anatomy.

The standard procedures of PVE are: contralateral transhepatic, ipsilateral transhepatic and laparotomic transileocolic. In the contralateral transhepatic approach, portal access is achieved through the parenchyma of the FRL [23]; in the case that right hepatectomy is planned, the catheter is introduced in the umbilical portion of the portal vein and advanced until the branches of the right portal system. This technique has the advantage of being simple since the catheterization of right portal branches is direct; its disadvantages are repre-sented by adverse events in 12.8%: migration of embolic material in the FLR, portal thrombosis, bleeding, (haemobilia, haemoperitoneum, subcapsular haematoma) and transient hepatic failure [24]. The complications of the con-tralateral approach, on the part of non-embolized liver that will remain, may be so significant that the planned resection may be more difficult or be abandoned [7,25]. The ipsilateral transhepatic approach described by Nagino [25] with the use of a dedicated two-way catheter and subsequently with traditional catheters [26] requires the puncture and catheterization of a peripheral portal branch of the lobe that will be resected. It presents the advantage that the FLR is not trau-matized, the risk of bleeding at catheter withdrawal is lower, but migration of embolic material into the portal system is still possible. The direct cannulation of the ileocolic vein and progression up to the portal branch for the emboliza-tion is the transileocolic approach [27]; it requires general anesthesia, laparoto-my, and is indicated whenever a staging operation or associated surgery are needed. It has the disadvantages of laparotomy risks and cannot take advantage of the assistance of the technical tools of an equipped radiologic room. The

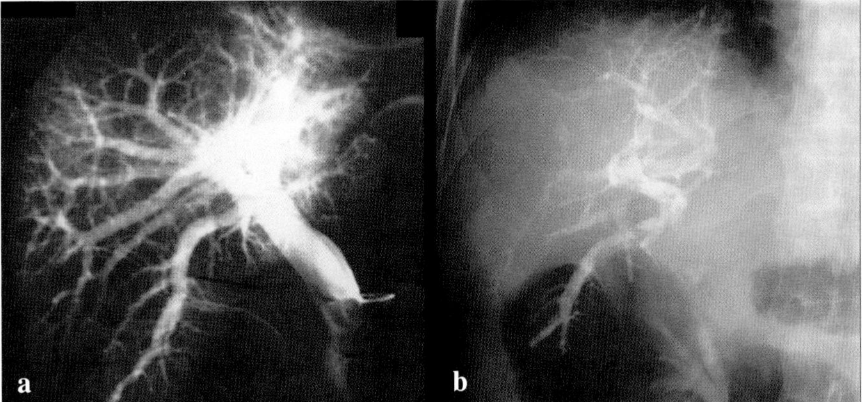

Fig. 2a,b Portal vein embolization: **a** Transparenchymal portography: the angiographic study allows defining the portal anatomy. **b** Radiological control after PVE shows embolic material (fibrin glue) in the right portal vein branches

experience in performing transjugular intrahepatic portosistemic shunts has allowed proposing the transjugular approach for PVE. The procedure requires the puncture of the right or left branch of portal vein from right, middle or left hepatic vein under ultrasound control; the positioning of the catheter to the portal bifurcation allows the right PVE. It is an initial experience that requires validation [28]. There are many agents with embolizing action that are utilized, sometimes associated with coils, and each one has its own characteristics. Development of new agents is very dynamic in the effort to guarantee a complete and permanent occlusion that can reduce recanalization after PVE and promote a prompt and adequate hypertrophy.

Results

Independently of the disease, technique, type of embolizing agents, and interval PVE-resection the results of the different series are similar. From Abdalla's review of 345 patients who underwent PVE, mean value in percentage of total liver volume resulted 26.6% before the procedure; after PVE the mean volume was 39.1% with a mean volume increase of 12.4%. From 2 to 20% of the cases PVE has been unable to stimulate a satisfactory hypertrophy [9]. The reasons for the unsuccessful augment have been vascular abnormalities due to recanalization of embolized segments and the presence of significant portal hypertension with porto-systemic shunts [19,29,30]. As abovementioned, diabetes and chronic hepatopathy reduce regenerative stimulus and can explain the ineffectiveness of PVE.

Post-PVE Course and Timing of Resection

PVE is usually followed by alteration of the hepatic functional parameters (particularly increased ALT, AST and bilirubinemia), leukocytosis and fever. These alterations are slight, transient and self-limiting. The entity of tissue necrosis after PVE is insignificant; therefore it is not related to considerable systemic symptoms as after arterial embolization. From 14 to 63 days after PVE a new hepatic volumetry is performed. If the expected hypertrophy of the FRL is noticed the patient is prepared for resection, when bilirubinemia returns within normal range [31]. The risk of portal recanalization induces the surgeon not to defer the operation.

Complications

Complications of the procedure (6–15%) [32] are represented by: (1) haemoperitoneum, haemobilia and subcapsular haematoma in the site of the hepatic access; (2) portal thrombosis; (3) migration of embolizing particles in the hepatic portion to be preserved; (4) intestinal obstruction in the transileocolic approach; (5) need for re-embolization. The planned hepatic resection was not performed due to complications (mainly hepatic thrombosis) of PVE in 0.5% of the cases [24].

Conclusions

Right extended hepatectomy or (less frequently) left extended hepatectomy are indicated in hilar cholangiocarcinoma. In case of right extended hepatectomy PVE is performed because the volume of segments II and III is often inadequate. PVE has an insignificant incidence of complications and gives a measurable hypertrophy of the non-embolized lobe. The preoperative increase in the volume and hepatic function of the FRL enlarges the pool of patient candidates for a curative resection and makes resection itself safer. Many surgical series confirm the low complication rate and postoperative failure after major hepatic resection [15,33–36]. PVE does not change long-term survival: 5-year survival was 40% in the resected group with previous PVE vs. 38% in the group that underwent resection alone [15]. The benefits of the procedure are validated by controlled randomized trials that are considered unethical. Indications for PVE are still unclear because of the few data regarding the minimal hepatic volume required to tolerate surgery without serious complications [21]. There are no evident data that define the minimal volume of hepatic parenchyma required for tolerating an extended hepatic resection; therefore it is possible that at present, PVE is overused [9,21].

References

1. Shirabe K, Shimada M, Gion T et al (1999) Postoperative liver failure after major hepatic resection for hepatocellular carcinoma in the modern era with special reference to remnant liver volume. J Am Coll Surg 188(3):304–309
2. Abdalla EK, Barnett CC, Doherty D et al (2002) Extended hepatectomy in patients with hepatobiliary malignancies with and without preoperative portal vein embolization. Arch Surg 137(6):675–680; discussion 680–681
3. Makuuchi M, Thai BL, Takayasu K et al (1990) Preoperative portal embolization to increase safety of major hepatectomy for hilar bile duct carcinoma: a preliminary report. Surgery 107(5):521–527
4. Black DM, Behrns KE (2002) A scientist revisits the atrophy-hypertrophy complex: hepatic apoptosis and regeneration. Surg Oncol Clin N Am 11(4):849–864
5. Yokoyama Y, Nagino M, Nimura Y (2007) Mechanisms of hepatic regeneration following portal vein embolization and partial hepatectomy: a review. World J Surg 31(2):367–374
6. Komori K, Nagino M, Nimura Y (2006) Hepatocyte morphology and kinetics after portal vein embolization. Br J Surg 93(6):745–751
7. Madoff DC, Abdalla EK, Vauthey JN (2005) Portal vein embolization in preparation for major hepatic resection: evolution of a new standard of care. J Vasc Interv Radiol 16(6):779–790
8. Nagino M, Nimura Y, Kamiya J (1995) Changes in hepatic lobe volume in biliary tract cancer patients after right portal vein embolization. Hepatology 21(2):434–439
9. Abdalla EK, Hicks ME, Vauthey JN (2001) Portal vein embolization: rationale, technique and future prospects. Br J Surg 88(2):165–175
10. Goto Y, Nagino M, Nimura Y (1998) Doppler estimation of portal blood flow after percutaneous transhepatic portal vein embolization. Ann Surg 228(2):209–213
11. Hemming AW, Reed AI, Howard RJ et al (2003) Preoperative portal vein embolization for extended hepatectomy. Ann Surg 237(5):686–691; discussion 691–693
12. Yigitler C, Farges O, Kianmanesh R et al (2003) The small remnant liver after major liver resection: how common and how relevant? Liver Transpl 9(9):S18-S25
13. Vauthey JN, Chaoui A, Do KA et al (2000) Standardized measurement of the future liver remnant prior to extended liver resection: methodology and clinical associations. Surgery 127(5):512–519
14. Kubota K, Makuuchi M, Kusaka K et al (1997) Measurement of liver volume and hepatic functional reserve as a guide to decision-making in resectional surgery for hepatic tumours. Hepatology 26(5):1176–1181
15. Azoulay D, Castaing D, Krissat J et al (2000) Percutaneous portal vein embolization increases the feasibility and safety of major liver resection for hepatocellular carcinoma in injured liver. Ann Surg 232(5):665–672
16. Farges O, Belghiti J, Kianmanesh R et al (2003) Portal vein embolization before right hepatectomy: prospective clinical trial. Ann Surg 237(2):208–217
17. Belghiti J (2004) Arguments for a selective approach of preoperative portal vein embolization before major hepatic resection. J Hepatobiliary Pancreat Surg 11(1):21–24
18. Imamura H, Shimada R, Kubota M et al (1999) Preoperative portal vein embolization: an audit of 84 patients. Hepatology 29(4):1099–1105
19. Cherqui D, Benoist S, Malassagne B et al (2000) Major liver resection for carcinoma in jaundiced patients without preoperative biliary drainage. Arch Surg 135(3):302–308
20. Nagino M, Nimura Y, Hayakawa N (1993) Percutaneous transhepatic portal embolization using newly devised catheters: preliminary report. World J Surg 17(4):520–524
21. Nagino M, Kamiya J, Nishio H et al (2006) Two hundred forty consecutive portal vein embolizations before extended hepatectomy for biliary cancer: surgical outcome and long-term follow-up. Ann Surg 243(3):364–372

22. Denys AL, Abehsera M, Sauvanet A et al (1999) Failure of right portal vein ligation to induce left lobe hypertrophy due to intrahepatic portoportal collaterals: successful treatment with portal vein embolization. AJR Am J Roentgenol 173(3):633–635

23. Kinoshita H, Sakai K, Hirohashi K et al (1986) Preoperative portal vein embolization for hepatocellular carcinoma. World J Surg 10(5):803–808

24. Di Stefano DR, de Baere T, Denys A et al (2005) Preoperative percutaneous portal vein embolization: evaluation of adverse events in 188 patients. Radiology 234(2):625–630

25. Nagino M, Nimura Y, Kamiya J et al (1996) Selective percutaneous transhepatic embolization of the portal vein in preparation for extensive liver resection: the ipsilateral approach. Radiology 200(2):559–563

26. Madoff DC, Hicks ME, Abdalla EK et al (2003) Portal vein embolization with polyvinyl alcohol particles and coils in preparation for major liver resection for hepatobiliary malignancy: safety and effectiveness study in 26 patients. Radiology 227(1):251–260

27. Liem MS, Liu CL, Tso WK et al (2005) Portal vein embolisation prior to extended right-sided hepatic resection. Hong Kong Med J 11(5):366–372

28. Perarnau JM, Daradkeh S, Johann M et al (2003) Transjugular preoperative portal embolization (TJPE) a pilot study. Hepatogastroenterology 50(51):610–613

29. Bruix J, Castells A, Bosch J et al (1996) Surgical resection of hepatocellular carcinoma in cirrhotic patients: prognostic value of preoperative portal pressure. Gastroenterology 111(4):1018–1022

30. Tanaka H, Hirohashi K, Kubo S et al (1999) Influence of histological inflammatory activity on regenerative capacity of liver after percutaneous transhepatic portal vein embolization. J Gastroenterol 34(1):100–104

31. Seyama Y, Kubota K, Sano K et al (2003) Long-term outcome of extended hemihepatectomy for hilar bile duct cancer with no mortality and high survival rate. Ann Surg 238(1):73–83

32. Kodama Y, Shimizu T, Endo H et al (2002) Complications of percutaneous transhepatic portal vein embolization. J Vasc Interv Radiol 13(12):1233–1237

33. Lee KC, Kinoshita H, Hirohashi K et al (1993) Extension of surgical indications for hepatocellular carcinoma by portal vein embolization. World J Surg 17(1):109–115

34. Shimamura T, Nakajima Y, Une Y et al (1997) Efficacy and safety of preoperative percutaneous transhepatic portal embolization with absolute ethanol: a clinical study. Surgery 121(2):135–141

35. Wakabayashi H, Yachida S, Maeba T, Maeta H (2000) Indications for portal vein embolization combined with major hepatic resection for advanced-stage hepatocellular carcinomas. A preliminary clinical study. Dig Surg 17(6):587–594

36. Tanaka H, Hirohashi K, Kubo S et al (2000) Preoperative portal vein embolization improves prognosis after right hepatectomy for hepatocellular carcinoma in patients with impaired hepatic function. Br J Surg 87(7):879–882

Prognostic Factors

Radical surgery is the only therapeutic option that can ensure a long-term survival; until now many aspects of this disease have not been well-known, such as pathogenesis, and clinical and histopathologic factors that determine survival. In this chapter we will analyze the main prognostic factors that influence survival: macroscopic aspect, local extent, lymph-node involvement and distant metastases. Histological characteristics and molecular factors related to prognosis will also be analysed.

Gross Type

Three different macroscopic forms have been described: sclerosing, nodular, and papillary. The sclerosing type represents about 70% of all hilar cholangiocarcinomas; it presents as a circumferential thickening of the biliary wall and is accompanied by important fibrotic and desmoplastic phenomena. The sclerosing type is characterized by compact masses that protrude into the lumens and are often associated with the infiltrative type. The papillary type represents 4–5 % [1,2] of all cholangiocarcinomas and is characterized by soft and friable lesion that occupies the bile duct lumen. In about 40% of papillary neoplasms a superficial spread is seen that extends up to 35 mm from the main lesion; this finding is defined as "bile duct carcinoma with superficial spread" [3].

Papillary neoplasms are usually associated with the early stage of the disease, TNM UICC/AJCC Stage <IIa, in more than 70% of the cases, with 4% of lymph-node metastases [4]. In general papillary forms are associated with a better prognosis than nodular-infiltrative, with median survival of 55 vs. 33 months [4]. Even when they are associated with advanced stages with lymph-node involvement, prognosis is better than nodular-infiltrative forms with 10-year survival rate of 12 vs. 5%, respectively [1].

A. Guglielmi, A. Ruzzenente, C. Iacono (eds.) *Surgical Treatment of Hilar and ICC.*
© Springer 2008

Microscopic Pattern

The main microscopic factors of hilar cholangiocarcinoma, that affect prognosis, are: cellular differentiation, perineural infiltration, lymphatic and microvascular infiltration.

Cellular differentiation is an important prognostic factor, and is directly associated with the stage of disease, percentage of curative resections and long-term prognosis.

Survival is significantly related to cellular differentiation: 34–41 months for G1–G2 and 14–20 months for G3 [5,6].

Jarnagin [4] has observed that 64% of well-differentiated hilar cholangiocarcinoma shows an early stage (TNM UICC/AJCC IIa), compared to only 25% of moderately or poorly differentiated types. Moreover, the percentage of curative R0 resection is related to cellular differentiation; Neuhaus reported [7] a radical resection in 75, 63 and 48% for well, moderately and poorly differentiated neoplasms, respectively.

Perineural infiltration is present in 60–80% of cases and is a further prognostic factor associated with stage and long-term survival [7,8]. Five-year survival rate in patients with perineural infiltration is significantly lower than that in patients without infiltration, 32 vs. 67%, respectively [8]. In addition, it is associated with a more advanced stage and a lower rate of R0 resections than in patients without perineural infiltration, 58 vs. 66% respectively [7].

Lymphangiosis carcinomatosa occurs in more than 70% of the neoplasms and survival is significantly higher in patients without this condition, 48 vs. 30% at 5 years. It is also associated with a larger number of non-curative resections for advanced stage of disease, 45 vs. 21% [7].

Microvascular invasion determines long-term survival, with 5-year survival rate of 40% in absence of microvascular invasion vs. 16% when it is present [9].

Biological and Molecular Prognostic Factors

In extrahepatic cholangiocarcinoma biological and molecular prognostic factors and pathological associations have not yet been analyzed in prospective studies.

More frequent genetic alterations comprehend oncogene and antioncogene mutations such as K-ras, p53, p27, of TGF-β, of HGF, of MDM2, of NMT, and the presence of microsatellite instability (MSI).

Of these, alteration of K-ras is highly variable, from 0 to 39%, and its prognostic significance has not been clarified.

The frequency of alteration of p53 expression in extrahepatic cholangiocarcinoma varies from 38 to 66% in the literature: these alterations are rare in early papillary tumours but their frequency increases progressively with the degree of cellular atypia grade. The expression of p53 correlates with cellular differentiation, stage and presence of N+ [10].

Overexpression of mdm2 is present in 79% of cases and it is correlated to a worse prognosis, with a median survival of 33 and 75 months in patients who are mdm2 positive and negative, respectively [11].

TGF-β is involved in alteration of cellular growth in the tumoral cell lines of the biliary extrahepatic tract, but its prognostic role has not yet been established.

Presence of MSI and TGFBR2 have been identified as potential prognostic factors but their role has not yet been clarified (Table 1).

Table 1 Biological and molecular prognostic factors in hilar cholangiocarcinoma. Adapted from [11–17]

Poor differentiation	Increased T stage	Increased lymphatic invasion	Increased nodal metastases	Distant metastases	Increased likelihood of recurrence	Decreased survival
–	p53	–	–	NMT+p53	–	NMT+p53
–	MDM2	–	–	NMD2	–	NMD2+p53
–	–	Cyclin D1	Cyclin D1	–	–	–
–	–	CD44	CD44	–	–	CD44
↓p27$^{\text{Kip1}}$	↓p27$^{\text{Kip1}}$	↓p27$^{\text{Kip1}}$	↓p27$^{\text{Kip1}}$	–	↓p27$^{\text{Kip1}}$	↓p27$^{\text{Kip1}}$
–	↓p27$^{\text{WAF/CIP1}}$	–	–	–	↑or↓p27$^{\text{WAF/CIP1}}$	↑or↓p27$^{\text{WAF/CIP1}}$
–	–	–	–	–	–	KRas

p27^{Kip1}, Cyclin-dependent kinase inhibitor; *p27$^{WAF/CIP1}$*, cyclin-dependent kinase inhibitor; *p53*, tumour suppressor gene; *Cyclin D1*, cell-cycle modulator; *CD44*, transmembrane protein with endothelial cell binding function; *NMD2*, oncoprotein that binds Tp53 and inhibits p53-mediated transactivation; *NMT*, N-myristoyltransferase, intracellular signal transduction modulator

T Category

The wall of the biliary duct is composed of biliary epithelium, submucosa surrounded by a dense fibromuscular layer (dense fibrous tissue with sparse smooth muscle fibers) organized around the lumen. Contiguously with the ductal wall there are the adipose tissue and the vessels of the hepatoduodenal ligament. TNM UICC/AJCC classification defines as T1 the neoplasms confined to the bile duct, whereas T2 neoplasm invades beyond the wall of the bile duct, T3 neoplasm invades the liver, gallbladder, unilateral branch of portal vein and hepatic artery, while in T4 the tumour invades other adjacent structures. According to TNM UICC/AJCC criteria the radial extent is not well defined, so some authors have proposed assessing the depth of invasion of the neoplasm in mm. T1 neoplasm shows a depth of invasion less than 5 mm in 87% of cases, while this rate falls to 51% for T2 tumour. The depth of invasion is related to a median survival of 61 months in the patients with an infiltration of less than 5 mm and of 23 months in the patient with an infiltration greater than 5 mm (Table 2) [18].

Table 2 Association between T classification and depth of invasion, lymph-node involvement and survival. Adapted from [18]

| | Depth of invasion | | |
	<5 mm	5–12 mm	>12 mm
T1	41 (87%)	6 (13 %)	0
T2	36 (51%)	29 (40%)	6 (10%)
T3	21 (22%)	57 (60%)	16 (18%)
T4	1 (10%)	3 (30%)	6 (60%)
N0	83 (54%)	58 (38%)	11 (8%)
N+	16 (16%)	17 (39%)	17 (61%)
Median survival (months)	61	23	17

T1

The neoplasm within the ductal wall is defined as early bile duct cancer; it represents about 10% of all cholangiocarcinoma and shows distinctive characteristics. In 52% of cases the neoplasms show a papillary aspect and in more than 60% are well differentiated. Lymph-node involvement is present in 0–2% of the cases and perineural invasion is present in 0–10% [19,20]. The prognosis is good with a 5-year survival rate of 78%. According to gross type the survival rate of papillary and infiltrative neoplasms is not significantly different. Recurrence is uncommon and occurs in about 13% of cases (Table 3).

Table 3 Prevalence of early bile duct cancer (T1 according to the 6th TNM AJCC/UICC) and 5-year survival

Author	Year	Total	Early cancer (T1)	5-Year survival
Mizumoto [21]	1993	171	14 (8%)	100%
Bhuiya [22]	1993	70	7 (10%)	-
Kurosaki [23]	1998	90	7 (8%)	86%
Hong [24]	2005	222	47 (21%)	53%
Cha [20]	2006	614	61 (10%)	78%

T2

The depth of the neoplastic invasion of the ductal wall is associated with relevant prognostic aspects such as vascular, lymphatic and perineural invasion. In T1 neoplasms Tabata did not observe vascular, perineural or lymphatic invasion, while in T2 neoplasms the invasion rate increased to 40, 56 and 31%, respectively [19] (Table 4).

In T2 neoplasms the survival is significantly worse than in T1 neoplasms; Hong noticed a 5-year survival rate of 30 and 53%, respectively [24]. Instead the difference between T2 and T3 neoplasms is not significant: 30–37 and 25–32%, respectively (Table 5) [24,25].

Table 4 Association between T stage and pathological factors. Adapted from [19]

T stage infiltration (5th edn)	Patients	Lymph nodes metastasis	Lymphatic permeation	Venous invasion	Perineural
T1	4 (5.3%)	0%	0%	0%	0%
T2	32 (42%)	31%	71%	40%	56%
T3	39 (52%)	61%	87%	59%	84%

Table 5 5-Year survival according to T-stage

Author	Patients	T1	T2	T3	T4
Nishio 2005 [25]	166	69%	37%	32%	10%
Hong 2005 [24]	222	53%	30%	25%	0%

T3

According UICC/AJCC classification, T3-stage neoplasm spreads beyond the ductal wall and involves adjacent structures: hepatic parenchyma, gallbladder, and diramations of portal vein and/or hepatic artery. As mentioned previously, the depth of ductal invasion is related with more aggressive neoplasms, with an increased frequency of lymph-node metastases (64.7% in T3 neoplasm; 33.3% in T2 neoplasm) [26].

The patients with T3 (6th edition TNM UICC/AJCC) neoplasms have a significantly worse prognosis than T1, with a 5-year survival rate of 32 vs. 69%, respectively, while the difference is not significant if compared with T2 neoplasms (survival rate 37%) [25].

Invasion of hepatic parenchyma is very frequent in hilar cholangiocarcinoma, but in the patients who undergo radical resection (R0) it does not represent a negative prognostic factor [6,24,32].

In the past, invasion of the portal vein was a major obstacle to resection of advanced cholangiocarcinoma; however, recent studies reported in the literature show that resection and reconstruction of the portal vein offer better long-term survivals compared to non-resected patients, with 5-year survival rate of 9.9 vs. 0%, respectively. However, portal invasion represents an important prognostic factor; 5-year survival rate in the patients with macroscopic infiltration of the portal vein is 9.9 vs. 36.8% of the patients without [9]. Other authors confirm the prognostic significance of portal vein involvement (Table 6).

Table 6 Survival in patients with portal vein involvement subjected to portal vein resection

Author	Patients	Portal involvement	5-Year survival	Median survival (months)
Launois 1999 [35]	40	17.5%	0%	–
Kosuge 1999 [32]	65	27.7%	–	23.9
Kondo 2004 [6]	40	30%	–	34.7
Nishio 2005 [25]	301	32%	11%	–

Infiltration of the hepatic artery is considered a criterion for unresectability in the majority of the cases; it is a negative prognostic factor and only recently some studies in the literature report the results of hepatic resection combined with resection and reconstruction of the hepatic artery [39,40]. Invasion of the hepatic artery is associated with an advanced stage of disease, lymph-node metastases in more than 70% of the cases, and perineural invasion in all of them [33]. Miyazaki reports a 3-year survival rate of 11% and no 5-year survival in a group of patients who underwent arterial resection and reconstruction [33].

According to Kosuge, transmural extension to gallbladder is a negative prognostic factor ($p=0.0023$). Neoplasms involving the gallbladder are usually associated with diffuse infiltration of the connective tissue of the hepatoduodenal ligament [32].

T4

According to the 6th edition of TNM UICC/AJCC, stage T4 is determined by the invasion of surrounding organs, or portal vein, or infiltration of the hepatic artery proper. These elements imply unresectability in the majority of the cases.

Stage T4 is correlated with poor prognosis, with a median survival of 13–17 months [24,25].

N Category

Lymph-node involvement is an important prognostic factor in hilar cholangio-carcinoma and it is present in 30–50% of patients who have undergone surgical resection [7,26–31].

The percentage of lymph-node involvement is closely related to T stage in accordance with UICC/AJCC criteria and the depth of invasion estimated in millimeters. Lymph-node involvement is present in 17.1% of T1 neoplasms, in 28.4% of T2, in 39.6% of T3 and in 60% of T4 [24].

Based on radial extent expressed in millimeters, the frequency of N+ was 16% in the neoplasms under 5 mm, 39% in neoplasms between 5 and 12 mm, and 61% in neoplasms over 12 mm [1].

Lymph-node metastases are also associated with vascular invasion: the rates are 55% and 39% in patients with and without vascular invasion [9].

Five-year survival rate is 45% in N0 patients, 16% in N1, 14% in non-regional node involvement defined as M1 according to the criteria of TNM UICC/AJCC. In the literature, different series show that the 5-year survival rate in patients with lymph-node metastases does not exceed 25% [7,25–29,32–34] (Table 7).

The prevalence of non-regional lymph-node metastases, defined as M1, is not well known in hilar cholangiocarcinoma since few authors performed a systematic dissection of non-regional lymph nodes; in Kitagawa's study [26], the prevalence of positive para-aortic lymph nodes (M1) was 17% [26]. The presence of non-regional lymph-node metastases is an important prognostic factor,

Table 7 Prevalence and survival for patients with positive lymph-node metastases (*N*+)

Author	Patients	N+ patients	Survival for N+ patients	
			Median (months)	Rate (%)
Launois 1999 [35]	40	15%	-	16.7%
Kosuge 1999 [32]	65	44%	26.4	-
Nagakawa 2002 [36]	1183	45%	-	15%
Kitagawa [26]	110	53%	-	16%
Kondo 2004 [6]	40	37.5%	26.6	-
Hemming 2005 [34]	80	-	-	21%
Lai 2005 [37]	36	35%	-	0%
Nishio 2005 [16]	301	49%	-	10%
Ramacciato 2006 [38]	23	34%	21	-
Dinant 2006 [5]	99	19%	18	-

with survival of less than 15% at 5 years [17]. The analysis of the characteristics of the patients with para-aortic lymph-node metastases showed that survival in patients with M1 nodes with a normal macroscopic aspect is significantly better than the group of patients with macroscopically positive nodes, with a 5-year survival rate of 28.6 vs. 0%, respectively [26].

Even the number of metastatic nodes represents an independent prognostic factor that is statistically significant ($p=0.017$). Patients with more than 5 positive lymph nodes have shown a shorter survival compared to patients with less than 4 metastatic lymph nodes, with a HR at univariate analysis of 2.95 and 1.7, respectively [1].

In a recent study, Schwartz [41] observed a correlation between survival and number of removed nodes in N0 patients. Median survival was 21 months in the patients with 1 to 2 total lymph nodes examined, and 34 months in patients with more than 10 lymph nodes examined, respectively. Also in N1 patients a difference in survival has been recognized in the patients with 1 to 2 lymph nodes examined vs. more than 10 nodes, with median values of 13 and 16 months, respectively.

Immunohistochemical techniques that utilize antibodies against cytokeratin can identify micrometastases that are not detected by haematoxylin-eosin staining. Micrometastases are detected in 24–39% of the patients with negative nodes [42,43]. The prognostic significance of micrometastases is still controversial. Yuchiro has not found significant differences in patients with or without microscopic lymph-node metastases, with 43.6 and 42.1% 5-year survival rates, respectively [42]. Conversely, in 28 patients in N0 stage Taniguchi identified a significant correlation between micrometastases, stage of disease and prognosis, with 5-year survival rates of 21 and 66%, respectively [43].

M Category

The presence of distant metastases is the most frequent cause of unresectability: about 30% of patients are excluded from surgical treatment during preoperative workup or at laparotomy [44].

The more common sites of metastases are: liver, peritoneum, lung and bone; the median survival of the patients with metastases is no longer than 11 months [35].

In presence of hepatic metastases, the resection has very few satisfactory results with a median survival of 6–12 months [32].

Prognostic Significance of TNM UICC/AJCC Classification

Until now, few reports have valued the prognostic significance of TNM classification for hilar cholangiocarcinoma. The new edition of TNM staging (6th edition of UICC/AJCC) focuses on two aspects: vascular invasion and the presence of lymph-node metastases [45].

The prognostic significance of staging grouping according to UICC/AJCC is still debated; in a recent study, Zervos did not show any correlation between stage and survival in 42 patients submitted to surgical resection [12]; nor did Hemming's study show any significant correlation between stage and prognosis [34].

However, other authors have shown a significant difference between stage and survival; in fact, in 222 patients Hong reported a median survival in stages Ib, IIa, IIb and III of 40 months, 39 months, 19 months and 13 months, respectively [24].

In 166 patients, Nishio also observed a correlation between stage and survival, with 5-year survival rate in stages Ia, Ib, IIa, IIb, III and IV of 75, 45, 43, 19, 13, and 14%, respectively [25] (Fig. 1).

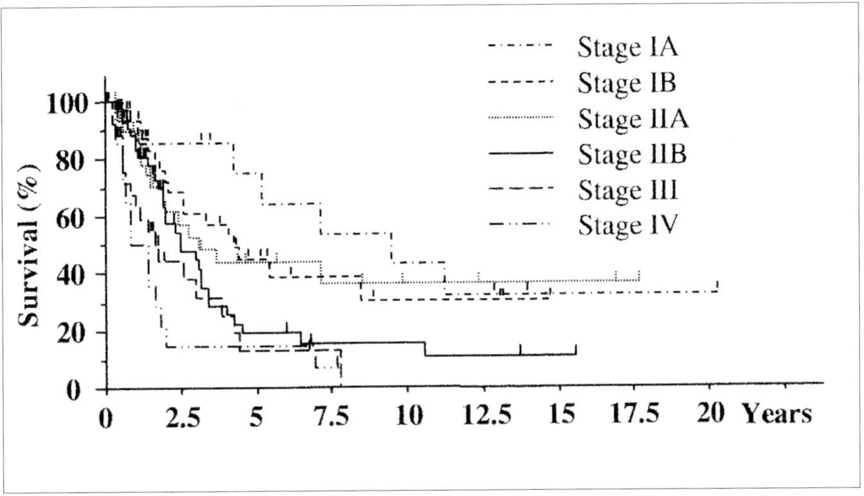

Fig. 1 Survival according to UICC/AJCC stage grouping. Adapted from [25]

References

1. Hoang MP, Murakata LA, Katabi N et al (2002) Invasive papillary carcinomas of the extrahepatic bile ducts: a clinicopathologic and immunohistochemical study of 13 cases. Mod Pathol 15(12):1251–1258
2. Albores-Saavedra J, Murakata L, Krueger JE, Henson DE (2000) Noninvasive and minimally invasive papillary carcinomas of the extrahepatic bile ducts. Cancer 89(3):508–515
3. Sakamoto E, Nimura Y, Hayakawa N et al (1998) The pattern of infiltration at the proximal border of hilar bile duct carcinoma: a histologic analysis of 62 resected cases. Ann Surg 227(3):405–411
4. Jarnagin WR, Bowne W, Klimstra DS et al (2005) Papillary phenotype confers improved survival after resection of hilar cholangiocarcinoma. Ann Surg 241(5):703–712; discussion 712–714

5. Dinant S, Gerhards MF, Rauws EA et al (2006) Improved outcome of resection of hilar cholangiocarcinoma (Klatskin tumour). Ann Surg Oncol 13(6):872–80

6. Kondo S, Hirano S, Ambo Y et al (2004) Forty consecutive resections of hilar cholangiocarcinoma with no postoperative mortality and no positive ductal margins: results of a prospective study. Ann Surg 240(1):95–101

7. Neuhaus P, Jonas S, Bechstein WO et al (1999) Extended resections for hilar cholangiocarcinoma. Ann Surg 230(6):808–818; discussion 819

8. Bhuiya MR, Nimura Y, Kamiya J et al (1992) Clinicopathologic studies on perineural invasion of bile duct carcinoma. Ann Surg 215(4):344–349

9. Ebata T, Nagino M, Kamiya J et al (2003) Hepatectomy with portal vein resection for hilar cholangiocarcinoma: audit of 52 consecutive cases. Ann Surg 238(5):720–727

10. Liu XF, Zhang H, Zhu SG et al (2006) Correlation of p53 gene mutation and expression of P53 protein in cholangiocarcinoma. World J Gastroenterol 12(29):4706–4709

11. Jarnagin WR, Klimstra DS, Hezel M et al (2006) Differential cell cycle-regulatory protein expression in biliary tract adenocarcinoma: correlation with anatomic site, pathologic variables, and clinical outcome. J Clin Oncol 24(7):1152–1160

12. Zervos EE, Osborne D, Goldin SB et al (2005) Stage does not predict survival after resection of hilar cholangiocarcinomas promoting an aggressive operative approach. Am J Surg 190(5):810–815

13. Itoi T, Shinohara Y, Takeda K et al (2000) Detection of telomerase activity in biopsy specimens for diagnosis of biliary tract cancers. Gastrointest Endosc 52(3):380–386

14. Abdalla EK, Vauthey JN (2001) Biliary tract cancer. Curr Opin Gastroenterol 17(5):450–457

15. Rajala RV, Radhi JM, Kakkar R et al (2000) Increased expression of N-myristoyltransferase in gallbladder carcinomas. Cancer 88(9):1992–1999

16. Cormier JN, Vauthey JN (2000) Biliary tract cancer. Curr Opin Gastroenterol 16(5):437–443

17. Rashid A, Ueki T, Gao YT et al (2002) K-ras mutation, p53 overexpression, and microsatellite instability in biliary tract cancers: a population-based study in China. Clin Cancer Res 8(10):3156–3163

18. Hong SM, Cho H, Moskaluk CA, Yu E (2007) Measurement of the invasion depth of extrahepatic bile duct carcinoma: an alternative method overcoming the current T classification problems of the AJCC staging system. Am J Surg Pathol 31(2):199–206

19. Tabata M, Kawarada Y, Yokoi H et al (2000) Surgical treatment for hilar cholangiocarcinoma. J Hepatobiliary Pancreat Surg 7(2):148–154

20. Cha JM, Kim MH, Lee SK et al (2006) Clinicopathological review of 61 patients with early bile duct cancer. Clin Oncol (R Coll Radiol) 18(9):669–677

21. Mizumoto R, Ogura Y, Kusuda T (1993) Definition and diagnosis of early cancer of the biliary tract. Hepatogastroenterology 40(1):69–77

22. Kurosaki I, Tsukada K, Watanabe H, Hatakeyama K (1998) Prognostic determinants in extrahepatic bile duct cancer. Hepatogastroenterology 45(22):905–909

23. Bhuiya MR, Nimura Y, Kamiya J et al (1993) Clinicopathologic factors influencing survival of patients with bile duct carcinoma: multivariate statistical analysis. World J Surg 17(5):653–657

24. Hong SM, Kim MJ, Pi DY et al (2005) Analysis of extrahepatic bile duct carcinomas according to the New American Joint Committee on Cancer staging system focused on tumour classification problems in 222 patients. Cancer 104(4):802–810

25. Nishio H, Nagino M, Oda K et al (2005) TNM classification for perihilar cholangiocarcinoma: comparison between 5th and 6th editions of the AJCC/UICC staging system. Langenbecks Arch Surg 390(4):319–327

26. Kitagawa Y, Nagino M, Kamiya J et al (2001) Lymph-node metastasis from hilar cholangiocarcinoma: audit of 110 patients who underwent regional and paraaortic node dissection. Ann Surg 233(3):385–392

27. Nakeeb A, Pitt HA, Sohn TA et al (1996) Cholangiocarcinoma. A spectrum of intrahepatic, perihilar, and distal tumours. Ann Surg 224(4):463–473; discussion 473–475

28. Sugiura Y, Nakamura S, Iida S et al (1994) Extensive resection of the bile ducts combined with liver resection for cancer of the main hepatic duct junction: a cooperative study of the Keio Bile Duct Cancer Study Group. Surgery 115(4):445–451

29. Iwatsuki S, Todo S, Marsh JW et al (1998) Treatment of hilar cholangiocarcinoma (Klatskin tumours) with hepatic resection or transplantation. J Am Coll Surg 187(4):358–364

30. Ogura Y, Kawarada Y (1998) Surgical strategies for carcinoma of the hepatic duct confluence. Br J Surg 85(1):20–24

31. Miyazaki M, Ito H, Nakagawa K et al (1999) Parenchyma-preserving hepatectomy in the surgical treatment of hilar cholangiocarcinoma. J Am Coll Surg 189(6):575–583

32. Kosuge T, Yamamoto J, Shimada K et al (1999) Improved surgical results for hilar cholangiocarcinoma with procedures including major hepatic resection. Ann Surg 230(5):663-671

33. Miyazaki M, Kato A, Ito H et al (2007) Combined vascular resection in operative resection for hilar cholangiocarcinoma: does it work or not? Surgery 141(5):581–588

34. Hemming AW, Reed AI, Fujita S et al (2005) Surgical management of hilar cholangiocarcinoma. Ann Surg 241(5):693–699; discussion 699–702

35. Launois B, Terblanche J, Lakehal M et al (1999) Proximal bile duct cancer: high resectability rate and 5-year survival. Ann Surg 230(2):266–275

36. Nagakawa T, Kayahara M, Ikeda S et al () Biliary tract cancer treatment: results from the Biliary Tract Cancer Statistics Registry in Japan. J Hepatobiliary Pancreat Surg 9(5):569–575

37. Lai EC, Lau WY (2005) Aggressive surgical resection for hilar cholangiocarcinoma. ANZ J Surg 75(11):981–985

39. Miyazaki M, Ito H, Nakagawa K et al (1998) Aggressive surgical approaches to hilar cholangiocarcinoma: hepatic or local resection? Surgery 123(2):131–136

40. Gerhards MF, van Gulik TM, de Wit LT et al (2000) Evaluation of morbidity and mortality after resection for hilar cholangiocarcinoma—a single center experience. Surgery 127(4):395–404

41. Schwarz RE, Smith DD (2007) Lymph node dissection impact on staging and survival of extrahepatic cholangiocarcinomas, based on U.S. population data. J Gastrointest Surg 11(2):158–165

42. Tojima Y, Nagino M, Ebata T et al (2003) Immunohistochemically demonstrated lymph node micrometastasis and prognosis in patients with otherwise node-negative hilar cholangiocarcinoma. Ann Surg 237(2):201–207

43. Taniguchi K, Tabata M, Iida T et al (2006) Significance of lymph node micrometastasis in pN0 hilar bile duct carcinoma. Eur J Surg Oncol 32(2):208–212

44. Jarnagin WR, Shoup M (2004) Surgical management of cholangiocarcinoma. Semin Liver Dis 24(2):189–199

45. Ramacciato G, Corigliano N, Mercantini P et al (2006) [Prognostic factors after surgical resection for hilar cholangiocarcinoma] Ann Chir 131(6-7):379–85, French

45. Sobin LH, Wittekind C (eds) (2002) TNM classification of malignant tumours, 6th edn. Wiley, New York

Staging Systems

Many staging systems have been proposed for hilar cholangiocarcinoma and none of them has been accepted unanimously.

Three different types of classification have been suggested:
- Classification based on macroscopic biliary involvement (Bismuth-Corlette)
- Histopathologic classification (TNM AJCC/UICC and Japanese Society for Biliary Surgery, JSBS)
- Classification based on biliary and vascular involvement (Gazzaniga and Memorial Sloan Kettering Cancer Center, MSKCC)

Bismuth-Corlette Classification

Bismuth-Corlette classification was introduced in 1975 and modified in 1992; it classifies lesions according to biliary longitudinal extent (Table 1) [1,2] into different anatomical groups based on radiological and operative findings (Fig. 1).

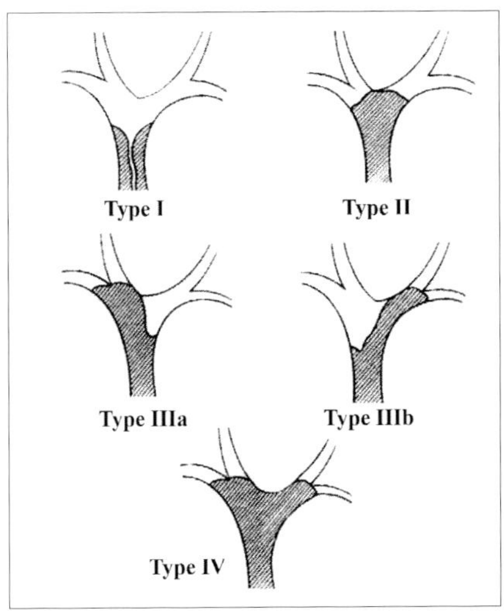

Fig. 1 Modified Bismuth-Corlette classification of the longitudinal extent of hilar cholangiocarcinoma (see also Table 1)

A. Guglielmi, A. Ruzzenente, C. Iacono (eds.) *Surgical Treatment of Hilar and ICC.*
© Springer 2008

Table 1 Bismuth-Corlette classification [1]

Type I	Neoplasm arises near the biliary confluence without involvement of the left and right biliary ducts
Type II	Neoplasm arises at the biliary confluence with extension to left and right ducts
Type IIIa	Neoplasm arises at the biliary confluence with extension to the right hepatic duct up to the second order ducts
Type IIIb	Neoplasm arises at the biliary confluence with extension to left biliary duct up to the second order ducts
Type IV	Neoplasm arises at the biliary confluence with bilateral extension to the second order biliary ducts

This classification considers only the extent of biliary involvement at preoperative workup. Bismuth's validation experience in 1992 [2] on 23 resected patients showed that this system can be used to tailor the surgical operation. In type I patients, resection of the biliary tract alone provides a curative resection. In type II the neoplasm involves the confluence, dividing the left and right ducts, and frequently the biliary ducts of the caudate lobe. In order to obtain a radical resection (R0) Bismuth suggests biliary resection associated with caudate lobe resection. In type IIIa and IIIb, resection of the biliary tract does not guarantee a curative resection and therefore major hepatic resection must be associated. In type IV the bilateral involvement of secondary ducts frequently precludes a radical resection despite extended hepatectomy. This staging system is still used to define the extent of the disease; nevertheless its use in therapeutic choice and prognostic evaluation is limited since important factors such as vascular invasion and lymph-node metastases are not considered. In a recent comparative study on 42 resected patients with hilar cholangiocarcinoma. Bismuth-Corlette classification failed to show a correlation with long-term survival [3].

TNM Staging System According to UICC/AJCC 6th Edition

The sixth edition of TNM classification by Internal Union Against Cancer (UICC) and the sixth edition of the Manual for Staging of Cancer edited by American Joint Committee on Cancer were published in 2002 and used the same TNM classification and subdivision in stages [4]. Local extent of disease (T), nodal involvement (N) and presence of distant organ involvement (M) are determined by preoperative, intraoperative and pathological findings.

T Category

T category evaluates local extent based on the degree of ductal wall involvement, portal vein and hepatic artery involvement and invasion of adjacent structures. T-category is divided into four types (Table 2).

Table 2 Evaluation of local extent according to UICC/AJCC [4]

T	Carcinoma in situ
T1	Tumour is confined to biliary duct
T2	Tumour invades through entire biliary duct wall
T3	Tumour invades liver, gallbladder, main branches of portal vein or hepatic artery (right or left)
T4	Tumour invades portal vein trunk, proper hepatic artery or other surrounding organs (colon, stomach, duodenum)

This staging system has been validated by a clinical study on 166 resected patients where T category showed a correlation with long-term survival: 5-year survival was 69% in T1, 37% in T2, 32% in T3 and 10% in T4 [5].

N Category

According to UICC/AJCC criteria, the regional lymph nodes are: cyst duct, pericholedochal, hilar, peripancreatic (head only), periduodenal, periportal, celiac, and superior mesenteric lymph nodes. The involvement of non-regional lymph nodes (aorto-caval and inferior peripancreatic) is defined as distant metastases (M1).

N category is defined in two stages (Table 3).

Table 3 Evaluation of lymph-node involvement according to UICC/AJCC [4]

N0	No lymph-node metastases
N1	Presence of regional lymph-node involvement

Many reports in the literature confirm the prognostic value of regional nodal involvement with 5-year survival of 30.5% in N0, and 14.7% in N1 (p=0.09). Kitagawa et al. have also proved the poor prognosis in non-regional node diffusion (M1) with a 5-year survival of 12.3% [6].

M Category

M category is based on the presence of metastases to other organs or non-regional lymph nodes. It is classified in Table 4.

Table 4 Evaluation of presence of metastases according to UICC/AJCC [4]

M0	No metastases
M1	Presence of metastases

Stage Grouping

The three categories T, N and M are arranged to classify patients in homogeneous groups. In the sixth edition of TNM classification of the UICC/AJCC seven groups are listed (Table 5).

Table 5 Staging system according to UICC/AJCC [4]

Stage 0	T	N0	M0
Stage IA	T1	N0	M0
Stage IB	T2	N0	M0
Stage IIA	T3	N0	M0
Stage IIB	T1, T2, T3	N1	M0
Stage III	T4	Any N	M0
Stage IV	Any T	Any N	M1

The grouping in stages defines neoplasms at the early stage as limited to the biliary duct (stage I), neoplasms at the intermediate stage involving hepatic parenchyma, vascular structures (hepatic artery or portal vein) or regional lymph nodes (stage II). Advanced tumours in stages III (diffusion to adjacent structures and/or regional lymph nodes) and IV (presence of metastases) rarely benefit from a surgical operation with intent to cure. Prognostic significance of this classification has been evaluated by several clinical studies; nevertheless there are no conclusive data available as yet. In a study of 40 patients who underwent resection for hilar cholangiocarcinoma, Liu et al. showed no significant difference in terms of survival between the groups of patients with stages I and II vs stages III and IV, with median survival of 17.6 and 21.2 months ($p=0.25$), respectively [7]. Hong reported a significant difference in survival for stages Ia, Ib, IIa, IIb and III, with a 5-year survival rate of 54, 35, 31, 7, 5 and 0%, respectively [8].

Comparison between 5th and 6th Edition of TNM UICC/AJCC

The last two staging editions of TNM, the 5th and 6th editions, present different criteria for classification of T and N categories. In the T category of the 5th edition all neoplasms involving adjacent structures were classified as T3; instead in the last edition T3 has been divided based on the structures involved: T3 for lesions that invade per contiguity the liver, gallbladder, pancreas, or the vessels unilaterally and T4 for the lesions invading other adjacent organs (colon, stomach and duodenum) or the main portal vein.

This new distinction has shown better accuracy in evaluating prognosis of patients who had undergone surgical resection. A comparative study between the 5th and 6th editions in 166 patients shows 5-year survival for T3 stage (5th edition) of 24% while for T3 of the 6th edition survival is 32% and 10% for T4, with a statistically significant difference [5]. The invasion of stomach, colon and duodenum is rare in hilar cholangiocarcinoma and the majority of T4 indicates invasion of main portal vein. The new formulation of T4 category emphasizes the value of vascular invasion which many reports have shown to be an important negative prognostic factor [9]. N category has been modified as well; in fact in the 5th edition lymph-node metastases were divided in N1 (hepatoduodenal ligament lymph nodes) and N2 (other regional lymph nodes); in the updated edition N category has been simplified in a single group of patients with metastatic regional lymph nodes. This new group of regional lymph nodes has gained validation in a clinical study on 110 patients in whom significant differences in long-term survival were not shown between patients with positive N1 versus N2 with median survival of 29 and 25 months respectively [6]. Both editions define as M1 the presence of non-regional lymph-node metastases.

Staging System According to JSBS

Classification of hilar neoplasm formulated by JSBS was published in English in its 2nd edition in 2004 [10]. As TNM of UICC/AJCC this classification is based on anatomic and pathological findings and analyzes the local extent of the neoplasm (T), its nodal extension, and involvement of other organs (M). Both TNM UICC/AJCC and JSBS classify hilar cholangiocarcinoma along with the other neoplasms of the extrahepatic biliary tract.

Macroscopic Growth Pattern

On macroscopic assessment neoplasms would be classified on the basis of the type of growth of the tumour inside the biliary duct:

– *Papillary type* (included pedunculated and sessile tumours thicker than 2 mm)
  Expanding pattern
  Infiltrating pattern
– *Nodular type*
  Expanding pattern
  Infiltrating pattern
– *Flat type*
  Expanding pattern
  Infiltrating pattern (flat type with infiltrating pattern entails diffuse infiltrating type)
– *Other types of growth*

T Category

Evaluation of the extent of the disease involves five different parameters: serosa, hepatic parenchyma, pancreas, portal vein and hepatic artery.

Involvement of serosa in this type of neoplasm is difficult to assess since only a portion of the hepatic hilum is lined by serosa (Fig. 2). In the portions lined by serosa it is defined by the infiltration of visceral peritoneum S(-) and the invasion beyond the serosa or of surrounding organs such as colon, stomach, abdominal wall or vena cava S(+).

Invasion of hepatic parenchyma is classified as Hinf1b if less than 5 mm, Hinf2 between 5 and 20 mm and Hinf3 if more than 20 mm.

Invasion of the pancreas is rare in hilar neoplasms and is defined according to the depth of invasion: less than 5 mm (Panc1b), between 5 and 20 mm (Panc2) and more than 20 mm (Panc3).

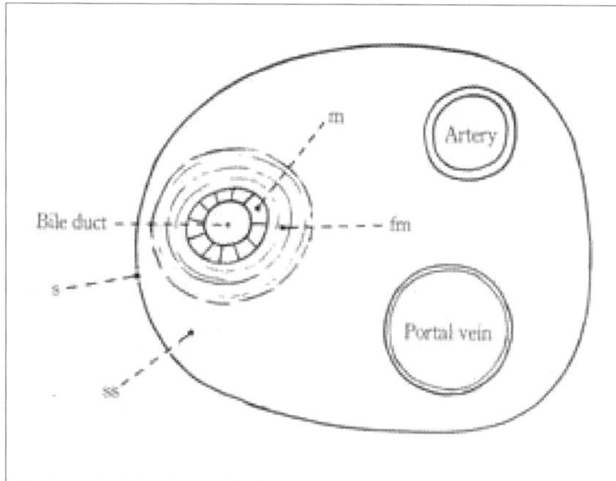

Fig. 2 Schematic representation of hepatic hilum; the different grades of infiltration of S-Stage are based on the involvement of ductal wall and visceral peritoneum. S(-): invasion of mucosa and fibro-muscular layer of biliary duct (*m* and/or *fm*); or invasion of subserosa (*ss*) S(+): invasion os serosa (*s*) and evidence of the tumour at visceral peritoneum (*se*), or invasion beyond serosa layer to other organs. Adapted from [10]

The invasions of portal and arterial structures are divided into adventitial infiltration (PV1 or A1), tunica media infiltration (PV2 or A2) or extended to tunica intima with stenosis and/or obstruction (PV3 or A3).

The division of T category on the basis of involvement of adjacent structures allows us to distinguish four categories (Table 6).

Table 6 Classification of T according to JSBS (Japanese Society of Biliary Surgery) [10]

T-stage	Serosa	Hepatic infiltration	Pancreatic infiltration	Portal infiltration	Arterial infiltration
T1	m, fm	Hinf0	Panc0	PV0	A0
T2	ss	Hinf1a	Panc1a	PV0	A0
T3	se	Hinf1b	Panc1b	PV0	A0
T4	any	Hinf2,3	Panc2,3	PV1–3	A1–3

Hinf, direct extent to hepatic parenchyma (0: no invasion; 1a: invasion beyond fibromuscular layer but not of parenchyma; 1b: <5 mm; 2: 5–20 mm; 3 invasion more than 20 mm); *Panc*, extent to pancreas (0: no invasion; 1a: invasion beyond fibromuscolar layer but not of parenchyma; 1b: <5 mm; 2: 5–20 mm; 3 more than 20 mm); *PV*, extent to portal vein (0: no invasion; 1: invasion of adventitia; 2: up to tunica media; 3: up to tunica intima with stenosis or obstruction); *A*, extent to hepatic artery (0: no invasion; 1: invasion of adventitia; 2: up to tunica media; 3: up to tunica intima with stenosis or obstruction). For serosa invasion, see Fig. 2

Classification of T according to JSBS includes prognostic factors that become evident from many clinical studies and permit precise classification of the extent of the disease. In literature no reported studies have validated this categorization of T category and due to its complexity it is not much used in clinical practice.

N Category

According to the Japanese classification, the lymph nodes for hilar hepatic neoplasms are divided into three levels: N1, N2 and N3. Lymph nodes of the hepatoduodenal ligament (station 12) belong to the first level (N1) and are categorized for their relationship with the biliary tract (12b), portal vein (12p) and proper hepatic artery (12a). Retropancreatic lymph nodes (13a) and those along the common hepatic artery (8) belong to the second level (N2). Para-aortic (16), celiac (9), mesenteric (14) or anterior-pancreatic (17) and inferior retropancreatic (13b) lymph node stations pertain to the third level (N3) (Figs. 3,4).

The division of lymph nodes for hilar hepatic neoplasms is shown in Table 7.

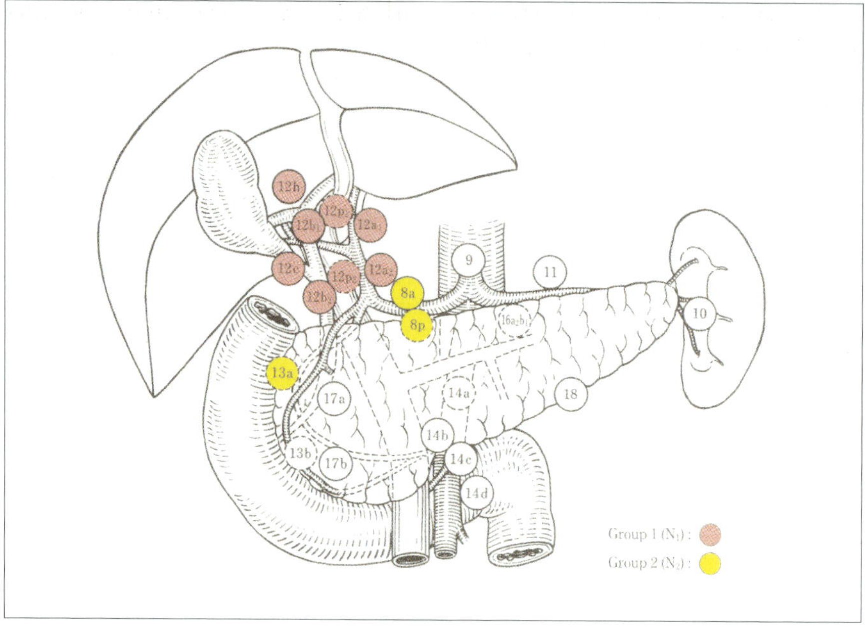

Fig. 3 Japanese classification of lymph node stations for hilar hepatic neoplasms. Adapted from [10]

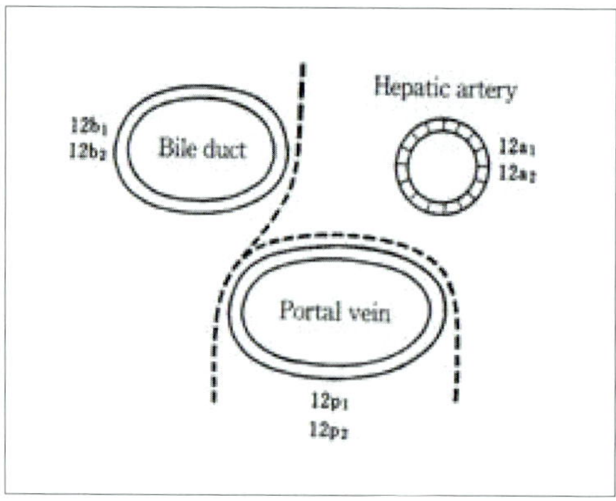

Fig. 4 The lymph nodes of the hepato-duodenal ligament are subdivided into three groups according to their relationship with biliary duct (*12b*), portal vein (*12p*), proper hepatic artery (*12a*). Adapted from [10]

M Category

In this category distant metastases are differentiated into hepatic, peritoneal and other organs. Hepatic metastases are differentiated according to number and site:
- H0: no hepatic metastasis
- H1: metastases limited to a single lobe (H1r metastases limited to right lobe, H1l metastases limited to left lobe)

Table 7 Division of lymph node stations for hilar hepatic neoplasms according to JSBS (Japanese Society of Biliary Surgery) [10]

Station	Site	Category
1	Right cardial	Optional
2	Left cardial	Optional
3	Gastric lesser curvature	Optional
4	Greater gastric curvature	Optional
5	Suprapyloric	Optional
6	Subpyloric	Optional
7	Left gastric artery	Optional
8a	Anterior hepatic artery	N2
8p	Posterior hepatic artery	N2
9	Celiac trunk	N3
10	Splenic hilum	Optional
11	Splenic artery	Optional
12h	Hepatic hilum	N1
12a1	Superior hepatic artery	N1
12a2	Inferior hepatic artery	N1
12p1	Superior portal vein	N1
12p2	Inferior portal vein	N1
12b1	Superior biliary duct	N1
12b2	Inferior biliary duct	N1
12c	Cystic duct	N1
13a	Superior retropancreatic	N2
13b	Inferior retropancreatic	N3
14a	Superior mesenteric artery	N3
14b	Inferior pancreaticoduodenal artery	N3
14c	Origin of middle colic artery	N3
14d	First jejunal branch	N3
15	Middle colic	Optional
16a1, b2	Superior and inferior para-aortic	N3
16a2, b1	Middle para-aortic	N3
17a	Anterior superior pancreatic	N3
17b	Anterior inferior pancreatic	N3
18	Inferior pancreatic	Optional

- H2: a few hepatic metastases in both lobes
- H3: many hepatic metastases in both lobes

Peritoneal metastases are also classified by site and number:

- P1: metastases adjacent to hepatic ducts
- P2: a few distant metastases
- P3: many distant metastases
  Diffusion to organs other than liver and peritoneum is defined:
- M-: no evidence of distant metastases (other than hepatic or peritoneal)
- M+: presence of distant metastases (other than hepatic or peritoneal)

Stage Grouping

The grouping of T, N and M categories allows subdivision of the neoplasms as in the following outline (Fig. 5).

This TNM staging is based on a precise classification of pathological findings; as TNM UICC/AJCC classification it is useless in preoperative evaluation and for defining resectability. In patients who undergo surgical exploration and resection with curative intent this classification permits precise assignment to classes with different prognoses. Unfortunately the complexity of this system has limited its use and as yet the literature has not reported any validation studies.

Early Cancer

Hilar cholangiocarcinoma is defined as "early" when the deepest invasion is limited to the mucosa or fibromuscolar layer of the bile duct, regardless of lymph-node metastasis. Macroscopically it can be classified according to the following types (Fig. 6):
- Protruded (p: pedunculated; s: sessile)
- Superficial (a: elevated; b: flat; c: depressed)
- Excavated

Gazzaniga Staging System

The classification proposed by Gazzaniga in 1985 was the first to consider biliary and vascular invasion [11]. Based on preoperative workup two elements are evaluated: extent of biliary involvement according to Bismuth-Corlette and portal and arterial vascular infiltration.

<table>
<tr><td></td><td colspan="4" align="center">H0, P0, M-</td><td align="center">H1-2-3, P1-2-3, M+</td></tr>
<tr><td></td><td align="center">pN0</td><td align="center">pN1</td><td align="center">pN2</td><td align="center">pN3</td><td></td></tr>
<tr><td>pT1</td><td align="center">I</td><td align="center">II</td><td></td><td></td><td rowspan="4" align="center">IVb</td></tr>
<tr><td>pT2</td><td align="center">II</td><td></td><td></td><td align="center">IVa</td></tr>
<tr><td>pT3</td><td></td><td align="center">III</td><td align="center">IVa</td><td></td></tr>
<tr><td>pT4</td><td></td><td align="center">IVa</td><td></td><td></td></tr>
</table>

Fig. 5 Staging system according to JSBS (Japanese Society of Biliary Surgery) [10]
H, Hepatic metastases (H0: absent; H1: limited to a lobe; H2 few metastases to both lobes, H3: many metastases to both lobes); *P*, peritoneal metastases (P0: absent, P1 adjacent to biliary ducts, P2: few distant metastases, P3: many distant metastases); *M*, metastases to other organs (M+: present, M- absent); *N*, lymph nodes metastases (N1: 1st level lymph nodes metastases, N2: 2nd level lymph nodes metastases, N3: 3rd level lymph nodes metastases

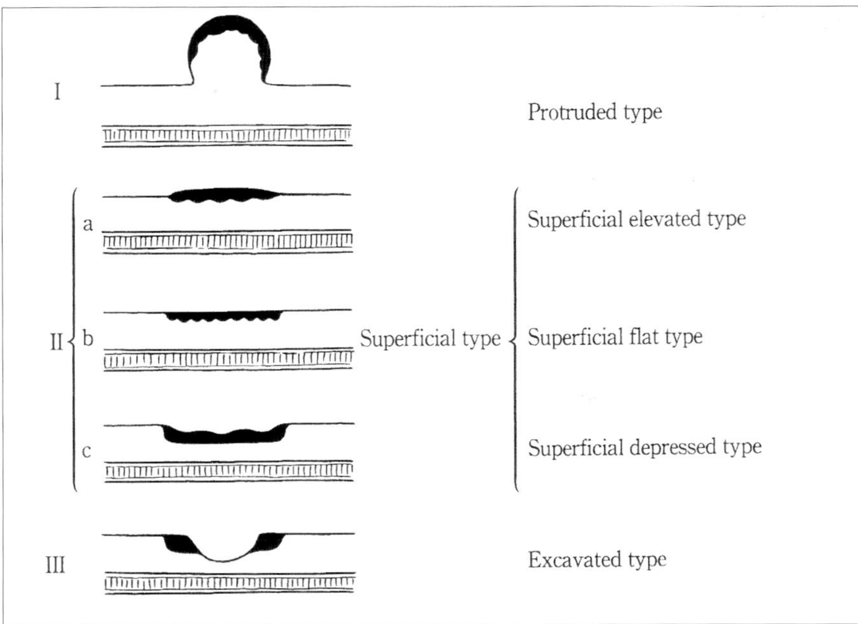

Fig. 6 Macroscopic types of early cancer

This classification divides patients into four categories with prognostic significance (Fig. 7, Table 8).

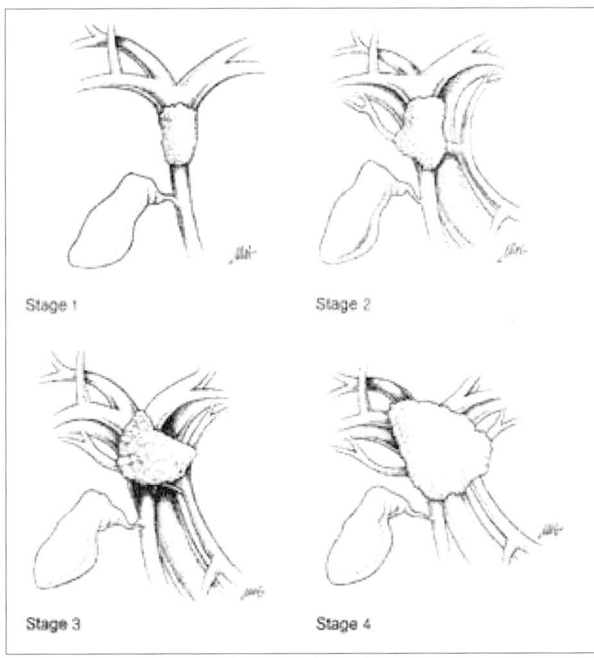

Fig. 7 Gazzaniga classification of hilar cholangiocarcinoma. It evaluates extent of biliary involvement and vascular infiltration (see also Table 8). Modified from [11]

Table 8 Gazzaniga staging system [11]

Stage I	Neoplasm of the proximal portion of the biliary tract with solely endoductal diffusion that arrives more than 2 cm from confluence
Stage II	Neoplasm with endoductal diffusion similar to stage I or with involvement of segmental and/or subsegmental branches of one lobe and with monolobar portal infiltration
Stage III	Neoplasm of the proximal portion of the biliary tract with endo- and extraductal diffusion extended to right or left lobar vascular pedicles and to a component of contralateral vascular pedicles
Stage IV	Neoplasm of the proximal portion of biliary tract with mono- or bilobar segmental biliary infiltration associated with bilobar portal infiltration or obstruction extended to segmental or subsegmental branches

The authors proposed an association between the stage of disease and the type of surgical approach: resection of the biliary tract alone for stage I, resection of the biliary tract associated with hepatic resection for stage II, hepatic and biliary resection associated with vascular resection and reconstruction for stage III and palliative non-surgical approach for stage IV. In a study of 159 patients Gazzaniga validated this classification and identified a correlation between stage and resectability: 43.5% for stage I, 45.6% for stage II and 10.9% for stage III.

Memorial Sloan-Kettering Cancer Center Staging

The classification proposed in 1998 and subsequently modified in 2001 by Memorial Sloan-Kettering Cancer Center (MSKCC) is based on preoperative imaging findings for three parameters [13,14]:
- Extent of the tumour along the biliary tract
- Portal vein involvement
- Presence of hepatic atrophy

This staging system was first proposed in 1998; 90 patients with hilar cholangiocarcinoma were analyzed and divided into four stages with prognostic significance. In 2001 the data of 225 patients with hilar cholangiocarcinoma were retrospectively analyzed and the classification was reviewed: the patients were grouped into three clinical stages with prognostic value and therapeutic indications (Table 9).

In a validation study on 225 patients clinical staging showed a statistically significant correlation with resectability that was 69% for stage 1, 31% for stage 2 and 0% for stage 3. Also long-term outcome was related to the stage, with a median survival of 20 months for stage 1, 13 months for stage 2 and 8 months for stage 3 [14].

Table 9 Memorial Sloan-Kettering Center staging system [13]

T1	Tumour involves biliary confluence ± unilateral extent to 2nd order ducts
T2	Tumour involves biliary confluence ± unilateral extent to 2nd order ducts and homo-lateral portal infiltration ± homolateral lobar atrophy
T3	Tumour involves biliary confluence + bilateral extent to 2nd order ducts, unilateral extent to 2nd order ducts with contralateral portal vein infiltration, unilateral extent to 2nd order biliary ducts with contralateral hepatic atrophy, or involvement of main portal trunk

In a recent study Zervos et al. did not confirm the correlation between the classification of MSKCC with resectability and long-term survival with a median survival of 45 months for T1, 90 months for T2, 43 months for T3 and 33 months for T4 [3].

This clinical classification offers an approach that has proved to be useful in defining resectability and prognosis. Unfortunately prognostic evaluation does not consider some factors such as lymph-node involvement which has been shown to be prognostically relevant.

Conclusions

There are various staging systems proposed for hilar cholangiocarcinoma and at present the choice of the best system is still under debate.

As noted previously, the classifications listed show different features and can be divided into two categories: clinical and pathological staging systems.

The clinical classifications [1,11,14] serve to define criteria of resectability, indicate the type of operation and estimate the prognosis of the disease.

Bismuth-Corlette classification divides patients only based on extent of biliary involvement and does not consider other important elements of the preoperative evaluation such as vascular involvement and lobar atrophy; therefore it cannot be used to assess resectability [1,2].

The Gazzaniga classification proposed in 1985 has added the degree of vascular involvement [11] to evaluation of extent of biliary involvement; however its diffusion in clinical practice is very limited.

The clinical classification proposed by MSKCC adds vascular involvement and hepatic atrophy evaluation of extent of biliary involvement according to the Bismuth-Corlette classification [13,14].

TNM UICC/AJCC [4] and JSBS [10] staging systems are based on histopathologic criteria and evaluate the local and distant extent after surgical operation. These classifications have mainly prognostic significance but are not useful for assessing resectability. The complexity of JSBS classification limits its use in clinical practice.

A classification of this disease that permits a complete evaluation of resectability and outcome is not available at present. It would be useful to have a staging system that combine biliary involvement, vascular invasion, local extent and lymph-node involvement.

References

1. Bismuth H, Corlette MB (1975) Intrahepatic cholangioenteric anastomosis in carcinoma of the hilus of the liver. Surg Gynecol Obstet 140(2):170–178
2. Bismuth H, Nakache R, Diamond T (1992) Management strategies in resection for hilar cholangiocarcinoma. Ann Surg 199 215(1):31–38
3. Zervos EE, Osborne D, Goldin SB et al (2005) Stage does not predict survival after resection of hilar cholangiocarcinomas promoting an aggressive operative approach. Am J Surg 190(5):810–815
4. Sobin LH, Wittekind C (eds) (2002) TNM classification of malignant tumours, 6th edn. Wiley, New York
5. Nishio H, Nagino M, Oda K et al (2005) TNM classification for perihilar cholangiocarcinoma: comparison between 5th and 6th editions of the AJCC/UICC staging system. Langenbecks Arch Surg 390(4):319–327
6. Kitagawa Y, Nagino M, Kamiya J et al (2001) Lymph-node metastasis from hilar cholangiocarcinoma: audit of 110 patients who underwent regional and paraaortic node dissection. Ann Surg 233(3):385–392
7. Liu CL, Fan ST, Lo CM et al (2006) Improved operative and survival outcomes of surgical treatment for hilar cholangiocarcinoma. Br J Surg 93(12):1488–1494
8. Hong S-M, Kim M-J, Pi DY et al (2005) Analysis of extrahepatic bile duct carcinomas according to the new American Joint Committee on Cancer Staging System focused on tumour classification problems in 222 patients. Cancer 104(4):802–810
9. Ebata T, Nagino M, Kamiya J et al (2003) Hepatectomy with portal vein resection for hilar cholangiocarcinoma: audit of 52 consecutive cases. Ann Surg 238(5):720–727
10. Japanese Society of Biliary Surgery (2004) Classification of biliary tract carcinoma. 2nd English edn. Kanehara, Tokyo
11. Gazzaniga GM, Faggioni A, Bonanza G et al (1984) Classificazione anatomo-chirurgica dei tumori dell'ilo epatico. Notiz Chir 5:128–129
12. Gazzaniga GM, Filauro M, Faggioni A et al (1986) Neoplasie primitive dell'ilo epatico: trattamento e risultati. Chir Epatobil 5:59–63
13. Burke EC, Jarnagin WR, Hochwald SN et al (1998) Hilar Cholangiocarcinoma: patterns of spread, the importance of hepatic resection for curative operation, and a presurgical clinical staging system. Ann Surg 228(3):385–394
14. Jarnagin WR, Fong Y, DeMatteo RP et al (2001) Staging, resectability, and outcome in 225 patients with hilar cholangiocarcinoma. Ann Surg 234(4):507–517; discussion 517–519

Surgical Anatomy of the Hepatic Hilus

The development of curative surgery for hilar cholangiocarcinoma is based on the precise knowledge of anatomy of the hepatic hilus and of the frequent anatomical variations that may be encountered. For these reasons it would be useful to point out some anatomical details, with particular regard to the anatomy of the hilar and caudate lobe area that are the crucial point of this surgery. Biliary ducts, arterial and portal vessels that are covered by connective tissue arising from the fusion of Glisson's capsule, in the intrahepatic portion, and peritoneum of the hepatoduodenal ligament, in the extrahepatic portion, constitute the plate system. In this space several lymphatic vessels, nerves and a small vascular network are present (Fig. 1).

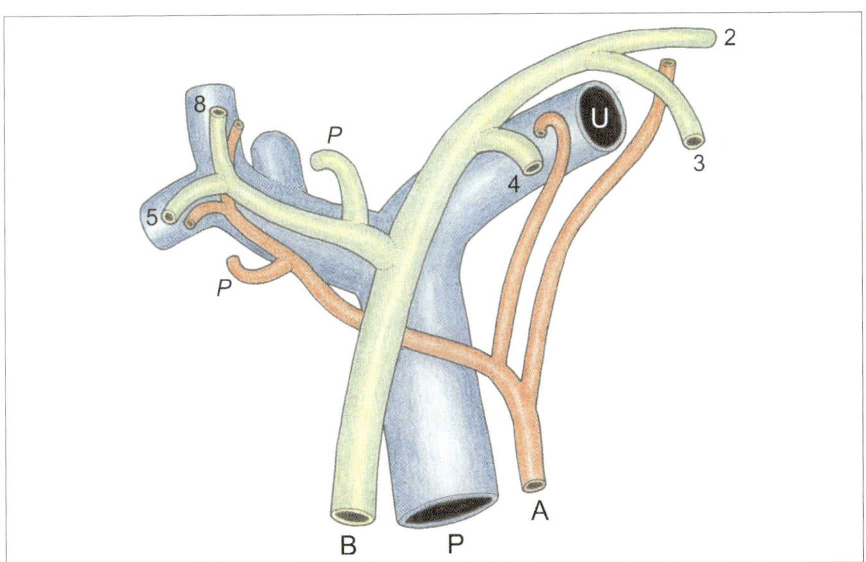

Fig. 1 Anatomy of hepatic hilus. *A*, Hepatic artery; *B*, bile duct; *P*, portal vein; *P*, posterior branch of hepatic artery and right biliary duct; *U*, umbilical portion. Modified from [1]

A. Guglielmi, A. Ruzzenente, C. Iacono (eds.) *Surgical Treatment of Hilar and ICC.*
© Springer 2008

The plate system is divided into three parts of connective thickening: the hilar plate that separates the biliary confluence from the inferior part of the quadrate lobe (S4a), the cystic plate that envelops the gallbladder and cystic duct and the umbilical plate that covers the umbilical portion of the portal vein.

Anatomy of the Bile Duct Branches

At the hepatic hilum the right and left hepatic ducts meet in the biliary confluence. Anatomical variants of the confluence are very common so that a regular anatomic confluence is present in no more than the two-thirds of cases.

The left lateral segmental ducts (B2 and B3) generally join at the level of the umbilical fissure situated posterior to the umbilical portion. Rarely (6% of cases) the duct for segment 3 (B3) runs caudally to the umbilical portion of the left portal vein with a direct outlet on the B4 biliary duct [1]. The recognition of this anatomic variation is important in case of right trisectionectomy, to avoid biliary injury and modify surgical technique with separate biliary reconstruction of B2 and B3. The left medial segment (B4) joins to form the left hepatic duct immediately on the right of Rex's recessus.

For the left intrahepatic bile duct Ohkubo [2] described four confluence patterns:
- Type 1 (78%): the left medial sectional bile duct (B4) enters the left lateral sectional bile duct
- Type 2 (4%): the left medial sectional bile duct (B4) enters just at the confluence of B2 with B3
- Type 3 (18%): B4 enters directly the B3
- Type 4 (2%): B4 enters the hepatic confluence (Fig. 2)

The merger of anterior and posterior ducts forms the right hepatic duct. At this point the anatomic variations are very common: in 50–70% of cases the anterior and posterior segmental ducts join to form the right hepatic duct, which in turn meets the left hepatic duct in the hilar confluence (common type); in 9–27% of the cases the posterior segmental duct joins the left hepatic duct; in 7–14% of the cases the posterior segmental duct joins the hilar confluence (three branch type); finally, in 6–9% the anterior segmental duct joins the left hepatic duct (Fig. 3).

Analysing the anatomic variations of the hepatic confluence in relation to the portal vein, based on the examination of surgical specimens, Ohkubo [2] described three confluence patterns of the right intrahepatic bile ducts according to the anatomic relationship between the right posterior sectional bile duct and the portal vein (Fig. 4):
- Supraportal pattern (81%) in which the right posterior bile duct (B6+B7) runs dorsally and cranially to the right portal vein and joins the right bile duct at its cranial side.

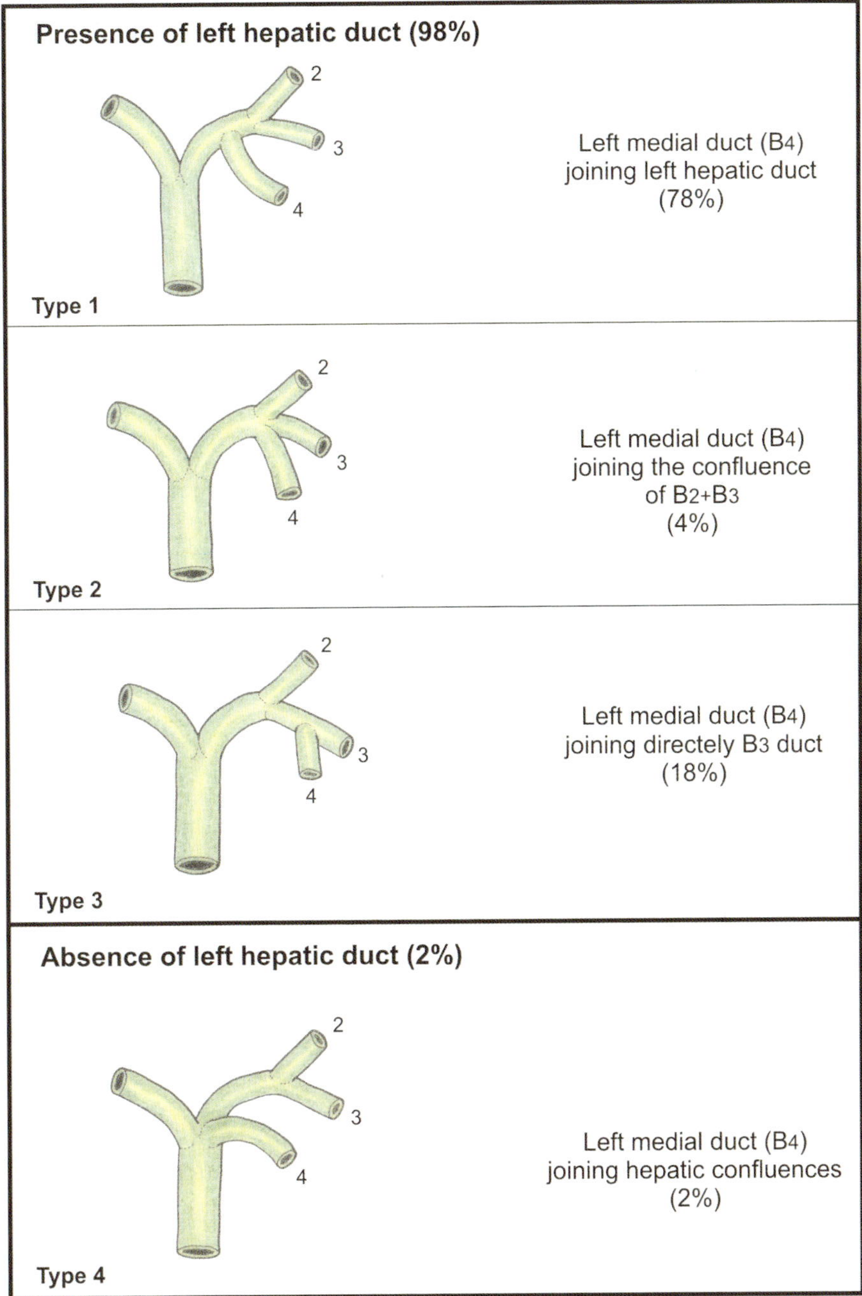

Fig. 2 Anatomical variations of the left hepatic bile duct. Numerals refer to Couinaud's segments. Modified from [2]

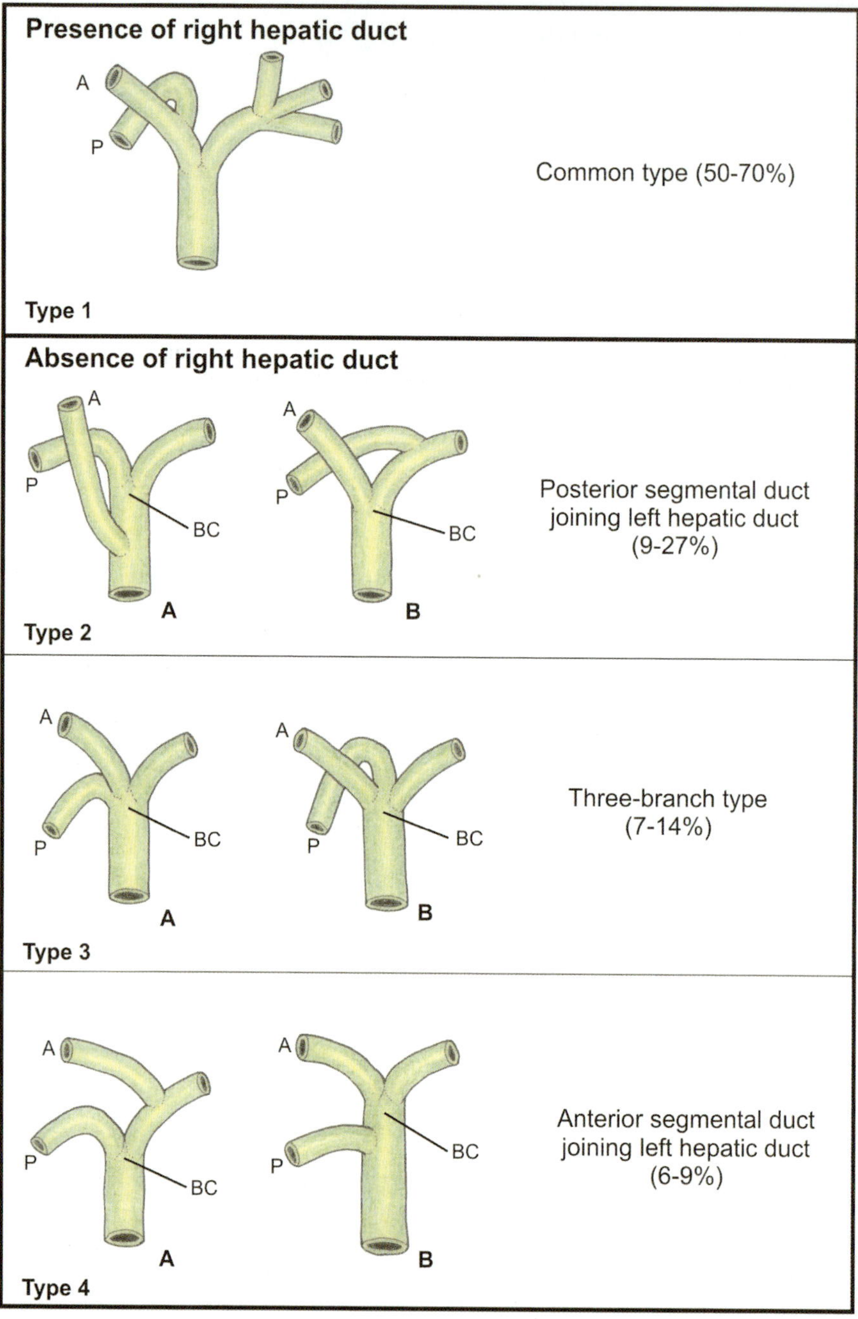

Fig. 3 Anatomical variation of the right hepatic bile duct. *A*, Anterior branch; *P*, posterior branch; *BC*, bile duct confluence. Modified from [2]

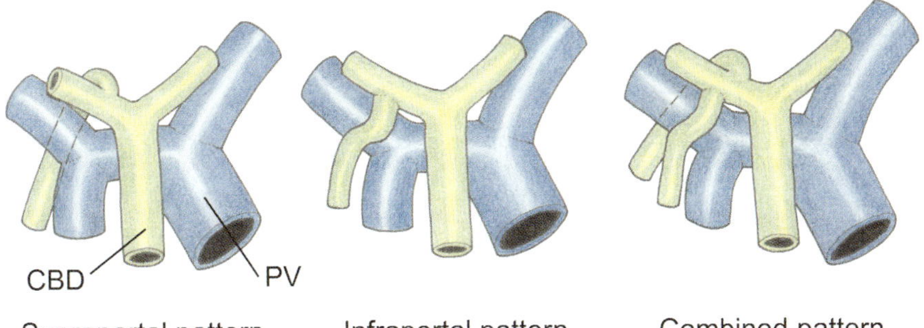

Fig. 4 Patterns of confluence of the right posterior bile duct in relationship to the right portal vein. *CBD*, Common bile duct; *PV*, Portal vein. Modified from [2]

- Infraportal pattern (12%) in which the right posterior bile duct (B6+B7) runs ventrally and caudally to the right portal vein and joins the right bile duct at its caudal side.
- Combined pattern (5%) in which the right posterior bile ducts drain separately into the right bile duct, supraportally and infraportally.

The knowledge of the subsegmental anatomy of the intrahepatic bile duct based on clinical cholangiograms, as reported by Nimura [3], is indispensable for the precise preoperative diagnosis of proximal tumour extension and for understanding the anatomical variations of the intrahepatic biliary tree. In addition, it is possible to arrange precisely the surgical plan and recognise subsegments during liver dissection.

On anteroposterior projection, the right anterior segmental branches overlap on the branches of posterior segments, making their identification difficult. Instead on right lateral projection it is easier to distinguish them, as the segmental branches of the anterior segment project cranially to the left while the posterior project caudally to the right [4] (Fig. 5).

Anatomy of the Portal Vein Branches

Usually few variants regard portal vein branches due to their early embryonic development during the gestation period. Three principal portal vein branching patterns in the hilar area are described by different authors:
- The common type (74–84%) in which the anterior segmental branch joins the posterior to form the right branch of the portal vein.
- The three branch type (8–12%) in which the anterior segmental branch joins the portal vein confluence.
- The left branch type (9–17%) in which the anterior segmental branch joins the left branch of the portal vein [5] (Fig. 6).

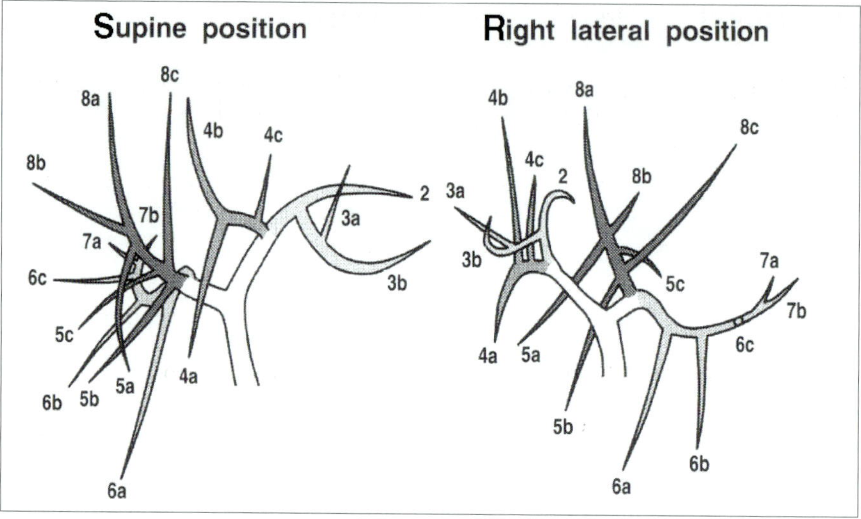

Fig. 5 Cholangiographic anatomy of the intrahepatic segmental bile duct according to patient's position. Numerals refer to Couinaud's segments. *3a*, superior branch; *3b*, inferior branch; *4a*, inferior branch; *4b*, superior branch; *4c*, dorsal branch; *5a*, ventral branch; *5b*, dorsal branch; *5c*, lateral branch; *6a*, ventral branch; *6b*, dorsal branch; *6c*, lateral branch; *7a*, ventral branch; *7b*, dorsal branch; *8a*, ventral branch; *8b*, lateral branch; *8c*, dorsal branch. Modified from [3]

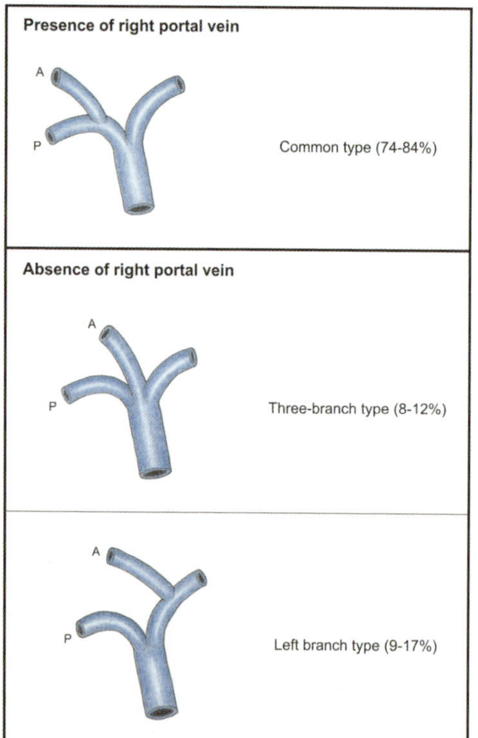

Fig. 6 Variations of the anatomy of the right branch of the portal vein. *A*, Anterior branch; *P*, posterior branch

Anatomy of the Hepatic Artery Branches

The left hepatic artery enters the liver on the left side of Rex's recessus; the middle hepatic artery, through the right side of Rex's recessus; the right hepatic artery more frequently runs between the portal vein and the bile duct, posterior to the confluence. The right hepatic artery divides into the anterior branch that runs between the bile duct and the portal vein, and posterior branch that turns caudally to the right portal vein and enters the liver (see Fig. 1) [3].

Variations of the hepatic artery are very common: more than 10 types of anatomic variants including the presence of accessory or replaced artery, have been described. The principal types of anatomic variants are:
- Type 1: the right, middle and left hepatic artery arise from the common hepatic artery (71–72%)
- Type 2: the right hepatic artery arises from the superior mesenteric artery (13–14%)
- Type 3: the left hepatic artery arises from the left gastric artery (11–12%)
- Type 4: the common hepatic artery arises from the superior mesenteric artery (2–5%) [5] (Fig. 7)

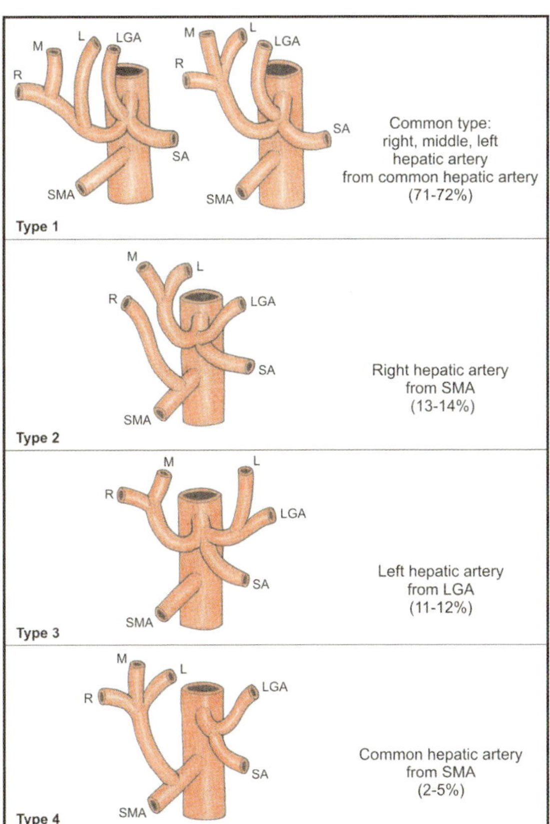

Fig. 7 Anatomical variations of the main hepatic artery. *R*, Right hepatic artery; *M*, middle hepatic artery; *L*, left hepatic artery; *SMA*, superior mesenteric artery; *LGA*, left gastric artery; *SA*, spleen artery

Regarding the relationship between proper hepatic artery, portal vein and biliary tract, the proper hepatic artery more frequently (76% of cases) runs behind the biliary tract and rarely (24% of cases) has an anterior course. Finally, in 9% of cases the right hepatic artery runs dorsally to the portal vein.

Surgical Anatomy of the Caudate Lobe

Knowledge of anatomy of the caudate lobe and its relationship with the porta hepatis area are mandatory for a correct surgical approach to hilar cholangiocarcinoma. In fact, the surgical treatment of this disease requires en-bloc resection of the caudate lobe.

Currently the caudate lobe is divided into three parts, according to Couinaud's definition [6]:

– Segment 1 (S1), or caudate lobe, in the strict sense of the word, which corresponds to the portion with left development
– Segment 9 (S9), corresponding according to Couinaud [7] to the portion with right development
– Caudate process, a small portion of parenchyma which represents the inferomedian extension of segment 9

Nimura [8] has proposed naming Segment 1 on the left: S1l; segment 9 on the right: S1r; caudate process: S1c (Fig. 8). The right and left caudate lobe are separated by the Arantius canal or ligamentum venosum, an embryonic vein coming from the base of the umbilical portion that enters the left hepatic vein, or the common trunk of the left and middle hepatic vein or directly into the inferior vena cava. The right lateral margin of S1r is on the left site of the right posterior portal vein, and the superior margin extends up towards the diaphragm, crossing middle and right hepatic veins.

The biliary branches of the caudate lobe are very variable. They join the left and right hepatic ducts and their confluence. According to Nimura [8], these branches are classified in four groups:

– B1ls, branches that come from the superior part of segment 1 and enter into left hepatic duct
– B1li, biliary branches coming from the inferior part of segment 1 and open into right posterior biliary duct
– B1r, biliary branches coming from segment 9 of Couinaud and open into both the right posterior segmental and the left ducts
– B1c: small biliary branches of the caudate process that join the right posterior duct (Fig. 9)

The small arteries for the caudate lobe originate directly from the right and left hepatic artery.

The portal component is variable: from two to six vessels come from the left portal vein, two or three small vessels come from the right portal vein, finally one or two vessels arise from the main trunk or portal bifurcation.

Venous drainage consists of short hepatic veins, variable in number and size (1–6 mm), that open into the vena cava, with a very short course of a few millimeters. Lastly, some small venous rami (two or three) coming from the right caudate lobe (S1r) directly join the middle hepatic vein.

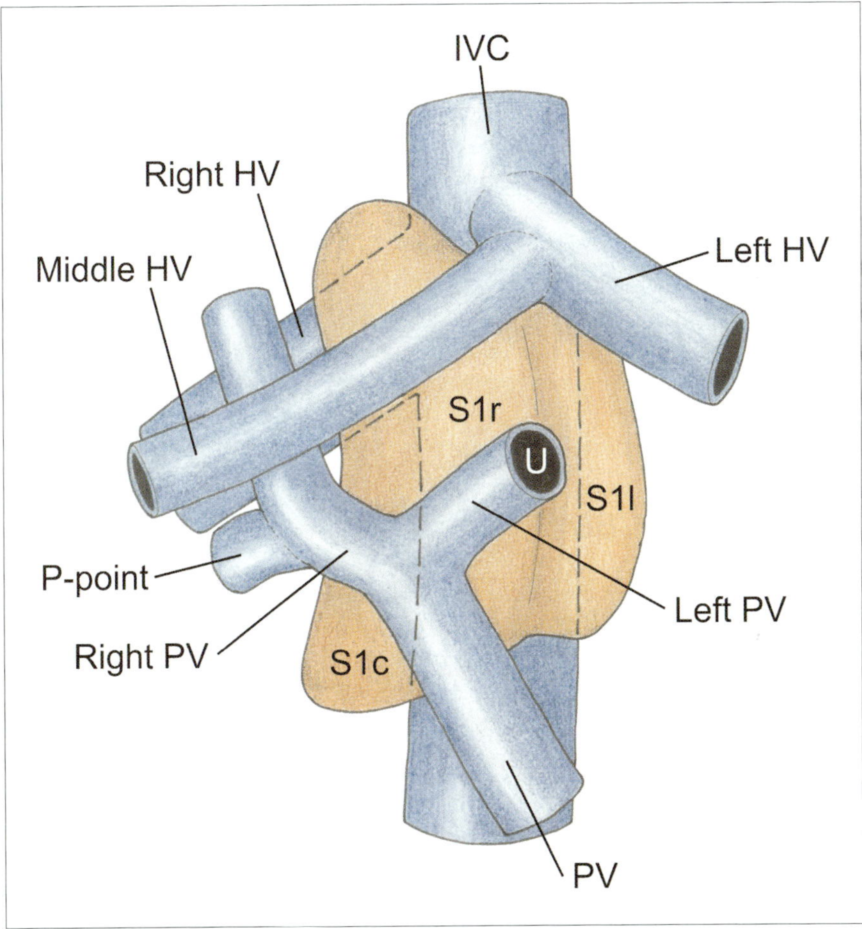

Fig. 8 Caudate lobe anatomy. The lobe is divided in three parts: left part (*S1l*); right part, or segment 9 according to Coinaud (*S1r*); caudate process (*S1c*). *HV*, Hepatic veins; *U*, umbilical portion

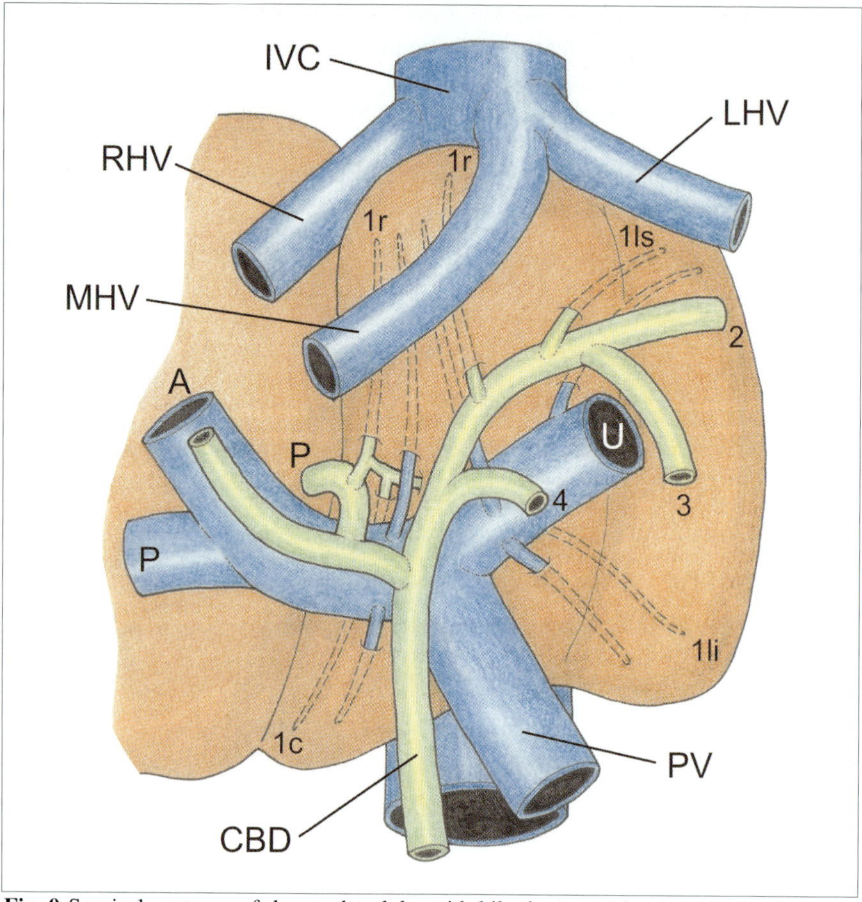

Fig. 9 Surgical anatomy of the caudate lobe with bile duct, portal vein and hepatic veins. *IVC*, Inferior vena cava; *RHV*, right hepatic vein; *MHV*, middle hepatic vein; *LHV*, left hepatic vein; *CBD*, common bile duct; *PV*, portal vein; *1 r*, biliary branch of the right caudate lobe; *1 ls*, superior biliary branch of the left caudate lobe; *1 li*, inferior biliary branch of the left caudate lobe; *1 c*, biliary branch of caudate process. Numerals refer to Couinaud's segmental anatomy

References

1. Ozden I, Kamiya J, Nagino M et al (2002) Clinicoanatomical study on the infraportal bile ducts of segment 3. World J Surg 26(12):1441–1445
2. Ohkubo M, Nagino M, Kamiya J et al (2004) Surgical anatomy of the bile ducts at the hepatic hilum as applied to living donor liver transplantation. Ann Surg 239(1):82–86
3. Nimura Y, Hayakawa N, Kamiya J et al (1995) Hilar cholangiocacinoma: surgical anatomy and curative resection. J Hepatobiliary Pancreat Surg 2:239–248
4. Nimura Y (1997) Surgical anatomy of the biliary ducts. In: Rossi P, Bezzi M (eds) Biliary tract radiology. Springer, Berlin, pp 21–30

5. Kawarada Y, Das BC, Taoka H (2000) Anatomy of the hepatic hilar area: the plate system. J Hepatobiliary Pancreat Surg 7(6):580–586
6. Couinaud C (1989) Surgical anatomy of the liver revisited. Couinaud, Paris
7. Couinaud C (1994) The paracaval segment of the liver. J Hep Bil Panc Surg 2:145–151
8. Nimura Y, Hayakawa N, Kamiya J et al (1990) Hepatic segmentectomy with caudate lobe resection for bile duct carcinoma of the hepatic hilus. World J Surg 14(4):535–543; Discussion 544

Surgical Treatment

The rationale for surgical treatment requires the knowledge provided by T-stage of radial and longitudinal neoplastic diffusion, and of N and M stages. As described in Chap. "Preoperative Assessment of Liver Function", a correct preoperative assessment is often difficult to achieve.

Significant data on lymph node diffusion and correlated prognosis are still lacking in the literature, except for few reports of Japanese institutions. Surgical choices are now determined mainly by local extension of disease. Nowadays resectability criteria differ from those of the past: portal and/or arterial infiltration are no longer an absolute contraindication to resection.

In the past, hilar cholangiocarcinoma was treated by biliary tract resection and limited hepatic resection. Recent data in the literature have shown that associated hepatic resection significantly increases the rate of R0 resection, with a better long-term outcome. Instead, the need to resect the caudate lobe systematically is still under debate.

Postoperative morbidity and mortality rates after major resection have decreased thanks to improvement of preoperative hepatic function (biliary drainage, portal embolisation), a better selection of patients and an upgrading of surgical techniques.

Surgical option is determined by stage and neoplastic diffusion, tailoring the type of operation that guarantees a better probability of curative resection and therefore a better prognosis.

General Principles

Hilar cholangiocarcinoma remains one of the most difficult management problems in terms of staging and radical treatment. It has long been recognised that surgical resection with complete removal of all cancer tissues offers the only chance for cure and long-term survival.

Several studies have confirmed the importance of hepatic resection as a means of achieving a margin negative resection (Table 1).

A. Guglielmi, A. Ruzzenente, C. Iacono (eds.) *Surgical Treatment of Hilar and ICC.*
© Springer 2008

Table 1 Resection rate of curative resection in patients with hilar cholangiocarcinoma

Author	Year	Patients (number)	Resection rate	Curative resections
Jarnagin [1]	2001	225	36%	78%
Launois [2]	2000	552	32%	–
Lee [3]	2000	151	85%	–
Neuhaus [4]	2003	133	–	60%
Nimura [5]	2000	177	80%	70%
Puhalla [6]	2003	88	42%	33%
Tsao [7] (Lahey)	2000	100	25%	28%
Tsao [7] (Nagoya)	2000	155	79%	78%
Uchiyama [8]	2003	57	58%	64%
Yi [9]	2004	197	61%	41%
Otto [10]	2007	99	71%	75%

There appears to be controversy regarding the selection of patients for whom extensive hepatic resection is indicated, the type of hepatectomy indicated, i.e. right- or left- sided hepatectomy, and whether routine caudate lobe resection is necessary.

The lack of consensus largely arises from the difficulty of diagnosing precisely the proximal tumour extension before surgical resection or even during laparotomy. The main purpose of surgical therapy of hilar cholangiocarcinoma is to achieve not only curative resection but also to apply the general rules of oncological surgery which must accomplish the following:

1. R0 resection of biliary tract and liver preserving a residual parenchyma, well-functioning not less than 30–40%
2. Broad tumour-free margin not less than 1 cm on proximal and distal biliary tract confirmed by frozen section
3. Caudate lobe resection, isolated or associated with extended hepatectomy
4. Dissection of the lymph nodes and connective tissues in the hepatoduodenal ligament (12a, 12p, 12b), posterior to the upper portion of the pancreatic head (superior retropancreatic 13a), and around the common hepatic artery (8a)
5. The decision of whether right- or left-sided hepatectomy is indicated, is made according to the predominant site of the lesion (longitudinal tumour extension)
6. No-touch technique to prevent neoplastic seeding
7. Avoid intra-operative open tumour biopsy
8. Keep the operative field clear of biliary contamination due to the risk of neoplastic cell spreading

The close relationship of the neoplasm with portal bifurcation, right hepatic artery and hepatic parenchyma makes it difficult to address the aforementioned principles without a careful evaluation of tumour extent.

Radial spread of the lesion to surrounding structures is facilitated by delayed diagnosis and by the absence of a muscular layer in the biliary duct; besides, infiltrative growth pattern is the most frequent in this neoplasm and determines a rapid periductal and perineural diffusion along the ducts and Glisson spaces. These are the reasons why surgical choice must follow the rule of obtaining an adequate free margin at least of 1 cm rather than limited resection.

Assessment of Resectability

Evaluation of patients with hilar cholangiocarcinoma is mainly an assessment of resectability, since resection is the only effective therapy. As a general rule, in presence of a resectable tumour an R0 resection must be carried out preserving a well-functioning and vascularised future remnant liver with adequate biliary drainage.

In the last 20 years the definition of resectability has changed and a standardised opinion has not yet been agreed upon, especially between Japanese and Western authors [7].

The following must be taken into consideration:
1. Physical status of the patient and liver function
2. Biliary extent of neoplasm
3. Vascular involvement
4. Presence of lobe atrophy
5. Lymph-node involvement
6. Presence of distant metastases

Patient Factors

First of all the surgeon must assess the patient's general condition and fitness for a major operation that usually includes hepatectomy. Resection is generally precluded if the patient is medically unfit or otherwise unable to tolerate a major operation, or in the presence of significant co-morbidity, chronic liver disease, hepatic cirrhosis and/or portal hypertension.

Biliary Extent of Neoplasm

The infiltration growth of hilar cholangiocarcinoma includes longitudinal and radial diffusion. Longitudinal diffusion is either mucosal or submucosal and is correlated to the macroscopic aspect of the neoplasm [11]. The former is more frequent in the papillary or nodular types and can spread 20 mm beyond the macroscopic margin of the lesion in 40% of cases; the latter is typical of invasive types and spreads on average 6 mm. Ebata [12] analysed 80 cases of resected specimens with microscopically positive margin and observed that the submucosal invasive type spread less than 10 mm in all the cases while the non-invasive superficial type (carcinoma in situ) is limited to within 20 mm in 90% of the cases. Considering these data, a macroscopic margin of 10 mm can be considered accurate for eradication of invasive extra-hepatic bile duct carcinoma. However this requires additional removal of any non-invasive component.

The presence of invasive carcinoma on the resected margin worsens the outcome while the presence of carcinoma in situ on the margin does not have a statistical significance on survival compared to negative margin cases [13]. When a margin is positive on frozen section it is advisable to extend biliary resection, if technically feasible; however, discriminating between carcinoma in situ and invasive carcinoma is clinically important.

If tumour extension is definitely thought to extend peripherally to the second segmental ramification of the second order intrahepatic biliary radicles bilaterally the patient is considered to be unresectable. In selected cases with Bismuth type IV neoplasm a left or right trisectionectomy can be performed if hepatic function and residual volume after PVE are at least 40%.

Radial diffusion extends to the hepatoduodenal ligament and to the perivascular connective tissue of the hepatic artery and portal vein that are close to the biliary tract. This aspect determines the choice of type of hepatectomy and likely associated vascular resection.

Vascular Involvement

Portal Vein

Portal invasion is generally associated with homolateral lobar atrophy but it is not a contraindication to surgical resection (Fig. 1). However, the results are different if we consider portal resection in advanced cases or in "en-bloc" portal resection during extended right hepatectomy.

Ebata [14] reported a study of 52 patients who underwent portal resection, and classified histological grades of portal infiltration in three levels:
- Grade 0: no involvement
- Grade I: cancer invasion limited to the tunica adventitia or media
- Grade II: cancer invasion arriving at the tunica intima.

Portal resection is a negative prognostic factor but it improves outcome compared with non-resected patients. Three and 5-year survival were 26 and 10%, respectively, in patients with hepatic and portal combined resection, and 54 and 37% in patients who underwent hepatic resection alone ($p<0.0001$), respectively.

Moreover, survival in patients with grade I or II portal invasion was similar to that of the group of patients without microscopic portal invasion (grade 0)

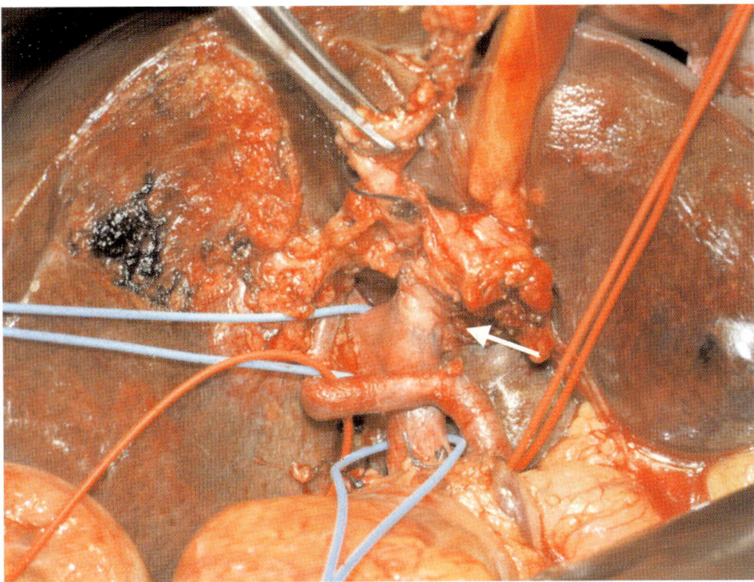

Fig. 1 Left portal vein infiltration (*left white arrow*) after complete lymph node dissection of the hepatoduodenal ligament and resection of the extra-hepatic bile duct

with 3-year survival of 22 vs. 36%, and 5-year survival of 10 vs. 18% (p=0.1506), respectively. At multivariate analysis, only macroscopic portal invasion is considered an independent prognostic factor (RR 2.18; p<0.02), while microscopic invasion is not.

The authors' conclusion was that portal invasion is not a contraindication to resection in hilar cholangiocarcinoma and that hepatectomy can be carried out safely in selected patients. Portal resection does not increase complications and mortality rate, which was about 10% [5,15].

More recently Kondo [16] reported a similar morbidity rate (48%) in patients who underwent combined portal resection vs. hepatic resection alone with no mortality using the "en-bloc resection" technique before hepatic dissection.

Neuhaus [15] reported 5-year survival of 65% in R0 cases after combined liver and portal vein resection using the "en-bloc resection" technique. This work has been criticised because microscopic portal invasion was confirmed in only 12% of resected cases (2/17). Although 60-day mortality (17%) and non-curative resection were excluded from this series, these results showed that portal resection associated with hepatectomy can improve the chances of long-term survival.

Concerning extension of portal invasion, the encasement or occlusion of the main portal vein proximal to its bifurcation, or bilateral portal venous encasement by cancer are a contraindication to resection.

Hepatic Artery

Data on arterial vascular resection are few. Recently there have been reported cases of hepatic artery resection, mainly right branch, during extended left hepatectomy for advanced hilar neoplasm. However, conclusive data on the prognostic value of such operations are still lacking. Reconstruction of the hepatic artery is performed less frequently than that of the portal vein; the reason is that this condition is often associated with very advanced neoplasm.

Jarnagin [17] maintained that invasion of proper hepatic artery or of the artery of remnant liver is a contraindication to surgical resection. Although recent reports of major hepatectomy with hepatic artery reconstruction show a low mortality (0–8%) and that it can be done safely, this operation is obviously more burdened by high morbidity and mortality rates than is hepatectomy without vascular reconstruction. For this reason, at present hepatic artery reconstruction associated with major hepatectomy is advisable only if the advanced tumour can be resected radically.

The study at Nagoya University showed that the only absolute contraindication for resection was bilateral hepatic arterial encasement by cancer [5].

Lobar Atrophy

Lobar atrophy is associated with occlusion of the portal trunk (Fig. 2) determined by neoplastic infiltration . It is not a contraindication to surgery unless the following conditions occur:

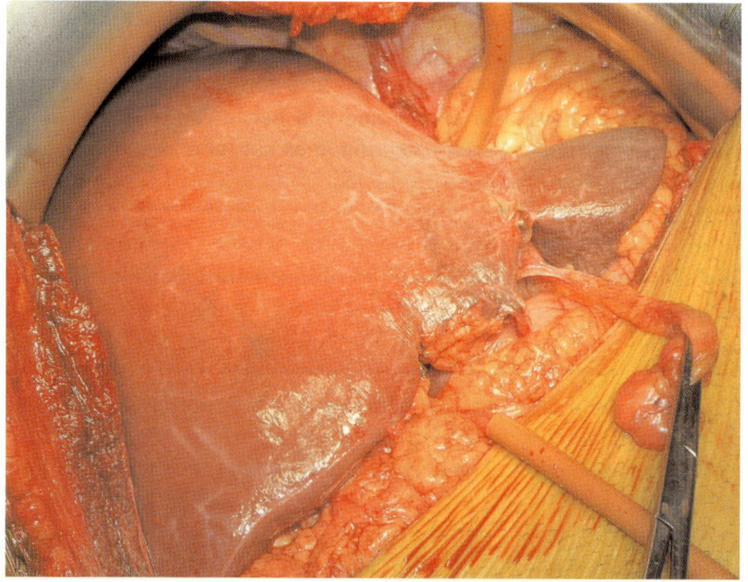

Fig. 2 Hilar cholangiocarcinoma with left portal vein infiltration and left lobar atrophy

- Atrophy of one hepatic lobe with contralateral portal vein branch encasement or occlusion
- Atrophy of one hepatic lobe with contralateral tumour extension to secondary biliary radicles
- Unilateral tumour extension to secondary biliary radicles with contralateral portal vein branch encasement or occlusion

Lymph-Node Involvement

The presence of lymph-node metastases is not rare in hilar cholangiocarcinoma patients. In a recent review, Kitagawa [18] reported N0 in 47% cases, regional N+ in 35% and para-aortic N+ in 17%. Survival was closely related to nodal involvement: 5-year survival in N0 patients was 31%, 15% in regional N+ and 12% in para-aortic N+ [18]. Considering carefully the outcome of patients with para-aortic positive nodes the author identified that survival was significantly better in patients with "macroscopically negative" nodes than in patients with "macroscopically positive" nodes, with a 5-year survival of 29 vs. 0%, respectively.

Kosuge [19] reported a mean and median survival of 79 months and 39 months, respectively, in N0 patients, 52 and 26 months in regional N+, and 15 and 14 months in N+ beyond regional. Five-year survival was 38% in N0, 30% in regional N+ (similar survival, not statistically significant) and 0% at 3-year survival in N+ beyond regional nodes.

To date, performing surgical resection in patients with wide and macroscopic involvement of non-regional lymph nodes does not appear justified. It has not yet been proved that extended lymphadenectomy guarantees improvement in survival in hilar cholangiocarcinoma but we believe a methodical regional nodal dissection must always be performed associated with R0 resection, at least until data are more consistent and conclusive.

According to Jarnagin at the MSKCC [20], pathological proven lymph-node metastases beyond the hepatoduodenal ligament (peripancreatic, periduodenal, celiac, superior mesenteric or posterior pancreaticoduodenal lymph nodes) was considered to represent disease not amenable to a potentially curative resection. In contrast, metastatic disease to cystic duct, pericholedochal, hilar or portal lymph nodes (i.e. within the hepatoduodenal ligament) did not necessary constitute a unresectable condition. At this time we perform lymphadenectomy of hepatoduodenal ligament and of the hepatic hilum (periportal, proper and common hepatic artery and retroduodenal lymph nodes) while peripancreatic, periduodenal, para-aortic and periceliac lymph nodes are sampled, if macroscopically suspect for staging.

Extrahepatic Disease

Adjacent extrahepatic organ invasion is not an absolute contraindication to resection. A concomitant pancreatic resection (hepatopancreatoduodenectomy HPD) is indicated if the tumour's longitudinal spread was considered to be in the lower intrapancreatic bile duct and/or massive peripancreatic head and pericholedochal lymph nodes metastases were suspected.

In presence of wide nodal infiltration, HPD indication is not the optimum as distant nodal metastases represent a negative prognostic factor. Nimura [21] first reported the results of this operation with an operative mortality of 35% and 5-year survival of 6%. Main causes of mortality were postoperative hepatic insufficiency and biliary leak. To decrease the risk of pancreatic fistula a two-stage operation with a delayed pancreo-jejunostomy was proposed [22].

Miyagawa [23] reported 12 cases treated with HPD and delayed pancreatic reconstruction, with 0% mortality rate.

Metastatic Disease

The presence of distant metastases (peritoneal, hepatic, pulmonary etc,) diagnosed preoperatively or intraoperatively stands for an absolute contraindication to surgical resection. The only exception can be the occurrence of hepatic metastases limited in the lobe to be resected; however, these cases there is no 5-year survival.

Indication for Surgical Resection

The indication of the type of surgical procedure is planned after a careful evaluation of the patient's physical status, hepatic function and neoplastic diffusion of the disease. The strategy of hepatic resection must be defined preoperatively based on exact knowledge of longitudinal and radial extension of the neoplasm.

Currently, there is no clinical staging system available that stratifies patients preoperatively into subgroups based on potential for resection. The modified Bismuth-Corlette classification [24] stratifies patients based only on the extent of biliary involvement by tumour, and the AJCC staging system is based largely on pathological criteria and has little applicability for preoperative staging or predicting resectability.

The preoperative staging system proposed recently by Jarnagin [1] is based on local tumour-related factors that determine resectability: biliary ductal involvement, vascular involvement, and lobar atrophy. This last staging system seems related to resectability (60% for T1, 30% for T2 and 0% for T3) and to the presence of extrahepatic disease (21% for T1, 43% for T2 and 41% for T3) [1]. Unfortunately it does not aid in establishing the type of resection to perform.

Surgical decision-making depends on the assessment of longitudinal infiltration of the biliary duct that determines which liver segments must be resected and the type of biliary reconstruction. The likely vascular invasion is useful for determining which type of hepatectomy to carry out, deciding which side, right or left. The extent of hepatic resection needs to be evaluated on the basis of the hepatic function and of the percentage of future remnant liver, which must not be less than 30–40%. Table 2 shows the indications for resection based on biliary segments involved by the disease.

Table 2 Cholangiogram-based strategy for resection. Modified from [7]

Cancer extent on cholangiogram	Recommended resection
Extrahepatic bile duct resections	
Common hepatic duct without obstruction of confluence	Extrahepatic bile duct alone
Caudate resections	
Hepatic duct confluence and caudate branches	Independent caudate lobectomy
Central resections	
Left medial (B4) segmental ducts	Left medial sectionectomy with caudate lobectomy
Right anterior (B5,B8) segmental ducts	Right anterior sectionectomy with caudate lobectomy
Right anterior (B5,B8) and left medial (B4) segmental ducts	Central hepatic bisegmentectomy with caudate lobectomy
Right resections	
Right anterior (B5,B8) and posterior (B6,B7) segmental ducts	Right hepatectomy with caudate lobectomy
Right anterior (B5,B8), posterior (B6,B7) and left medial (B4) segmental ducts	Right trisectionectomy with caudate lobectomy
Left resections	
Left lateral (B2,B3) and medial (B4) segmental ducts	Left hepatectomy with caudate lobectomy
Left lateral (B2,B3), medial (B4) and right anterior (B5,B8) segmental ducts	Left trisectionectomy with caudate lobectomy

Isolated Extrahepatic Bile Duct Resection

Isolated extrahepatic resection of the biliary tract is indicated for treatment of Bismuth-Corlette types I and II. Numerous criticisms have been raised regarding this indication and the procedure must be considered oncologically ineffi-

cient concerning long-term results, based on the following considerations:
- Cholangiography is not accurate enough to provide precise information about longitudinal cancer extension
- Hilar bile duct cancers often show submucosal tumour extension at their proximal margins, which might not be visualised by cholangiography
- Skip type lesions render assessment by imaging and biopsy modalities difficult

Moreover, in the group of patients who undergo margin-negative resections, hepatic resection is the only independent predictor of improved survival on multivariate analysis, suggesting that a more limited resection is ineffective for complete tumour clearance [1].

In the series reported by MSKCC there were no 5-year survival rates among patients who had undergone biliary resection alone [20]. Analogous results have been reported by Miyazaki [25] with 5-year survival of 0% in patients with biliary tract resection alone vs. 27% in patients with additional hepatic resection. A larger series is described by Nimura [5] who reported 8 cases of isolated R0 biliary tract resection, compared with 100 cases of associated hepatic resection. All the patients who had undergone isolated biliary tract resection died within 65 months. These data are confirmed by Neuhaus [4] who reported 5-year survival of 0 vs. 35% in patients who had undergone R0 biliary tract resection alone vs. additional hepatic resection, respectively.

Moreover, this type of operation has a high percentage of recurrence, up to 76%, mainly on the proximal resection margin [26].

The indications are therefore limited to surgical high-risk patients with tumour in an early stage (T1 and T2) and accompanied by poor hepatic function. It is no longer a good indication even as palliative treatment, since endoscopic and percutaneous drainages are preferred.

Independent Caudate Lobectomy (S1)

Resection of caudate lobe is always indicated in association with hepatectomy when the tumour involves biliary confluence, due to the high frequency of involvement of biliary branches varying from 48% [27] to 96% [28]. Neoplastic infiltration follows three pathways:
- Infiltration along the epithelium of biliary duct
- Direct infiltration of caudate parenchyma
- Periductal diffusion in interstitial tissue of caudate lobe

The importance of caudate lobe resection associated with hepatectomy was first underlined by Nimura [28] and it is now largely accepted. The clinical worth of caudate lobe resection was reported for the first time by Sugiura [29], who presented a 5-year survival of 46% with additional hepatectomy to caudate resection, and 12% without caudate resection.

Isolated resection of caudate lobe associated with resection of extrahepatic biliary tract finds few indications and is limited to the cases with neoplasm that grows at the biliary bifurcation and is confined between the right and left hepatic ducts with the sole involvement of the branches to caudate lobe. The results of isolated caudate lobectomy seem worse than those of more extended hepatic resections: Kondo [30] reported a 3-year survival of 30% after isolated caudate lobectomy vs. 75% after right hepatectomy (p=0.013).

Central Hepatic Resections

Central hepatectomies consisting of left medial sectionectomy with caudate lobectomy (S1+S4), right anterior sectionectomy with caudate lobectomy (S1+S5, S8) and central hepatic bisegmentectomy with caudate lobectomy (S1+S4, S5, S8), are proposed mainly by Japanese authors [5,31,32].

These "parenchyma-preserving" hepatectomies find their premise in limited hepatic resection to minimise postoperative risk of hepatic failure in high-risk patients, still maintaining a potentially curative R0 resection. These procedures have been criticised at times: resection is generally difficult since it required two parenchymal section lines and caudate resection, with increased postoperative morbidity (bile leakage); it is not possible to obtain an adequate length of margin on the biliary tract. Moreover, the need to maintain the portal bifurcation, and especially the right and left hepatic arteries, leads to oncological problems of radicality, above all regarding the right hepatic artery which runs just ventrally and very close to the biliary confluence. The reconstruction of bilio-digestive anastomosis is more complex and requires a greater number of anastomoses.

Shimada [32] compared the results of major hepatectomies with those of parenchyma-preserving hepatectomy. Curability rate (R0:R1) was 77% for the former and 54% for the latter, very similar to that of biliary resection alone (50%). The percentage of complications was comparable (47 vs. 54%), but biliary leaks were more frequent in parenchyma-preserving hepatectomy (27 vs. 3%), caused either by the wider raw surface of resection or by the greater number of bilio-jejunostomies (4.8±1.8). Mortality rate was nil in parenchyma-preserving hepatectomy and 13% in major hepatectomy, and 5-year survival were 15 and 25%, respectively.

The reasons for non-curative resection in parenchyma-preserving hepatectomy are almost always determined by microscopical infiltration of proximal biliary margin [33] or by residual tumour on portal bifurcation or hepatic artery [7].

Therefore parenchyma-preserving hepatectomy should be limited strictly to high-risk patients in whom the tumour is confined longitudinally to the right or left hepatic duct, does not invade any of segmental hepatic ducts or transversely invades an adjacent organ.

Extended Right Resections

If the predominant site of involvement is the right hepatic duct or when both hepatic ducts are invaded equally (Bismuth-Corlette types I, II, IIIa, IV), extended right hepatectomy or trisectionectomy are indicated.

In cases with hilar infiltration involving right intrahepatic ducts without extension to segment 4, an extended right hepatectomy with caudate lobectomy (S1+S5, S6, S7, S8) is indicated; instead, in presence of infiltration for contiguity of segment 4 a right trisectionectomy with caudate lobectomy (S1+S4, S5, S6, S7, S8) is indicated.

These operations are believed by most authors to guarantee the higher radicality rate and the best long-term results, especially if the principles of "no-touch technique" and portal resection "de principio" are applied [4].

Right hepatectomy is more likely to be associated with a negative resection margin than is left hepatectomy, based on the following anatomic considerations:

- The common bile duct is on the right side of the hepatoduodenal ligament, with the right hepatic artery passing behind its proximal portion. Therefore the right hepatic artery is frequently invaded by cancer at this site, whereas the left and middle hepatic artery runs along the left side of the hepatoduodenal ligament and is not associated with the bile duct until the end of the transverse portion (extratumoural course at the left margin of the hepatoduodenal ligament).
- It is not necessary to dissect any structure near the tumour, the portal bifurcation may be resected and thus does not need to be dissected. An end-to-end anastomosis of the portal trunk to the left portal vein branch will result in a more stretched course of this vessel and may avoid the kinking that sometimes occurs after right-sided resections.
- Generally liver dissection between the left lateral or left medial section will result in a small parenchymal surface.
- The extrahepatic part of the left hepatic duct is longer, with a more distant segmental ramification, than that of the right hepatic duct.
- Systematic caudate lobectomy can be carried out more easily in patients undergoing right-sided rather than left-sided hepatectomy.
- When portal vein resection is necessary for tumour invasion, it is easier to perform venous reconstruction with the left than with the right portal vein, due to the long extrahepatic portion of the transverse portion of the left part.

Neuhaus [4], utilising the principle of "no-touch technique" with right trisectionectomy and portal resection, reported a 5-year survival of 72% in R0 resected patients with portal vein resection vs. 52% in R0 patients who had undergone right trisectionectomy but without portal resection, and 23% in patients treated with simple right hepatectomy.

Extended Left Resections

The "extended left resections" are indicated when the neoplasm involves the hilar bifurcation and spreads preferentially towards left intrahepatic ducts (extended left hepatectomy with caudate lobectomy S1+S2, S3, S4) or when the neoplasm involves the entire left lobe and extends to the anterior segment (left trisectionectomy with caudate lobectomy S1+S2, S3, S4, S5, S8).

Left resections require a greater parenchymal dissection compared to right ones. Furthermore right portal pedicles are shorter, determining a more demanding portal resection. Ultimately the right hepatic artery that lies close to hilar neoplasm, may facilitate a microscopic local seeding during its mobilisation. The right biliary duct has a shorter course (about 5 mm) before its segmental bifurcation; this may make it difficult to obtain resection with an adequate margin. For all these reasons, many authors report 5-year survival that is worse in left hepatectomies than right ones (28 vs. 50% [7] and 34 vs. 44% [28]). Kondo [24] confirmed these results with significantly better survivals in right than left hepatectomies ($p>0.0013$).

References

1. Jarnagin WR, Fong Y, DeMatteo RP et al (2001) Staging, resectability, and outcome in 225 patients with hilar cholangiocarcinoma. Ann Surg 234(4):507–517; discussion 517–519
2. Launois B, Reding R, Lebeau G, Buard JL (2000) Surgery for hilar cholangiocarcinoma: French experience in a collective survey of 552 extrahepatic bile duct cancers. J Hepatobiliary Pancreat Surg 7(2):128–134
3. Lee SG, Lee YJ, Park KM et al (2000) One hundred and eleven liver resections for hilar bile duct cancer. J Hepatobiliary Pancreat Surg 7(2):135–141
4. Neuhaus P, Jonas S, Settmacher U et al (2003) Surgical management of proximal bile duct cancer: extended right lobe resection increases resectability and radicality. Langenbecks Arch Surg 388(3):194–200
5. Nimura Y, Kamiya J, Kondo S et al (2000) Aggressive preoperative management and extended surgery for hilar cholangiocarcinoma: Nagoya experience. J Hepatobiliary Pancreat Surg 7(2):155–162
6. Puhalla H, Gruenberger T, Pokorny H et al (2003) Resection of hilar cholangiocarcinomas: pivotal prognostic factors and impact of tumour sclerosis. World J Surg 27(6):680–684
7. Tsao JI, Nimura Y, Kamiya J et al (2000) Management of hilar cholangiocarcinoma: comparison of an American and a Japanese experience. Ann Surg 232(2):166–174
8. Uchiyama K, Nakai T, Tani M et al (2003) Indications for extended hepatectomy in the management of stage IV hilar cholangiocarcinoma. Arch Surg 138(9):1012–1016
9. Yi B, Zhang BH, Zhang YJ et al (2004) Surgical procedure and prognosis of hilar cholangiocarcinoma. Hepatobiliary Pancreat Dis Int 3(3):453–457

10. Otto G (2007) Diagnostic and surgical approaches in hilar cholangiocarcinoma. Int J Colorectal Dis 22(2):101–108

11. Sakamoto E, Nimura Y, Hayakawa N et al (1998) The pattern of infiltration at the proximal border of hilar bile duct carcinoma: a histologic analysis of 62 resected cases. Ann Surg 227(3):405–411

12. Ebata T, Watanabe H, Ajioka Y et al (2002) Pathological appraisal of lines of resection for bile duct carcinoma. Br J Surg 89(10):1260–1267

13. Wakai T, Shirai Y, Moroda T et al (2005) Impact of ductal resection margin status on long-term survival in patients undergoing resection for extrahepatic cholangiocarcinoma. Cancer 103(6):1210–1216

14. Ebata T, Nagino M, Kamiya J et al (2003) Hepatectomy with portal vein resection for hilar cholangiocarcinoma: audit of 52 consecutive cases. Ann Surg 238(5):720–727

15. Neuhaus P, Jonas S, Bechstein WO et al (1999) Extended resections for hilar cholangiocarcinoma. Ann Surg 230(6):808–818; discussion 819

16. Kondo S, Katoh H, Hirano S et al (2003) Portal vein resection and reconstruction prior to hepatic dissection during right hepatectomy and caudate lobectomy for hepatobiliary cancer. Br J Surg 90(6):694–697

17. Jarnagin WR, Bowne W, Klimstra DS et al (2005) Papillary phenotype confers improved survival after resection of hilar cholangiocarcinoma. Ann Surg 241(5):703–712; discussion 712–714

18. Kitagawa Y, Nagino M, Kamiya J et al (2001) Lymph-node metastasis from hilar cholangiocarcinoma: audit of 110 patients who underwent regional and paraaortic node dissection. Ann Surg 233(3):385–392

19. Kosuge T, Yamamoto J, Shimada K et al (1999) Improved surgical results for hilar cholangiocarcinoma with procedures including major hepatic resection. Ann Surg 230(5):663–671

20. Jarnagin WR, Shoup M (2004) Surgical management of cholangiocarcinoma. Semin Liver Dis 24(2):189–199

21. Nimura Y, Hayakawa N, Kamiya J et al (1990) Hepatic segmentectomy with caudate lobe resection for bile duct carcinoma of the hepatic hilus. World J Surg 14(4):535–543; discussion 544

21. Nimura Y, Hayakawa N, Kamiya J et al (1991) Hepatopancreatoduodenectomy for advanced carcinoma of the biliary tract. Hepatogastroenterology 38(2):170–175

22. Kubota K, Makuuchi M, Takayama T et al (2000) Appraisal of two-staged pancreatoduodenectomy: its technical aspects and outcome. Hepatogastroenterology 47(31):269–274

23. Miyagawa S, Makuuchi M, Kawasaki S et al (1996) Outcome of major hepatectomy with pancreatoduodenectomy for advanced biliary malignancies. World J Surg 20(1):77–80

24. Bismuth H, Nakache R, Diamond T (1992) Management strategies in resection for hilar cholangiocarcinoma. Ann Surg 215(1):31–38

25. Miyazaki M, Ito H, Nakagawa K et al (1998) Aggressive surgical approaches to hilar cholangiocarcinoma: hepatic or local resection? Surgery 123(2):131–136

26. Mittal B, Deutsch M, Iwatsuki S (1985) Primary cancers of extrahepatic biliary passages. Int J Radiat Oncol Biol Phys 11(4):849–854

27. Ogura Y, Kawarada Y (1998) Surgical strategies for carcinoma of the hepatic duct confluence. Br J Surg 85(1):20–24

29. Sugiura Y, Nakamura S, Iida S et al (1994) Extensive resection of the bile ducts combined with liver resection for cancer of the main hepatic duct junction: a cooperative study of the Keio Bile Duct Cancer Study Group. Surgery 115(4):445–451

30. Kondo S, Hirano S, Ambo Y et al (2004) Forty consecutive resections of hilar cholangiocarcinoma with no postoperative mortality and no positive ductal margins: results of a prospective study. Ann Surg 240(1):95–101

31. Kawarada Y, Isaji S, Taoka H et al (1999) S4a+S5 with caudate lobe (S1) resection using the Taj Mahal liver parenchymal resection for carcinoma of the biliary tract. J Gastrointest Surg 3(4):369–373

32. Shimada H, Endo I, Sugita M et al (2003) Is parenchyma-preserving hepatectomy a noble option in the surgical treatment for high-risk patients with hilar bile duct cancer? Langenbecks Arch Surg 388(1):33–41
33. Tashiro S, Tsuji T, Kanemitsu K et al (1993) Prolongation of survival for carcinoma at the hepatic duct confluence. Surgery 113(3):270–278

Surgical Technique

Surgical resection for hilar cholangiocarcinoma is usually a challenging operation. Correct accomplishment of a R0 resection must be planned with a careful preoperative evaluation that considers longitudinal and radial extent of neoplasms, the presence of lymph-node involvement, vascular infiltration and anatomic variants.

Surgical resection entails exeresis of the biliary tract, associated with hepatic resection and regional lymphadenectomy. Reconstructive phase follows with bilioenteric anastomosis with Roux-en-Y jejunal loop.

Position of the Patient

The patient is placed on the table in supine position, with left arm secured at right angles and right arm at the site. It may be helpful to place an inflatable support at the base of the thorax at D9-D10 level to expose the liver optimally. The skin is cleansed higher than the nipples and down to the pubis, and laterally to middle axillary lines. It may be useful to apply a crossing bar or similar device fixed on the table, which later holds a self-retaining retractor to elevate the costal margin.

Incision

In most cases a right subcostal incision which can be extended to the left and in the midline toward the xiphoid provides a good exposure. It is advisable to begin with a small right subcostal incision that permits one to explore the abdominal cavity and judge the resectability of the neoplasm.

In particular cases requiring biliary tract resection alone or limited left hepatic resection, a midline incision is made.

A. Guglielmi, A. Ruzzenente, C. Iacono (eds.) *Surgical Treatment of Hilar and ICC.*
© Springer 2008

Intraoperative Exploration

Abdominal inspection is a preliminary and fundamental phase in which staging is completed and resectability accurately established.

During this phase an initial exploration of the perihilar area is performed by manual palpation, checking for peritoneal or lymph-node metastases. Then the search for distant peritoneal or lymph-node metastases is performed, calling for frozen sectioning if indicated.

It should be kept in mind that a correct and complete evaluation of resectability is obtained only at a more advanced point in the operation when hepatic pedicle dissection and isolation of its elements are completed. Only at this time is a correct evaluation of portal and arterial vascular infiltration possible. Staging phase is then accomplished in all the cases with intraoperative ultrasound of the liver as previously described.

Hepatic Pedicle Dissection and Lymphadenectomy

Dissection of the hepatic pedicle usually begins with isolation of the artery followed by the biliary tract and portal vein.

Arterial dissection begins at the common hepatic artery which is freed, and a blood vessel loop is passed around it for traction. Its dissection allows removal of perineural and lymphatic structures of stations 8 and 12a. The isolation continues towards the hepatic hilum (Fig. 1) with dissection of the proper hepatic artery, gas-

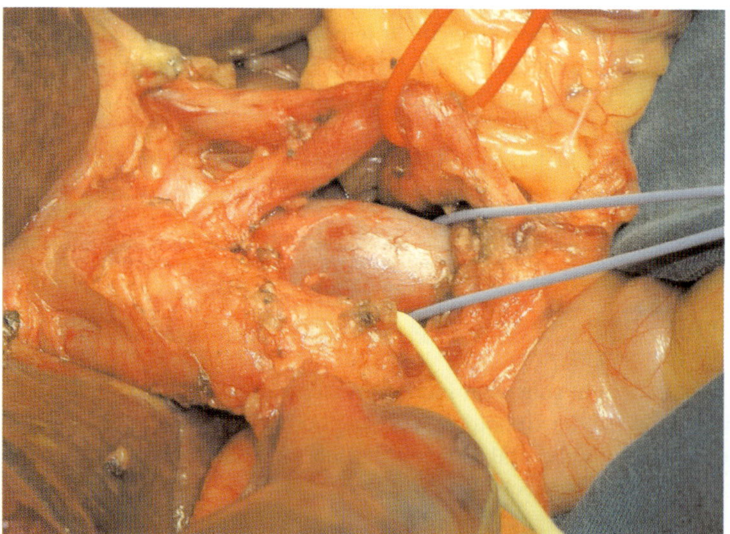

Fig. 1 Hepatic hilus after lymph node dissection of the hepatoduodenal ligament

troduodenal artery and subsequently of first order arterial branches (right, middle and left hepatic artery). Scrupulous attention must be paid at this point to find accessory arterial branches or anatomic variants which occur quite frequently.

Biliary dissection is begun at this stage, with duodenal mobilization and cholecystectomy. Then lymph node clearing of 12b and 13 stations is performed. Biliary tract is passed on tape and before dividing the distal bile duct it is appropriate to conclude the dissection of hepatoduodenal ligament with portal vein isolation and lymph nodal clearance of station 12p. Only at this time can a definitive statement on possible vascular infiltration and resectability of the disease be achieved. A potential portal involvement above the bifurcation can be accurately assessed with appropriate traction manoeuvres on the biliary tract and artery. In presence of portal or arterial vascular infiltration, hepatic resection can be associated with vascular resection and reconstruction as described later in the chapter.

Pedicle dissection ends with division and closure of the distal biliary stump at the suprapancreatic level, being careful to avoid spillage of bile possibly containing viable cancer cells. The margin of distal bile duct resection is sent for frozen section histology.

After completing lymphadenectomy of all stations of hepatoduodenal ligament and hepatic hilum, it is advisable to explore the pancreaticoduodenal and paraaortic lymph nodes that are resected for staging only if macroscopically suspected positive.

At this point the surgical management changes according to the planned operation.

Bile Duct Resection Alone

This operation is rarely indicated nowadays and only when the primary tumour is located exactly in the middle of the common hepatic duct with no invasion or spread, without portal or arterial involvement. It is also an option for high-risk patients who cannot tolerate hepatic resection due to the presence of cirrhosis or severe co-morbidities. It is considered a minimally invasive, less radical surgical treatment. After completion of lymph node dissection of hepatic pedicle and division of distal bile duct at the supraduodenal level, right and left Glisson pedicles are more exteriorized thanks to posterior access at the hilum that allows en-bloc resection of Glisson sheath and intrahepatic biliary ducts. Particular attention must be paid to dissect biliary confluence from portal vascular plane and right hepatic artery that runs behind biliary bifurcation. Whenever the right and left hepatic ducts are exposed, they are divided upon positioning a stay suture. The section of the left duct is usually farther from bifurcation as the left duct is longer than the right. On the right, given the shortness of the duct, the section line is on the bifurcation of anterior and posterior ducts. On the posterior aspect of the biliary confluence several biliary ducts are found that arise from the caudate lobe and can be either tied or anastomosed to the digestive tract (Fig. 2).

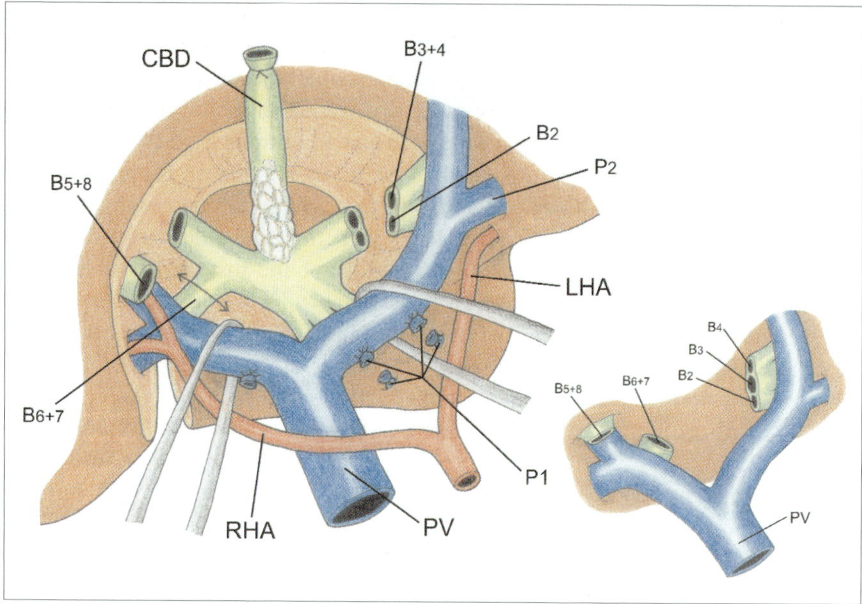

Fig. 2a,b Isolated resection of bile duct. **a** The common bile duct is turned cranially to expose the bile ducts branches of right posterior and caudate lobe. **b** Surgical field at the end of resection with bile ducts of the left and right side. Numbers refers to Couinaud's segments. *PV*, Portal vein; *CBD*, common bile duct; *RHA*, right hepatic artery; *LHA*, left hepatic artery

Restoration of digestive continuity is realised with a 50–60 cm Roux-en-Y jejunal loop anastomosed to right and left biliary ducts with interrupted or continuous PDS® 5/0 stitches.

Independent Caudate Lobectomy (S1)

The isolated resection of the caudate lobe associated with resection of the extrahepatic biliary tract represents a fairly rare indication and is limited to cases with neoplasm confined clearly inside the confluence between right and left ducts with involvement of caudate branches. The resection of the caudate lobe due to its position always requires the complete mobilization of the liver.

The operation begins with hepatoduodenal ligament dissection, lymph node clearing and transection of the suprapancreatic bile duct as described before. Subsequently ligation and section of arterial and portal branches to the caudate lobe are carried out. The caudate lobe is therefore mobilised from the vena cava with lesser omentum division and ligation of the Arantius duct that allows the mobilisation of the cranial portion of the caudate lobe. From the left, after having lifted and dislocated the caudate lobe towards the right, all the small acces-

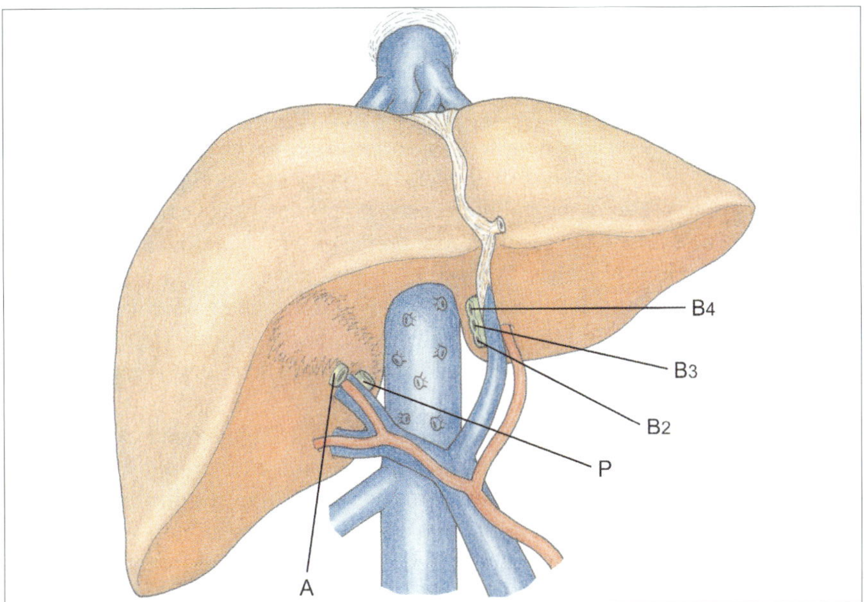

Fig. 3 Independent caudate lobectomy. The left bile duct is resected on the right side of the umbilical plate (*B4-B3-B2*); on the right side, at the origin of right anterior and posterior bile duct

sory hepatic veins are tied and divided; in this way the anterior surface of the vena cava is exposed up to the confluence with the left hepatic vein that represents the upper limit of the caudate lobe.

The right portion of caudate lobe is still connected to segment 7 by the caudate process, a thin parenchymal bridge which is easily divided. The biliary tract is transected on the left at level of S2, S3, and S4 ducts and on the right at the level of the anterior and posterior ducts (Fig. 3).

Bilio-digestive continuity is difficult and challenging due to the large number of anastomoses to be performed and the depth of operative field.

Right Hepatectomy with Caudate Lobectomy (S4a, S5, S6, S7, S8 + S1)

Right hepatectomy with caudate lobectomy is indicated for tumours involving the right anterior and posterior sectorial bile ducts with sparing of the left medial segmental bile duct to segment 4.

The resection entails the right hepatic lobe, caudate lobe and, if indicated, the caudal portion of segment 4 (4a) to obtain an adequate margin of biliary ducts.

After mobilisation of duodenum and retropancreatic lymph node dissection, the distal bile duct is transected in its suprapancreatic portion and sent for frozen section to obtain a histologic free margin. After lymph node dissection of the hepatoduodenal ligament, vascular isolation is performed in the hepatic hilus. Anatomic variations of hepatic artery or accessory branches are looked for and identified. First order branches of the hepatic artery are carefully isolated with particular care to preserve the middle hepatic artery that runs ventrally to the left portal vein. The caudate lobe is therefore prepared with isolation and section of its arterial and portal branches. Arterial branches, sometimes hard to visualise, arise from the right and left hepatic artery. Portal branches arise in a variable number from 2 to 6 from the left portal vein, 2 or 3 from the right one and 2 directly from the bifurcation. Subsequently right hepatic artery and right portal branch are tied and divided.

The left hepatic lobe is mobilised with section of triangular and coronary ligaments and lesser epiploon. If an accessory left hepatic artery is detected, it must be preserved. At this stage it is advisable to ligate the Arantius duct near its confluence into the left hepatic vein or vena cava. This manoeuvre is essential for achieving complete mobilisation of the caudate lobe and its removal en-bloc with the right hepatic lobe.

Complete mobilisation of the right hepatic lobe with section of triangular and coronary ligaments is performed. All the short hepatic veins, which enter the inferior vena cava, are doubly ligated and divided. The caudate lobe is completely detached from the cava. The right hepatic vein is then isolated, transected and sutured with a vascular stapler or prolene suture.

After ultrasound confirmation of the course of the middle hepatic vein, parenchymal section is carried out along the demarcation of Cantlie line on the cranial side and advanced just to the right side of the falciform ligament in the caudal part of segment 4 (segment 4a), to achieve a free bile duct surgical margin. The middle hepatic vein is seen during liver resection, and the proximal half of the vessel that drains the left medial superior segment (4b) should be preserved (Fig. 4).

At this point the caudate lobe can be turned and pulled ventrally from behind the left lateral segment. Finally the biliary duct is transected after placing a stay suture and the right hepatic lobe is resected en bloc with the caudate lobe and extrahepatic bile duct. The transected biliary duct stumps for segment 4, segment 3 and segment 2 are located just to the right of the umbilical portion of the left portal vein (Fig. 4).

Biliary-enteric continuity is established using a Roux-en-Y jejunal loop. The loop is brought up retrocolic-antegastric or retrocolic-retrogastric.

The anastomosis is created using interrupted or continuous absorbable monofilament 5–0 suture. It is advisable to place a biliary drainage tube across the anastomosis through the jejunal loop.

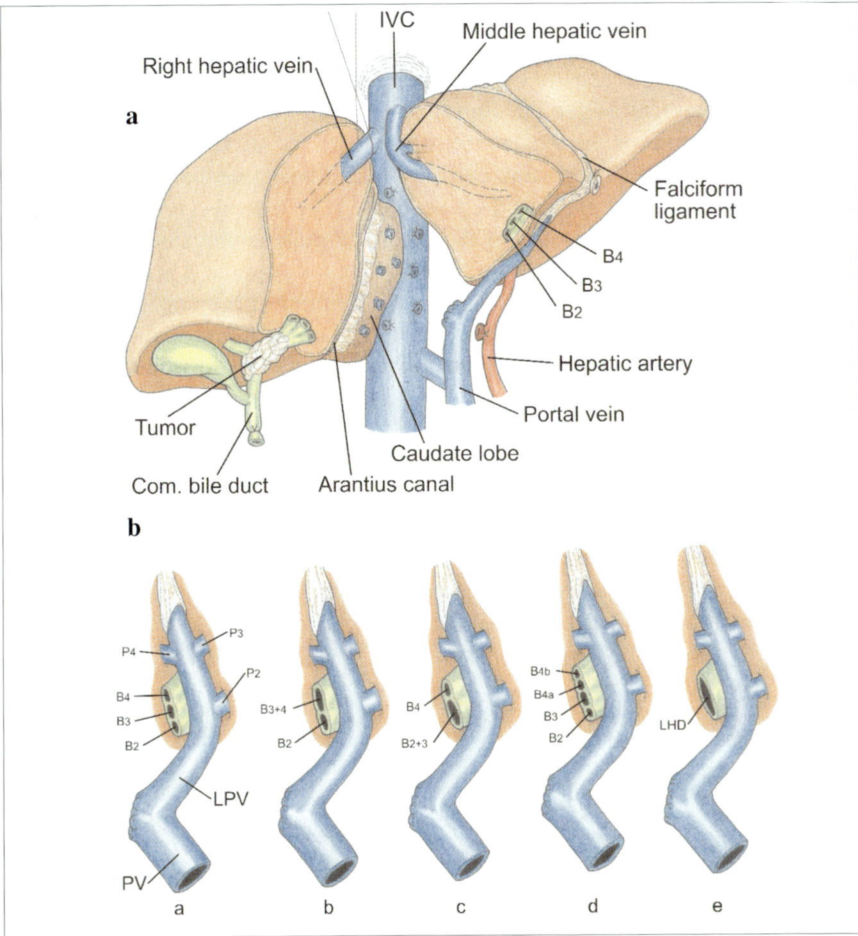

Fig. 4a,b Right hepatectomy with caudate lobectomy. **a** The caudal part of transaction line is advanced just to the right side of the falciform ligament to achieve a free surgical margin on bile ducts. **b** Variation of left bile ducts at the end of resection

Right Trisectionectomy with Caudate Lobectomy (S4, S5, S6, S7, S8 + S1)

The right trisectionectomy with caudate lobectomy is indicated for hilar cholangiocarcinoma that involves the right intrahepatic bile duct in continuity with the left medial segmental duct (segment 4).

The phases of retropancreatic and hepatoduodenal ligament lymph node dissection, of distal bile duct section and mobilization of caudate lobe are similar to the abovementioned for right hepatectomy. Right and middle hepatic artery and right portal vein are ligated and divided. Mobilisation of right hepatic lobe is completed and right hepatic vein is divided and sutured as previously reported.

Section line of the hepatic parenchyma is conducted along the right margin of falciform ligament. When the umbilical portion of the portal vein is reached, the biliary branches of the left lateral segment will be exposed just to the right and cranially to umbilical portion and are divided with free margins (Fig. 5).

In case of infiltrated margins the resection can be extended to the left side of the umbilical portion. Exposure of the umbilical plate is obtained through cautious isolation and section of all portal branches for segment 4 arising from the cranial side of the umbilical portion. Finally ligation of the cranial side of the Arantius canal consents the complete detachment of the left portal vein from the umbilical plate. Section of the biliary duct can be then performed on the left margin of the umbilical plate, on the ducts for S2 and S3, separately. This operation has been described by Nagino [1] as "anatomic right trisectionectomy" (Figs. 6,7).

Parenchymal section continues posteriorly up to the onset of middle hepatic vein that is divided and sutured at the origin with 4–0 prolene suture.

The previous section of Arantius duct allows at this point to pull out segment 1 ventrally, together with the right hepatic lobe and the left medial segment en bloc with extrahepatic bile duct. Bilioenteric continuity is re-established with a Roux-en-Y loop as previously described.

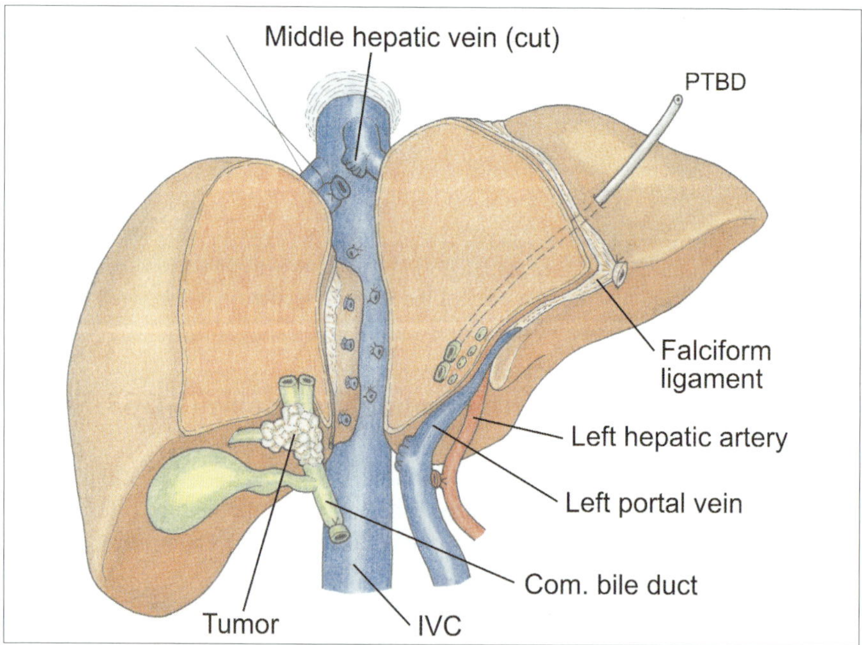

Fig. 5 Right trisegmentectomy with caudate lobectomy. The transaction plane is close to the right margin of falciform ligament

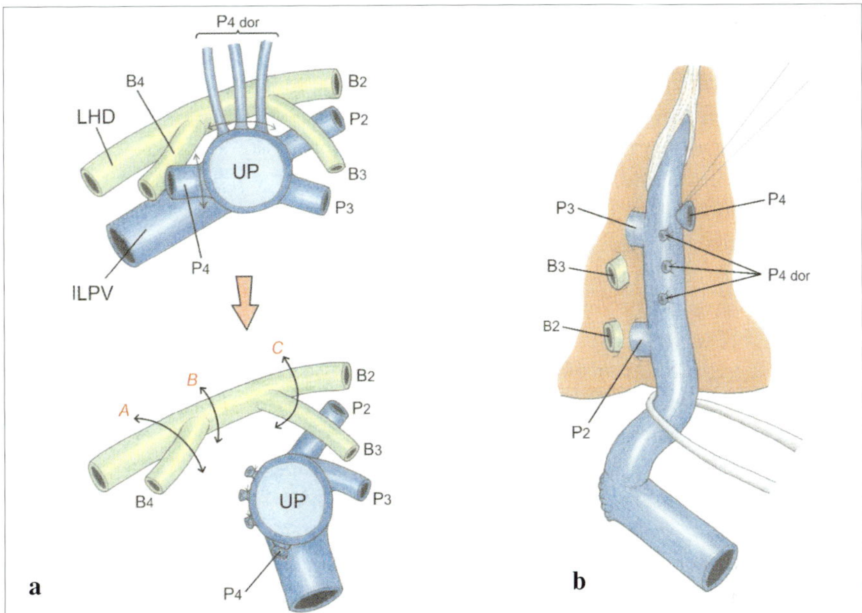

Fig. 6a,b a Complete dissection of the umbilical plate with ligation of the small branches of segment 2 (*P4 dor*). The resection line can be performed on segment B2 and B3 separately. The three lines indicate resection line of the left bile duct in right hepatectomy (*A*), right trisectionectomy (*B*), and anotomic right trisectionectomy (*C*). **b** Numerals indicate the segment bile duct (*B*) and portal branch (*P*) according to Couinaud's hepatic segment. *UP*, Umbilical portion

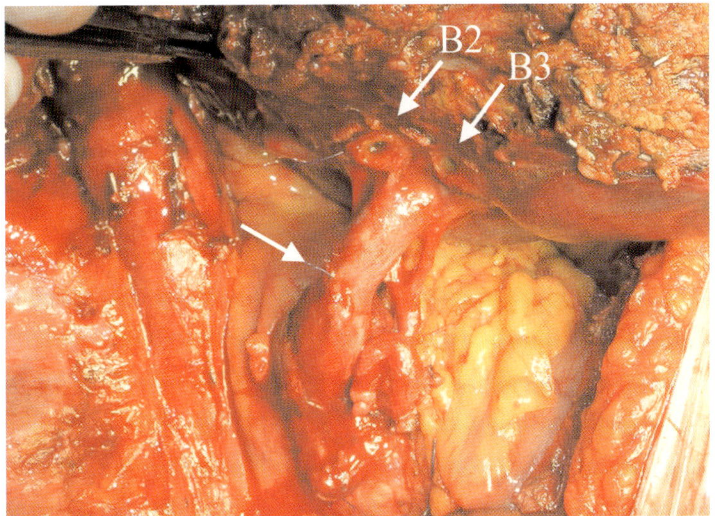

Fig. 7 Right trisectionectomy with portal resection (*white arrow*). *B2,B3*, bile duct for segment 2 and segment 3

Left Hepatectomy with Caudate Lobectomy (S2, S3, S4 + S1)

The extended left hepatectomy with caudate lobectomy finds its indication in neoplasms of the biliary confluence that extend to the left intrahepatic bile duct.

After hilar preparation and ligation of arterial and portal branches for caudate lobe, the left and middle hepatic artery and left portal vein are tied.

The left lobe is completely mobilised with section of left triangular and coronary ligaments. The lesser omentum is incised and the left part of the caudate lobe is mobilised from down upward until the confluence of the Arantius canal with the left hepatic or vena cava where it is tied. The caudate lobe is then completely mobilised from the vena cava after ligation and division of left and middle hepatic veins.

At this point hepatic parenchyma section is carried out along the Cantlie line. The line of section is slightly toward right anterior sector with exposure on resection line of the anterior segmental ducts (S5 and S8). The segmental anterior bile ducts are transected after placing a stay suture, with free margin distant from the tumour.

Hepatic dissection carries on behind where posterior segmental ducts (S6 and S7) are exposed on the cranial side of the right portal vein, and are transected after placing a stay suture, with free margin (Fig. 8).

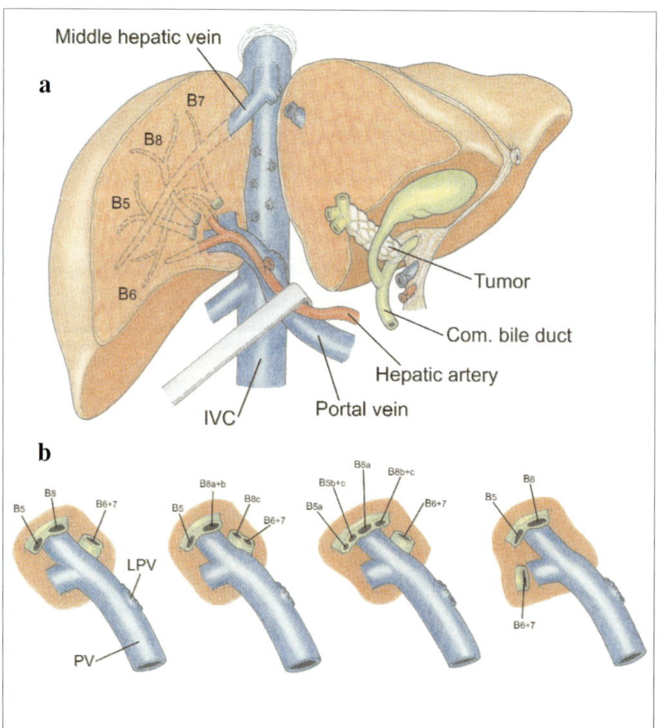

Fig. 8a,b a Left hepatectomy with caudate lobectomy. The plan of liver dissection is along the demarcation of Cantlie line. *IVC*, Inferior vena cava. b The right anterior and posterior bile duct are divided on free margin with different possibilities of anastomoses, in relation to anatomical variation. *LPV*, left portal vein. *PV*, portal vein. Numerals indicate the segment bile duct according to Couinaud's hepatic segment

Parenchymal section is completed with the section between right posterior segment and caudate lobe that begins down along the ischemic demarcation line of the caudate process and advances upward along the right margin of the vena cava. Dissection and division of caudate from segment 7 is completed.

The left hepatic lobe is then removed together with the caudate lobe and extrahepatic bile duct.

Bilioenteric continuity is re-established with a Roux-en-Y jejunal limb anastomosed with biliary ducts (Fig. 9).

Left Trisectionectomy with Caudate Lobectomy (S2, S3, S4, S5, S8 + S1)

The left trisectionectomy with caudate lobectomy is indicated for hilar cholangiocarcinoma that involves the left intrahepatic bile ducts in continuity with the duct to the right anterior sector (S5 and S8).

After concluding dissection of hepatoduodenal ligament as previously described, the left and middle hepatic arteries are tied and divided at their origins. The right artery is isolated very gently up to its second order bifurcation for anterior and posterior sectors. The branch for anterior sector and the small

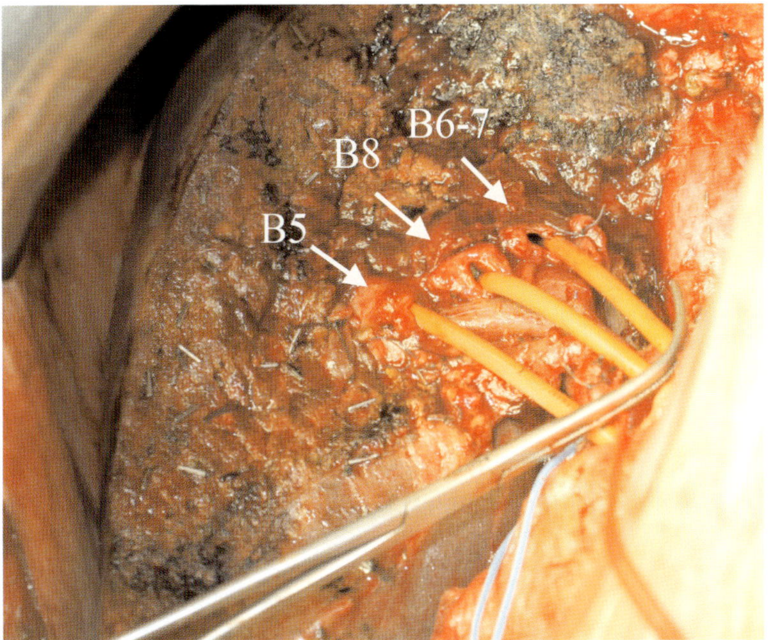

Fig. 9 Left hepatectomy. At the end of liver resection three different bile ducts for segments B5, B8 and B6+7 are identified

branches for caudate are divided and tied. Subsequently the left and right anterior sectorial portal branches are divided and ligated as well. The section of small portal branches to the caudate lobe, which arise from the right portal vein and bifurcation, is completed.

The left and caudate lobes are retracted to the right and the short retrohepatic caudate veins are ligated and divided beginning on the left caudally and progressing cranially.

At this point the Arantius duct (ligamentum venosum) is isolated and divided at its origin when it opens into the left hepatic or vena cava.

The left and middle hepatic vein are then isolated and divided either with a vascular stapler or running suture with 4–0 prolene. At this point the caudate and left lobes are completely detached from the inferior vena cava.

Parenchymal section begins along the line of demarcation that runs in the right portal scissura between the right anterior and posterior sectors. The plane of parenchymal section has to carefully regard the right hepatic along its entire course. The section ends with detachment of the caudate lobe from segment 7 with section of the parenchyma along the right side of the caudate process that advances cranially along the right margin of the inferior vena cava.

The right posterior sectorial bile duct is exposed on the cranial margin of the right portal vein and transected with histologic free margin after placing a stay suture. The left hepatic lobe and the right anterior sectors are then removed together with caudate lobe and extrahepatic bile duct. Bilio-enteric continuity is reconstructed with a Roux-en-Y jejunal loop anastomosed with the biliary ducts of S6 and S7 (Figs. 10,11).

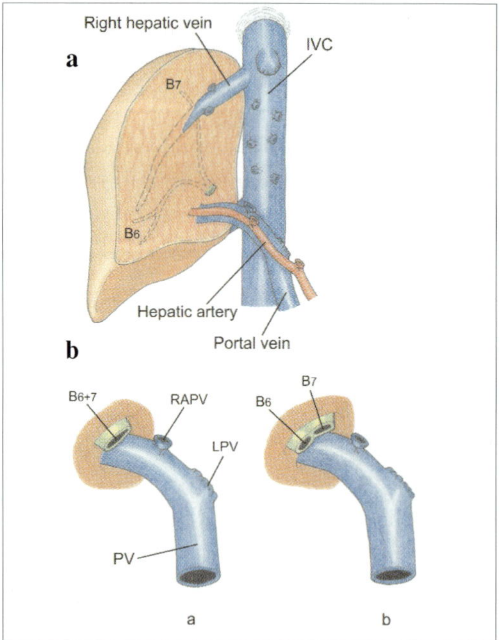

Fig. 10a,b a Left trisectionectomy and caudate lobectomy. b According to the anatomical variations the posterior segmental ducts (*B6, B7*) may be unique or separated

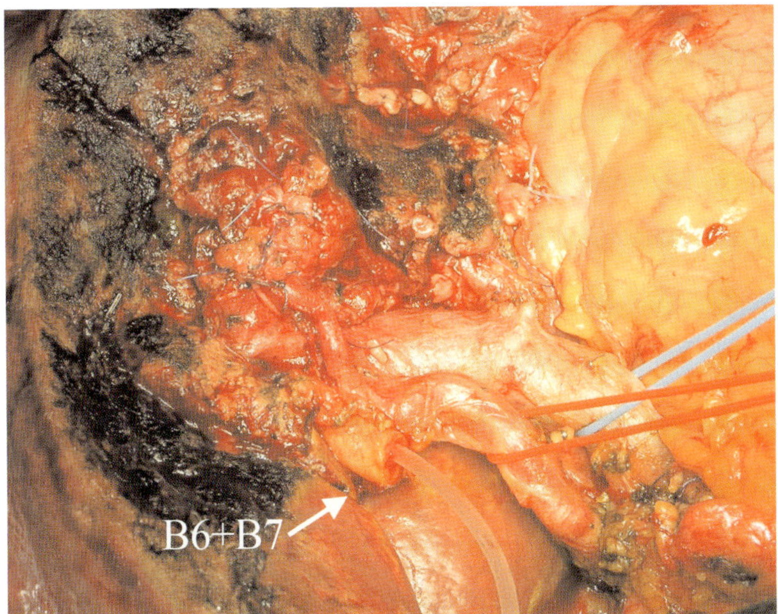

Fig. 11 Left trisectionectomy. Bile duct (*B6+B7*) for posterior hepatic segment are identified caudally to the portal branches

Central (Preserving) Hepatectomy

Central hepatectomy with total caudate lobectomy is rarely indicated in special cases of hilar cholangiocarcinoma that involves the confluence and segment 4 (Left medial sectionectomy with caudate lobectomy S4 + S1), the confluence and the right anterior sector (Right anterior sectionectomy with caudate lobectomy S5, S8 + S1) or the confluence and both left medial segment (S4) in continuity with right anterior sector (Central hepatic bisectionectomy with caudate lobectomy S4, S5, S8 + S1) .

Left Medial Sectionectomy with Caudate Lobectomy (S4 + S1)

The operation begins with hilar time, complete mobilisation of the liver and caudate lobe as described in the isolated caudate lobectomy.

The parenchymal dissection is performed with anatomic resection of caudate lobe and segment 4. Transection of the left biliary duct is immediately on the right of the falciform ligament on segment S2 and S3 while on the right side falls just on the two biliary ducts: the anterior and the posterior. The bilioenteric continuity is restored with multiple bilioenteric anastomoses on both the right and left sides that is very demanding and complex due to the high number of anastomoses to perform.

Right Anterior Sectionectomy with Caudate Lobectomy (S5, S8 + S1)

This operation also begins with the hilar phase, complete mobilisation of the liver and caudate lobe as described before. The arterial and portal branches to the caudate lobe that arise from the main right and left branches are ligated. After cholecystectomy and transection of the distal bile duct on free margin, the biliary tract is reflected upward and the right vascular elements are isolated up to the bifurcation in anterior and posterior branches. The arterial braches for the right anterior sector (S5 and S8) are dissected and divided. At this point a cyanotic demarcation line of the right anterior segment is evident. The next step is mobilisation of the liver with complete detachment of the caudate lobe from the vena cava. Parenchymal dissection begins on the left along the line of demarcation with segment 4. The right collaterals of the middle hepatic vein are divided, while it is advisable to preserve the main trunk in order to avoid vascular congestion of segment 4. The Arantius duct is divided next to the left hepatic vein or vena cava. This manoeuvre allows complete mobilisation of the caudate lobe that is dislocated ventrally in the resection plane. Transection of the left biliary tract is accomplished on the clear margin.

The second section line begins from the line of demarcation between the right anterior and posterior sectors that is now more evident after the vascular occlusion of the paramedian branches at the hilar time. The section line runs along the right lateral fissure, with scrupulous preservation of the right hepatic vein. Dissection between the caudate lobe and right posterior sector is accomplished from down upward after division of the right posterior biliary duct.

The operation ends with bilio-digestive reconstruction on the biliary ducts of segments S2, S3, S4 and S6+S7.

Central Hepatic Bisectionectomy with Caudate Lobectomy (S4, S5, S8 + S1)

Lymph node and connective tissue dissection of the hepatoduodenal ligament is performed first. The middle artery and right anterior arterial and portal branch are tied as well. The next step is the ligation of arterial and portal branches to the caudate lobe that arise from right and left main branches. Then the complete mobilisation of the right and left liver with separation of the caudate lobe from cava plane is achieved.

The parenchymal dissection of the liver begins on the right margin of the falciform ligament and umbilical portion, with complete separation of segment 4 from left lateral segment. The dissection starts caudally with sectioning of biliary ducts for segment 2 and 3, advancing upward along the right margin of the falciform ligament up to the origin of the middle hepatic vein that is then divided and sutured. The Arantius duct is also divided next to the left hepatic or vena cava. This phase allows to completely mobilise the caudate lobe that is pulled out from the section plane. The second section line follows the line of demarcation between right anterior and posterior sectors, and it is now enhanced by the occlusion of the anterior paramedian vascular branches. The section plane runs along the right lateral fissure with meticulous conservation of the right hepatic vein. The dissection between caudate lobe and right posterior sector is completed from down upward after transection of the right posterior biliary duct (Fig. 12).

The bilioenteric reconstruction is performed with left anastomoses on the ducts for segments 2 and 3 and on the right with the duct of posterior segment (S6 and S7) (Fig. 13).

Hepatectomy with Portal Resection and Reconstruction

The infiltration of portal bifurcation is not so rare in hilar cholangiocarcinoma, due to the close relationship of the biliary confluence with the portal system. In these cases the use of hepatectomy with en-bloc portal vein resection has been advocated by several authors, to increase the curative resections. When curative resection was achieved using portal resection and reconstruction, patients survived significantly longer than unresected patients [2].

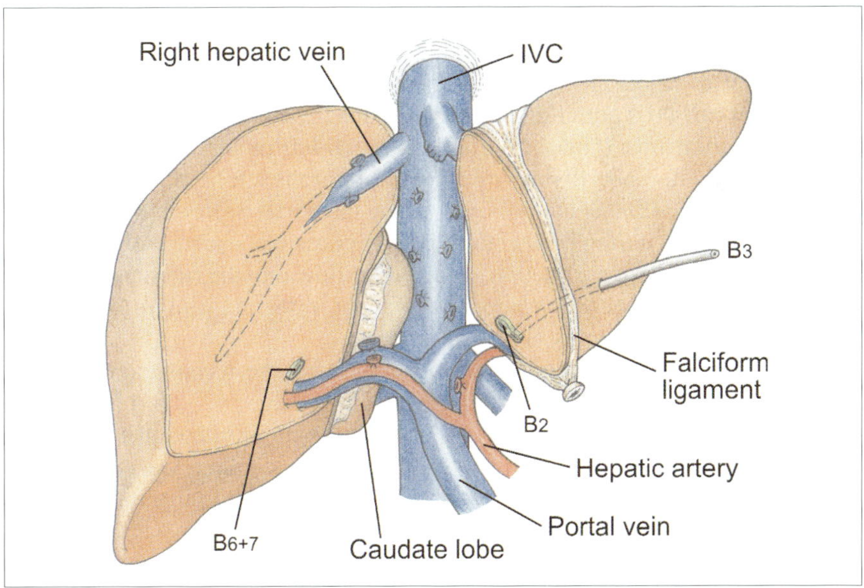

Fig. 12 Central hepatic bisectionectomy. The left medial (S4) and right anterior (S5+S8) segments are resected together with caudate lobe (S1)

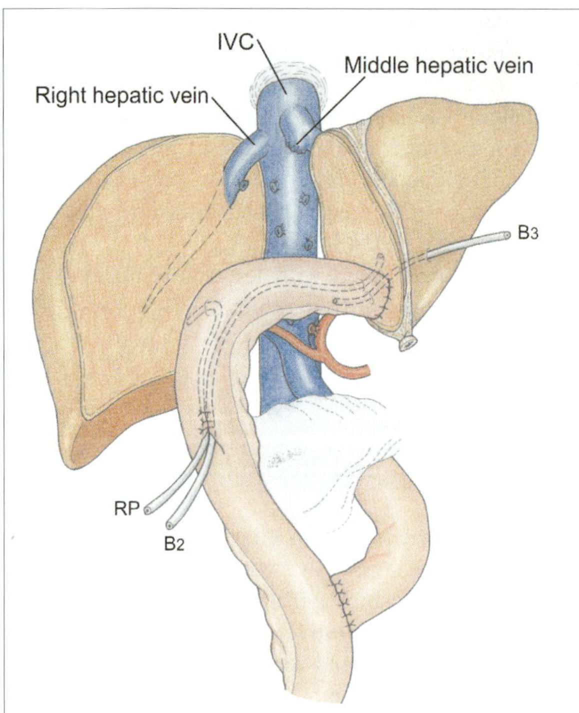

Fig. 13 Central hepatic bisegmentectomy. The bilio-enteric anastomosis are performed separately on left segments B2 and B3 and on the right posterior segmental duct (*B6+B7*)

The surgical attitude changes on the basis of the extent of portal infiltration and the type of hepatectomy to be performed. During right hepatectomy it is advisable to carry out portal resection before the hepatic dissection. The technical reasons are many: (1) right portal infiltration left in site makes the hepatic resection difficult, especially during the division of the left hepatic duct near the umbilical portion; (2) it is not possible to stop the portal inflow to the right liver to control bleeding during hepatectomy; (3) it is possible, during mobilization of the right liver, to cause obstruction of the portal flow into the future remnant left liver. These problems are avoided with portal resection and reconstruction before the right hepatectomy (Fig. 14).

Usually, given the length of the left portal trunk the reconstruction is performed end-to-end without any interposed venous graft.

To obtain a good anastomosis it is important to mobilise completely the left portal branch up to the base of the umbilical portion, dividing venous branches for the caudate lobe and Arantius canal. Also, the main portal trunk has to be freed completely up to the spleno-mesenteric confluence. This wide dissection facilitates the end-to-end portal anastomosis. The section line on the left portal trunk can be slightly oblique to achieve a comparable size. The suture is carried out with intraluminal suturing technique for the posterior wall and with an over-and-over method for the anterior wall (Fig. 15).

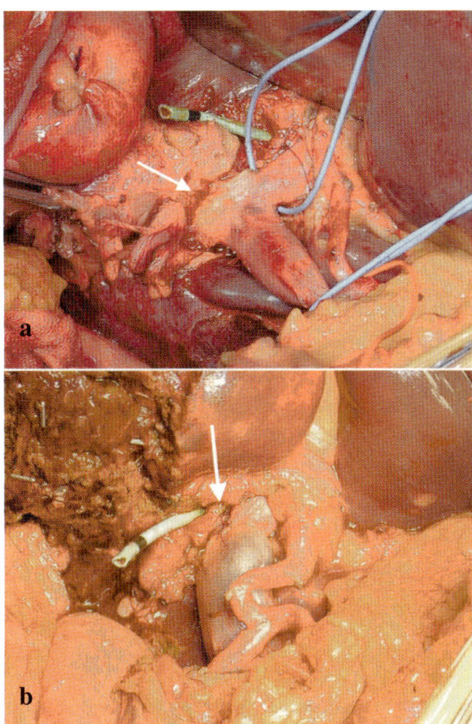

Fig. 14a,b a Right portal vein involvement (*white arrow*). **b** End-to-end anastomosis after portal vein resection (*white arrow*)

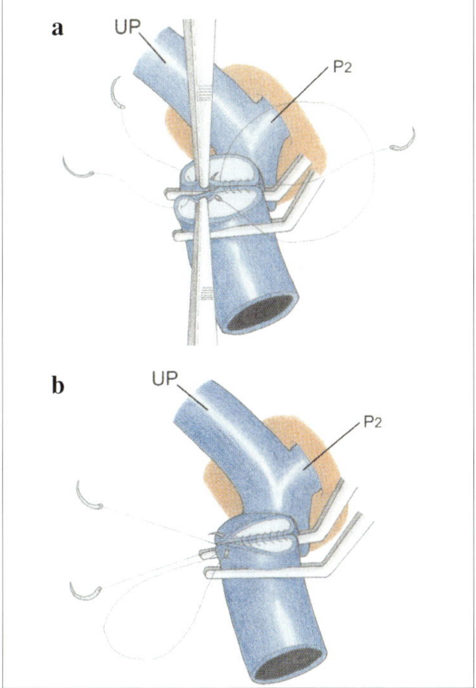

Fig. 15a,b Portal vein resection and reconstruction with intraluminal suturing technique for the posterior wall (**a**) and with over-and-over method for the anterior wall (**b**). *UP*, Umbilical portion; *P2*, portal branch for segment 2

Portal resection and reconstruction in left hepatectomy is usually more demanding due to the shortness of the right portal trunk that divides early into the two anterior and posterior branches with limited possibility of mobilisation of the right portal branch. For this reason some authors suggest carrying out resection and reconstruction after liver transection [3].

It is generally required to interpose a venous graft between the right portal branch and the main portal trunk. A graft of external iliac vein is habitually utilised, since it has an adequate size and length; as an alternative jugular vein, left renal vein or cryopreserved allograft can be used (Fig. 16).

If the portal bifurcation is not invaded by tumour circumferentially, a wedge resection can be performed [4]. After dissection of the common portal trunk and of the right posterior and anterior portal branches, a wedge resection of the portal bifurcation is carried out, taking care to secure a clear surgical margin. Portal reconstruction is performed with a continuous transverse suture, after placing two guy-sutures at the dorsal and ventral edges of the vein (Figs. 17,18).

If the defect is wide and cannot be repaired with direct suturing, a small interposed venous patch can be applied [5].

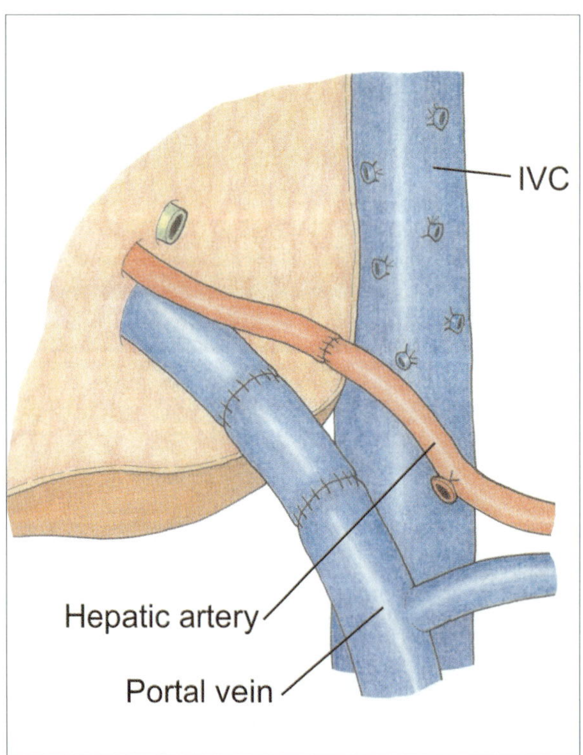

Fig. 16 Portal vein resection and reconstruction with interposition of iliac graft, and reconstruction of right hepatic artery

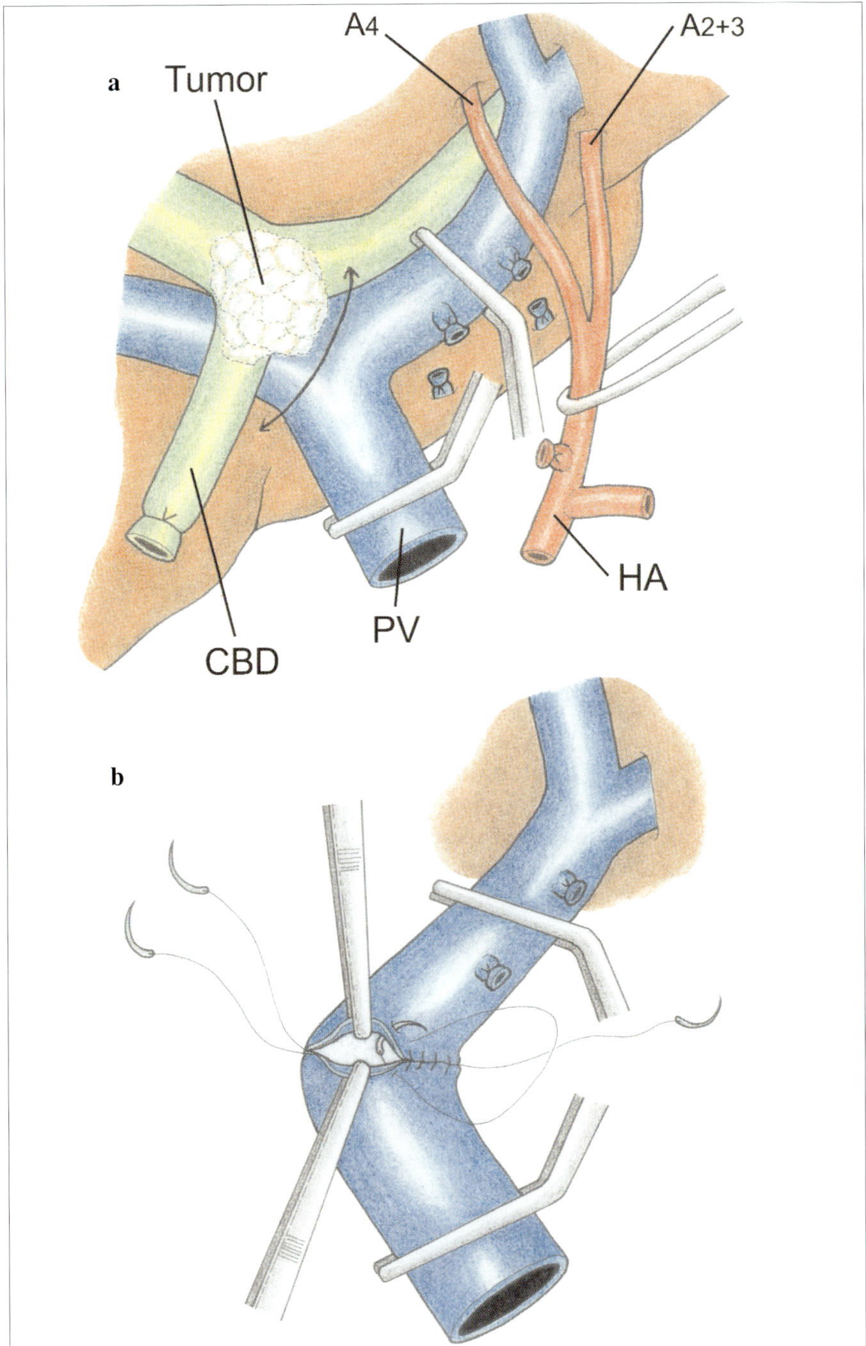

Fig. 17a,b a Wedge resection of the portal vein bifurcation when the tumour does not circunferentially invade the vein. **b** Reconstruction with a continuous transverse suture

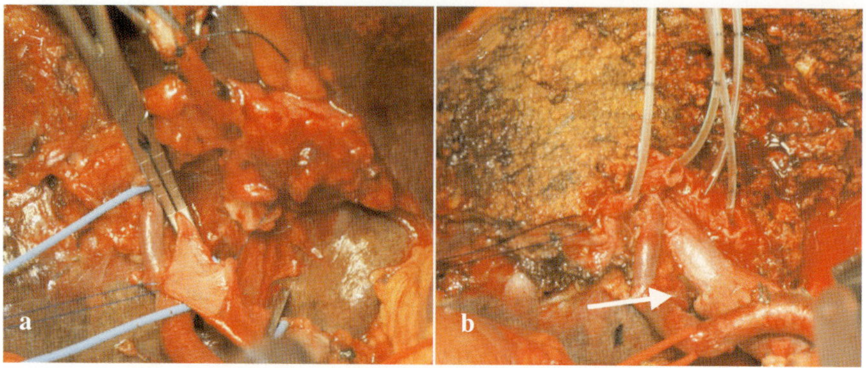

Fig. 18a,b a Wedge resection of portal vein bifurcation. **b** Reconstruction with a continuous transverse suture (*white arrow*)

Hepatectomy with Arterial Resection and Reconstruction

Unilateral arterial invasion has been a contraindication to surgical resection. Today many works report cases with portal and arterial vascular resection combined with left or right hepatectomy, even if the clinical significance of hepatic artery resection and reconstruction has not yet been resolved [6].

The indication for vascular reconstruction depends on the condition of vascular invasion shown by CT imaging, angiography, intraoperative echography, macroscopic inspection and palpation.

Hepatic artery reconstruction is performed less frequently than the portal, as it is often associated with advanced and unresectable disease. In fact arterial reconstruction is more often performed on the right hepatic artery, since it runs behind and very close to the biliary bifurcation and therefore is frequently involved by the disease even in the case of neoplasms that are locally advanced (Fig. 19).

Instead, the left hepatic artery runs farther from bifurcation and its neoplastic involvement represents a sign of extended infiltration of the hepatoduodenal ligament and generally a condition of unresectability.

Usually after adequate mobilisation of the artery an end-to-end anastomosis with direct microsurgical suture is performed (Fig. 16). Alternatively, a graft of the left radial artery can be used. Introduction of microsurgical reconstruction by means of a microscope has allowed achieving patent anastomosis at a rate of about 100% [7].

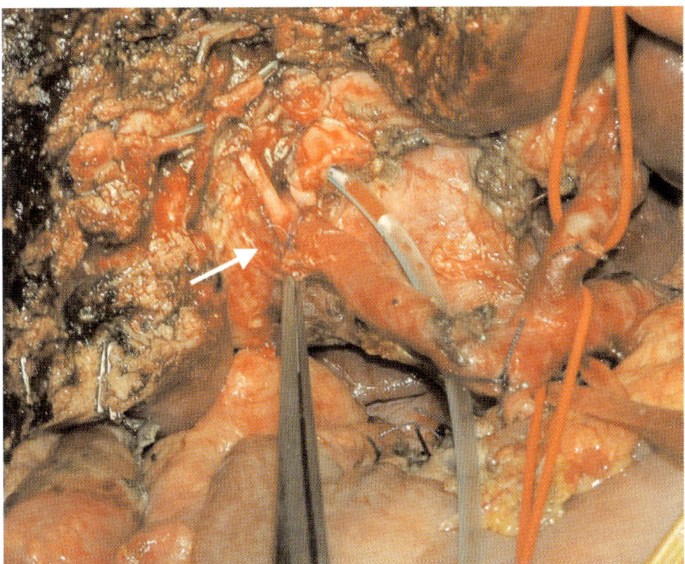

Fig. 19 Right hepatic artery reconstruction (*white arrow*) in left hepatectomy

Hepatopancreatoduodenectomy (HPD)

In presence of longitudinal tumour spread from the hepatic duct to the intrapancreatic bile duct or massive lymph-node metastases along the bile duct and behind the pancreatic head, HPD has been proposed to achieve surgical radicality. If massive lymph node infiltration occurred, HPD is not indicated due to the poor prognostic significance of lymph node invasion. In the first reported experiences, mortality and morbidity rates of HPD were very high because of postoperative liver failure and leakage of pancreatojejunostomy [8]. For this reason a two-stage operation in which reconstruction of the pancreatic duct is deferred to a second stage was proposed. This technique, associated with preoperative biliary drainage and PVE, has reduced complications and mortality significantly. Miyagawa [9] reported a consecutive series of 12 patients without mortality.

Biliary Anastomosis

Reconstruction of biliary-digestive continuity is performed with one or more anastomoses between segmental or subsegmental ducts and a Roux-en-Y jejunal loop. The first phase requires accurate identification of all the biliary ducts previously transected. Given the difficulty of detecting the biliary ducts on the raw surface of resection, it is advisable to indicate them before their division with a stay suture. The section margin of the duct has to be negative at frozen sectioning; it needs a regular line of section and should be well vascularised. When two ducts of similar size are nearby, ductoplasty can be carried out with the advantage of performing a single bilio-digestive anastomosis.

The Roux-en-Y procedure is used after preparing a 50–60 cm jejunal loop; the arm of the distal segment of jejunum is transposed into the supramesocolic area and brought to the liver retrocolic-antegastric or retrocolic-retrogastric. Therefore one or more jejunostomies are performed using the artifice of resecting any mucosal surplus. Bilioenteric anastomosis is performed with 5–0 absorbable monofilament in interrupted or running single layer suture, first on the posterior side and then on the anterior (Fig. 20).

A trans-anastomotic PTC tube of 6 Fr is placed in every anastomosis through the jejunal loop or transhepatically, to decompress the biliary tree and carry out postoperative cholangiographic control. In presence of dilated and large biliary ducts the anastomoses are performed without stent.

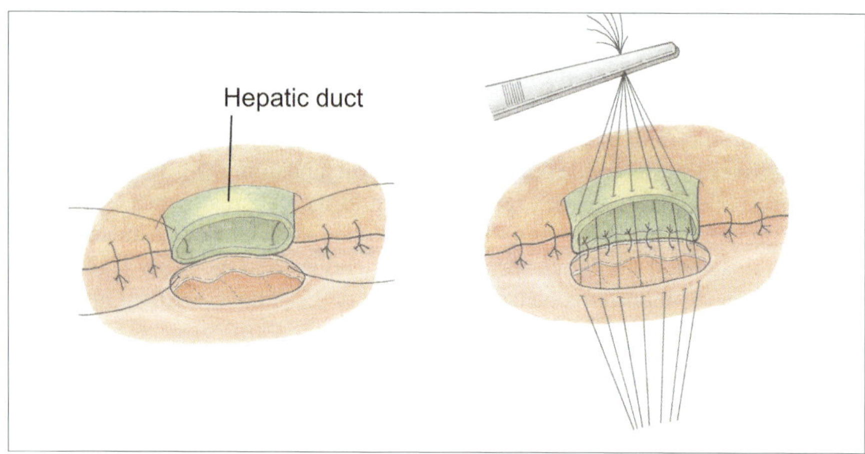

Fig. 20 Hepatic-jejunal anastomosis with one layer interrupted suture

References

1. Nagino M, Kamiya J, Arai T et al (2006) "Anatomic" right hepatic trisectionectomy (extended right hepatectomy) with caudate lobectomy for hilar cholangiocarcinoma. Ann Surg 243(1):28–32
2. Kondo S, Nimura Y, Hayakawa N et al (2002) Extensive surgery for carcinoma of the gallbladder. Br J Surg 89(2):179–184
3. Nimura Y, Kamiya J, Kondo S et al (2000) Aggressive preoperative management and extended surgery for hilar cholangiocarcinoma: Nagoya experience. J Hepatobiliary Pancreat Surg 7(2):155–162
3. Nagino M, Nimura Y (2006) Perihilar cholangiocarcinoma with emphasis on presurgical management. In: Blumgart LH (ed) Surgery of the liver, biliary tract, and pancreas, 4th edn. Saunders Elsevier, Philadelphia, pp 804–814
4. Kondo S, Katoh H, Hirano S et al (2002) Wedge resection of the portal bifurcation concomitant with left hepatectomy plus biliary reconstruction for hepatobiliary cancer. J Hepatobiliary Pancreat Surg 9(5):603–606
5. Nimura Y, Hayakawa N, Kamiya J et al (1991) Combined portal vein and liver resection for carcinoma of the biliary tract. Br J Surg 78(6):727–731
6. Seyama Y, Makuuchi M (2007) Current surgical treatment for bile duct cancer. World J Gastroenterol 13(10):1505–1515
7. Shimada H, Endo I, Sugita M et al (2003) Hepatic resection combined with portal vein or hepatic artery reconstruction for advanced carcinoma of the hilar bile duct and gallbladder. World J Surg 27(10):1137–1142
8. Nimura Y, Hayakawa N, Kamiya J et al (1991) Hepatopancreatoduodenectomy for advanced carcinoma of the biliary tract. Hepatogastroenterology 38(2):170–175
9. Miyagawa S, Makuuchi M, Kawasaki S et al (1996) Outcome of major hepatectomy with pancreatoduodenectomy for advanced biliary malignancies. World J Surg 20(1):77–80

Results of Surgery

Morbidity and Mortality

Long-term survival after surgery of hilar cholangiocarcinoma is related to patient status, tumour stage and proper treatment selection.

Principles of surgery for hilar cholangiocarcinoma have changed over the last 20 years. Early surgical experiences in the treatment of this disease were limited to isolated bile duct resection. The high recurrence rate (>70%) after this operation forced a change in the principles of the surgical management [1].

Current management of hilar cholangiocarcinoma includes resection of the extrahepatic biliary tract associated with major hepatic resection, and the results have improved during the last 20 years with a significant decrease in morbidity and mortality (Table 1).

The main reasons for these improvements are: accurate patient selection, optimization of liver function before surgery with preoperative biliary drainage and portal vein embolization, better surgical and anaesthesiological techniques and postoperative management.

Morbidity after surgical resection of hilar cholangiocarcinoma is still high; major complications occur in about 50% of patients and perioperative mortality ranges from 5 to 18%. Moreover, in recent series no mortality has been reported [2,3] (Table 1).

In a retrospective study in 105 patients Nagino observed 81% morbidity rate and 9.4% mortality rate after an aggressive surgical approach (including extended hepatectomies, vascular resections and associated pancreaticoduodenenctomies). Minor complications occurred in 37.1% of patients and 43.8% of patients suffered from major complications (Table 2).

Several factors are related to postoperative morbidity: jaundice, malnutrition, extent of hepatectomy, complexity of surgical procedure, associated procedures (pancreaticoduodenectomy), blood loss and operative time [2–6].

The relationship between jaundice and postoperative morbidity and mortality is still matter of debate as previously described, but several authors reported a higher incidence of postoperative complications in patients with jaundice and/or cholangitis [3,7,8]. Cherqui observed that the postoperative complication rate was 50% in jaundiced patients and 15% in the control group [7].

A. Guglielmi, A. Ruzzenente, C. Iacono (eds.) *Surgical Treatment of Hilar and ICC*.
© Springer 2008

Table 1 Morbidity and mortality in a series of hepatectomies for hilar cholangiocarcinoma in recent literature

Author	Year	Resections (number)	MHx	PV (%)	HA (%)	PD (%)	Morbidity (%)	Mortality (%)
Klempnauer [9]	1997	151	111	26	1	NA	NA	9.9
Neuhaus [10]	1999	95	66	24	NA	NA	59	9
Miyazaki [11]	1999	93	66	26	9	3	38	10
Kosuge [12]	1999	65	52	5	5	5	37	9.2
Nimura [13]	2000	142	114	30	NA	14	49	9
Gerhards [5]	2000	112	32	9	8	NA	65	18
Tabata [14]	2000	75	36	7	3	8	38	12
Lee [15]	2000	128	101	26	4	16	48	5.5
Seyama [16]	2002	67	58	13	NA	13	43	0
Kawasaki [17]	2003	79	69	6	3	16	14	1.3
Nagino [4]	2005	100	96	38	12	12	67	3
Hemming [18]	2005	53	52	43	6	8	40	9
Jarnagin [19]	2005	106	87	9	NA	2	62	7.5
Sano [3]	2006	102	102	22	5	7	50	0

MHx, Major hepatic resection; *PV*, portal vein resection; *HA*, hepatic artery resection; *PD*, pancreatoduodenectomy

Table 2 List of complications described in 105 patients. Data from [5]

Complication	Patients (number of occurrences)	%
Minor complications		
Pleural effusion	66	(62.9%)
Wound infection	39	(37.1%)
Bile leakage from liver stump	5	(4.8%)
Major complications		
Liver failure	29	(27.6%)
Renal failure	9	(8.6%)
Respiratory failure	7	(6.7%)
Gastrointestinal failure	6	(5.7%)
Haematological failure	6	(5.7%)
Bacteremia	18	(17.1%)
Intra-abdominal abscess	13	(12.4%)
Intra-abdominal bleeding	12	(11.4%)
Insufficiency of hepaticojejunostomy	10	(9.5%)
Insufficiency of pancreatojejunostomy	2	(20%)
Pyothorax	1	(1%)
Portal vein thrombosis	1	(1%)
Portal vein obstruction and kinking	1	(1%)

Bilirubin level and cholangitis in the preoperative period are significantly associated with postoperative liver failure; Fujii noticed that jaundice at admission was present in 71% of patients with postoperative liver failure and only in 25% of patients without postoperative liver failure [20]. Half of the patients with postoperative liver failure presented preoperative cholangitis, compared to 4% of patients without liver failure [20].

Postoperative liver failure is related to the volume of the remnant liver: the failure rate is 16.7% in patients with resection of less than 50% of liver volume but it increases to 36.8% for resection of more than 50% [21].

The extensive use of portal vein embolisation (PVE) can reduce the rate of this complication after major hepatic resection. In literature the reported rates of liver failure after major hepatectomy without PVE range from 0 to 30%, whereas with PVE they range from 0 to 5% [5,9,11,16–19,22–23].

Another frequent postoperative complication is anastomotic leak of hepaticojejunostomy which is associated with infectious complications, intra-abdominal bleeding, liver failure and postoperative death [31]. Incidence in literature varies between 1 and 22% [5,6,17,18,27,32,33]. Factors related to the occurrence of these complications are still under investigation; De Castro underlined the importance of the number of reconstructed bile ducts, and the incidence of anastomotic leak was significantly higher in segmental duct anastomosis (14%) compared to common hepatic duct anastomosis (1.8%) [34]. In other experiences these finding were not confirmed; Nagino did not observe any relationship between rate of anastomotic leak and number of reconstructed bile ducts. However, the author identified a relationship between the rate of anastomotic leak, patient age and intraoperative blood loss, in particular the incidence of anastomotic leak was significantly higher in patients with intraoperative blood loss >5 l (17 vs. 5.1%, respectively) [31].

Patients with advanced tumours require major hepatic resection associated with resection and reconstruction of vessels, such as the portal vein and hepatic artery, or associated with pancreatico-duodenenctomy.

The results of major liver resection combined with portal vein resection and reconstruction are still controversial. In the literature the rate of portal vein resection and reconstruction varies from 5 to 43% (Table 1).

Morbidity and mortality rates of major hepatic resection with portal vein resection and reconstruction are not different compared to patients who underwent major hepatic resection without vascular reconstruction, with a morbidity rate of 38 and 36%, and a mortality rate of 3 and 5%, respectively [35].

The impact of portal vein resection on long-term survival is less clear. Two different indications for portal vein resection are described in the literature.

Some authors choosed portal vein resection only for patients with advanced disease and tumour involvement; in these series the rate of invasion of portal vein is high (more than 70%) and long-term survival does not exceed 20% (Table 3). However long-term results showed higher survival rate in comparison to unresected patients with a 5-year survival of 9.9 vs. 0%, respectively [36].

Other authors also performed portal vein resection in patients without clear vascular involvement in order to increase the radicality of surgery, applying the "no touch technique" proposed by Neuhaus [10]. This strategy entails a low rate of histologically proven portal vein involvement and 5-year survival rate reaches 65% (Table 3).

The results of the two different strategies depend on different patient selection and are therefore difficult to compare (Table 3).

Table 3 Portal vein resection for hilar cholangiocarcinoma in previous report

Author	Year	Patients (number)	Histologically proven portal vein involvement (%)	5-year survival (%)
Neuhaus [10]	1999	23	12%	65%
Ebata [36]	2003	52	69%	9.9%
Hemming [18]	2005	26	38%	39%
Miyazaki [35]	2007	34	80%	16%

Few studies in the literature evaluate the role of hepatic artery resection and reconstruction. In surgical series less than 10% of patients were subjected to this type of vascular reconstruction and there is no consensus regarding the criteria of resectability for patients requiring hepatic artery resection or combined hepatic artery and portal vein resection and reconstruction. The postoperative morbidity and mortality for patients submitted to hepatic artery reconstruction is high. Miyazaki observed a 78% morbidity rate in the hepatic artery resection group compared to 38% in patients with portal vein resection alone and 36% in patients without vascular resection [35]. In this series, 77% of the patients who underwent hepatic artery resection had combined resection of the portal vein.

The high operative mortality rate after hepatic artery resection (30–50%) can be justified by the advanced stage of the tumours and the complexity of surgical interventions [5,33,35]. However, in other recent studies hepatic artery resection and reconstruction were carried out with postoperative mortality lower than 10% [37–39]. Long-term survival after hepatic artery resection for hilar cholangiocarcinoma is still under evaluation. In 9 patients Miyazaki reported 1- and 3- year survival rates of 11 and 0% [35].

The association of liver resection with pancreaticoduodenectomy (PD) increases the rate of surgical complications; Sano observed postoperative complications in more than 85% of patients with associated PD, and Nagino reported an incidence of liver failure of 50% in patients with combined PD in comparison to 25% in patients without PD [3,10]. Two stage strategies with delayed pancreaticoduodenectomy have been shown to reduce significantly the morbidity of this procedure with 0% postoperative mortality [40].

Long-term Results

Survival after resection of hilar cholangiocarcinoma has improved in the last decades with a 5-year survival rate ranging from 12 to 40% (Table 4).

Several prognostic factors have been identified after surgical resection of hilar cholangiocarcinoma: gross type, local extent, lymph-node involvement, distant metastases, vascular invasion, perineural invasion and radicality of surgery. Among these, R0 resection is the strongest factor identified in both univariate and multivariate analyses [10,12,19,27].

Neuhaus reported 5-year survival rate in R0 resections of 39%, compared with 9, and 0% for R1 and R2 resections. In R2 resection no patients survived more than 22 months. In a large series of 400 patients, Nishio confirmed these data and reported a 5-year survival rate of 27 and 2% for curative and non-curative resection, respectively [41].

To achieve radicality with safe margin, resection of the bile duct associated with hepatectomy, caudate lobectomy and regional lymphadenectomy are required.

Table 4 Hilar cholangiocarcinoma: R0 resection rate in literature and overall 5-year survival

Author	Year	Total	Resection R0 (%)	5-year survival rate (%)
Pichlmayr [23]	1996	125	73	26
Klempnauer [9]	1997	151	78	32
Nagino [24]	1998	138	78	25
Burke [42]	1998	30	83	45
Kosuge [12]	1999	65	52	35
Neuhaus [10]	1999	95	61	22
Launois [26]	1999	40	80	12
Miyazaki [11]	1999	93	70	36
Todoroki [27]	2000	98	14	28
Jarnagin [19]	2001	80	78	39
Seyama [16]	2002	67	64	40
Kawasaki [17]	2003	79	68	40
Kondo [28]	2004	40	95	40[a]
Rea [29]	2004	NA	80	26
Hemming [18]	2005	53	80	35
Nishio [41]	2005	301	77	22

[a] Three-year survival

The frequency of R0 resection depends on the type of surgery and the extent of liver resection (Table 5). To obtain R0 resection removal of the caudate lobe resection is required, due to the high rate of involvement (30–98%) [43]. Consequently curative resection rate is significantly higher in patients with associated resection of the caudate lobe (66 and 21%, respectively) [13].

Table 5 Relationship between rate of hepatectomy and negative margin resection

Author	Year	Patients (number)	Hepatectomy (%)	R0 (%)
Cameron [44]	1990	39	20	15
Su [6]	1996	49	57	49
Jarnagin [19]	2001	80	78	78
Lanois [26]	2000	40	62	80
Ebata [36]	2003	188	92	82

The type of hepatic resection contributes to determining curative rate and long-term outcome; Neuhaus reported a significantly higher rate of curative resection in patients submitted to right-sided hepatectomy in comparison with left hepatectomy, 71 vs. 33% [10]. Moreover, Kondo confirmed these results with a significantly higher survival rate for patients submitted to right hepatectomy in comparison to left hepatectomy, isolated caudate lobe resection and isolated bile duct resection [28].

Evaluation of the margin of the biliary duct is an important issue of curative surgery for hilar cholangiocarcinoma. A positive ductal margin influences the survival; in presence of negative margin 5-year survival rate is 46–56% vs. no 5-year survivors in presence of positive margin [45,46]. However, the presence of non-invasive carcinoma at the surgical margin does not influence long-term outcome, with 5- and 10-year survival rates of 69 and 23% [45].

Diffusion of the disease to regional lymph nodes is frequent in hilar cholangiocarcinoma (30–50%) and is one of the main determinants of prognosis after surgical resection [10,11,25,47–50].

Node-negative patients show 5-year survival rate of 31%, compared with 10% for those with regional lymph-node metastases [41]. Metastases to para-aortic lymph nodes can be found in 17% of patients; survival for these patients is significantly lower than for negative-lymph node patients, with 5-year survival rate of 12 and 30%, respectively.

Recurrence

Recurrence of the disease is frequent (22–60%) and is usually the cause of death [3,13,17,28]. The most frequent sites of recurrence are the peritoneum (50%), the remnant liver (22%) and, less frequently, local lymph nodes [28,51]. The median disease-free survival time is short (19 months).

The recurrence rate after curative surgery is higher in patients subjected to isolated resection of the bile duct (75%) in comparison to associated biliary and liver resection (52%) [13] (Table 6).

Anastomotic recurrence occurs in 8% of cases after curative resection and is related to the length of biliary tumour-free resection margin: Sakamoto described a recurrence rate of 18% for a tumour-free resection margin <2.5 mm, and of 10% for margins 2.5–5 mm; furthermore, he did not observe anastomotic recurrences when the margin was >5 mm [52].

Table 6 Site of recurrence after curative surgery. Data from [13]

Site of recurrence	Hepatectomy (N=100)	Bile duct resection (N=8)
Peritoneum	15	2
Liver	13	3
Retroperitoneum	7	-
Local	7	1
Bone	6	-
Drainage tract	5	-
Lymph nodes	3	2
Total	52 (52%)	6 (75%)

N, Number of patients

References

1. Mittal B, Deutsch M, Iwatsuki S (1985) Primary cancers of extrahepatic biliary passages. Int J Radiat Oncol Biol Phys 11(4):849–854
2. Seyama Y, Makuuchi M (2007) Current surgical treatment for bile duct cancer. World J Gastroenterol 13(10):1505–15
3. Sano T, Shimada K, Sakamoto Y et al (2006) One hundred two consecutive hepatobiliary resections for perihilar cholangiocarcinoma with zero mortality. Ann Surg 244(2):240–247
4. Nagino M, Kamiya J, Arai T et al (2005) One hundred consecutive hepatobiliary resections for biliary hilar malignancy: preoperative blood donation, blood loss, transfusion, and outcome. Surgery 137(2):148–155
5. Gerhards MF, van Gulik TM, de Wit LT et al (2000) Evaluation of morbidity and mortality after resection for hilar cholangiocarcinoma: a single center experience. Surgery 127(4):395–404
6. Su CH, Tsay SH, Wu CC et al (1996) Factors influencing postoperative morbidity, mortality, and survival after resection for hilar cholangiocarcinoma. Ann Surg 223(4):384–394
7. Cherqui D, Benoist S, Malassagne B et al (2000) Major liver resection for carcinoma in jaundiced patients without preoperative biliary drainage. Arch Surg 135(3):302–308
8. Kanai M, Nimura Y, Kamiya J et al (1996) Preoperative intrahepatic segmental cholangitis in patients with advanced carcinoma involving the hepatic hilus. Surgery 119(5):498–504
9. Klempnauer J, Ridder GJ, von Wasielewski R et al (1997) Resectional surgery of hilar cholangiocarcinoma: a multivariate analysis of prognostic factors. J Clin Oncol 15(3):947–954
10. Neuhaus P, Jonas S, Bechstein WO et al (1999) Extended resections for hilar cholangiocarcinoma. Ann Surg 230(6):808–818; discussion 819
11. Miyazaki M, Ito H, Nakagawa K et al (1999) Parenchyma-preserving hepatectomy in the surgical treatment of hilar cholangiocarcinoma. J Am Coll Surg 189(6):575–583
12. Kosuge T, Yamamoto J, Shimada K et al (1999) Improved surgical results for hilar cholangiocarcinoma with procedures including major hepatic resection. Ann Surg 230(5):663–671
13. Dinant S, Gerhards MF, Rauws EA et al (2006) Improved outcome of resection of hilar cholangiocarcinoma (Klatskin tumour). Ann Surg Oncol 13(6):872–880
14. Tabata M, Kawarada Y, Yokoi H et al (2000) Surgical treatment for hilar cholangiocarcinoma. J Hepatobiliary Pancreat Surg 7(2):148–154
15. Lee SG, Lee YJ, Park KM et al (2000) One hundred and eleven liver resections for hilar bile duct cancer. J Hepatobiliary Pancreat Surg 7(2):135–141

16. Seyama Y, Makuuchi M, Sano K et al (2002) Intermittent total vascular exclusion in removing caudate lobe tumour with tumour thrombus in the vena cava. Surgery 131(5):574–576

17. Kawasaki S, Imamura H, Kobayashi A et al (2003) Results of surgical resection for patients with hilar bile duct cancer: application of extended hepatectomy after biliary drainage and hemihepatic portal vein embolization. Ann Surg 238(1):84–92

18. Hemming AW, Reed AI, Fujita S et al (2005) Surgical management of hilar cholangiocarcinoma. Ann Surg 241(5):693–699; discussion 699–702

19. Jarnagin WR, Fong Y, DeMatteo RP et al (2001) Staging, resectability, and outcome in 225 patients with hilar cholangiocarcinoma. Ann Surg 234(4):507–517; discussion 517–519

20. Fujii Y, Shimada H, Endo I et al (2003) Risk factors of posthepatectomy liver failure after portal vein embolization. J Hepatobiliary Pancreat Surg 10(3):226–232

21. Nagino M, Kamiya J, Uesaka K et al (2001)Complications of hepatectomy for hilar cholangiocarcinoma. World J Surg 25(10):1277–1283

22. Miyagawa S, Makuuchi M, Kawasaki S (1995) Outcome of extended right hepatectomy after biliary drainage in hilar bile duct cancer. Arch Surg 130(7):759–763

23. Pichlmayr R, Weimann A, Klempnauer J et al (1996) Surgical treatment in proximal bile duct cancer. A single-center experience. Ann Surg 224(5):628–638

24. Nagino M, Nimura Y, Kamiya J et al (1998) Segmental liver resections for hilar cholangiocarcinoma. Hepatogastroenterology 45(19):7–13

25. Ogura Y, Kawarada Y (1998) Surgical strategies for carcinoma of the hepatic duct confluence. Br J Surg 85(1):20–24

26. Launois B, Terblanche J, Lakehal M et al (1999) Proximal bile duct cancer: high resectability rate and 5-year survival. Ann Surg 230:266–275

27. Todoroki T, Kawamoto T, Koike N et al (2000) Radical resection of hilar bile duct carcinoma and predictors of survival. Br J Surg 87(3):306–313

28. Kondo S, Hirano S, Ambo Y et al (2004) Forty consecutive resections of hilar cholangiocarcinoma with no postoperative mortality and no positive ductal margins: results of a prospective study. Ann Surg 240(1):95–101

29. Rea DJ, Munoz-Juarez M, Farnell MB et al (2004) Major hepatic resection for hilar cholangiocarcinoma: analysis of 46 patients. Arch Surg 139(5):514–523; discussion 523–525

30. Seyama Y, Makuuchi M (2007) Current surgical treatment for bile duct cancer. World J Gastroenterol 13(10):1505–1515

31. Nagino M, Nishio H, Ebata T et al (2007) Intrahepatic cholangiojejunostomy following hepatobiliary resection. Br J Surg 94(1):70–77

32. Miyazaki M, Ito H, Nakagawa K et al (1998) Aggressive surgical approaches to hilar cholangiocarcinoma: hepatic or local resection? Surgery 123(2):131–136

33. Madariaga JR, Iwatsuki S, Todo S et al (1998) Liver resection for hilar and peripheral cholangiocarcinomas: a study of 62 cases. Ann Surg 227(1):70–79

34. de Castro SM, Kuhlmann KF, Busch OR et al (2005) Incidence and management of biliary leakage after hepaticojejunostomy. J Gastrointest Surg 9(8):1163–1171; discussion 1171–1173

35. Miyazaki M, Kato A, Ito H et al (2007) Combined vascular resection in operative resection for hilar cholangiocarcinoma: does it work or not? Surgery 141(5):581–588

36. Ebata T, Nagino M, Kamiya J et al (2003) Hepatectomy with portal vein resection for hilar cholangiocarcinoma: audit of 52 consecutive cases. Ann Surg 238(5):720–727

37. Yamanaka N, Yasui C, Yamanaka J et al (2001) Left hemihepatectomy with microsurgical reconstruction of the right-sided hepatic vasculature. A strategy for preserving hepatic function in patients with proximal bile duct cancer. Langenbecks Arch Surg 386(5):364–368

38. Sakamoto Y, Sano T, Shimada K et al (2006) Clinical significance of reconstruction of the right hepatic artery for biliary malignancy. Langenbecks Arch Surg 391(3):203–208

39. Shimada M, Hamatsu T, Yamashita Y et al (2001) Characteristics of multicentric hepatocellular carcinomas: comparison with intrahepatic metastasis. World J Surg 25(8):991–995

40. Miyagawa S, Makuuchi M, Kawasaki S et al (1996) Outcome of major hepatectomy with pancreatoduodenectomy for advanced biliary malignancies. World J Surg 20(1):77–80

41. Nishio H, Nagino M, Nimura Y (2005) Surgical management of hilar cholangiocarcinoma: the Nagoya experience. HPB 7:259–262
42. Burke EC, Jarnagin WR, Hochwald SN et al (1998) Hilar cholangiocarcinoma: patterns of spread, the importance of hepatic resection for curative operation, and a presurgical clinical staging system. Ann Surg 228: 385–394
43. Dinant S, Gerhards MF, Busch OR et al (2005) The importance of complete excision of the caudate lobe in resection of hilar cholangiocarcinoma. HPB 7:263–267
44. Cameron JL, Pitt HA, Zinner MJ et al (1990) Management of proximal cholangiocarcinomas by surgical resection and radiotherapy. Am J Surg 159(1):91–97; discussion 97–98
45. Nimura Y, Kamiya J, Kondo S et al (2000) Aggressive preoperative management and extended surgery for hilar cholangiocarcinoma: Nagoya experience. J Hepatobiliary Pancreat Surg 7(2):155–162
46. Wakai T, Shirai Y, Moroda T et al (2005) Impact of ductal resection margin status on long-term survival in patients undergoing resection for extrahepatic cholangiocarcinoma. Cancer 103:1210–1216
47. Nakeeb A, Pitt HA, Sohn TA et al (1996) Cholangiocarcinoma. A spectrum of intrahepatic, perihilar, and distal tumours. Ann Surg 224(4):463–473; discussion 473–475
48. Sugiura Y, Nakamura S, Iida S et al (1994) Extensive resection of the bile ducts combined with liver resection for cancer of the main hepatic duct junction: a cooperative study of the Keio Bile Duct Cancer Study Group. Surgery 115(4):445–451
49. Iwatsuki S, Todo S, Marsh JW et al (1998) Treatment of hilar cholangiocarcinoma (Klatskin tumours) with hepatic resection or transplantation. J Am Coll Surg 187(4):358–364
50. Kitagawa Y, Nagino M, Kamiya J et al (2001) Lymph-node metastasis from hilar cholangiocarcinoma: audit of 110 patients who underwent regional and paraaortic node dissection. Ann Surg 233(3):385–392
51. Liu CL, Fan ST, Lo CM et al (2006) Improved operative and survival outcomes of surgical treatment for hilar cholangiocarcinoma. Br J Surg 93(12):1488–1494
52. Sakamoto E, Nimura Y, Hayakawa N et al (1998) The pattern of infiltration at the proximal border of hilar bile duct carcinoma: a histologic analysis of 62 resected cases. Ann Surg 227(3):405–411

The Role of Liver Transplantation

Indications and Results

Curative resection is the only treatment that produces good results in hilar cholangiocarcinoma. Hepatic transplantation has the theoretical premise of increasing surgical radicality and offers a treatment with curative intent for patients who are excluded from surgical treatment due to advanced stages of the disease or the presence of hepatic disease that contraindicates hepatic resection.

The indications for transplantation are not clearly defined in the literature since the studies are limited to a few cases in each institution and at present no absolute indications for this disease are ascertained (Table 1).

In the early studies, transplantation was performed in very advanced neoplasms with poor results: 3-year survival was 20% and recurrence rate was 57% [1]. Even more recent experiences report similar results: at the Cincinnati Transplant Tumour Registry, in 207 patients Meyer observed 5-year survival of 23% with a recurrence rate of more than 50% of the transplanted patients [2]. In a Spanish multicenter survey Robles reported 3-year survival of 30% with a 5-year disease-free survival of 30% [3].

Incidental cholangiocarcinoma revealed during transplantation for primary sclerosing cholangitis (PSC) represents about 8% of all the transplanted cases for PSC [4]. The localization is in the extrahepatic biliary tract in more than 80% of the cases [5].

The results of transplantation for patients with incidental hilar cholangiocarcinoma seem to be better than those for patients with a preoperative diagnosis of cholangiocarcinoma. Goss has described 10 cases with 1-year, 3-year and 5-year survival of 100, 83 and 83%, respectively, while none of the three patients with preoperative diagnosis survived more than 3 years [4]; other studies confirm these reports. Abu-Elmagd shows a 2-year survival of 55% for incidental cholangiocarcinoma, compared to 29% of the cases ascertained preoperatively [6].

Many prognostic survival factors have been identified in the literature. The depth of invasion of the biliary duct, determined by T-stage according to the UICC (5th edition), is related to prognosis; Iwatsuki reports a median survival

A. Guglielmi, A. Ruzzenente, C. Iacono (eds.) *Surgical Treatment of Hilar and ICC.*
© Springer 2008

Table 1 Results of liver transplantation for hilar cholangiocarcinoma

Author	Year	Institution	Patients	Survival			DFS		
				1-year	3-year	5-year	1-year	3-year	5-year
O'Grady [7]	1988	King's College	13	30	10	10	-	-	-
Pichlmayr [8]	1996	Hannover	25	60	21	17	-	-	-
Iwatsuki [9]	1998	Pittsburgh	27	60	36	36	-	-	-
Iwatsuki* [9]	1998	Pittsburgh	11	54.6	9.1	9.1	-	-	-
Shimoda [5]	2001	UCLA	9	86	31	-	57	57	-
Neuhaus** [10]	2000	Berlin	14	-	-	30 (4y)	-	-	-
Robles [3]	2004	Spanish survey	36	82	53	30	77	53	30
Zheng [11]	2005	Zhejang	5	80	80	-	-	-	-
Sudan*** [12]	2002	Nebraska	11	55	45	-	-	-	-
De Vreede*** [13]	2000	Mayo Clinic	11	100	100	92	-	-	-
Heimbach*** [14]	2004	Mayo Clinic	28	88	-	82	-	-	-
Rea*** [15]	2005	Mayo Clinic	38	92	82	82	100	95	88
Heimbach*** [16]	2006	Mayo Clinic	65	91	76	-	-	60	-

*, Cluster transplantation; **, Liver trasplantation + pancreatoduodenectomy; ***, Neoadjuvant radiotherapy + chemotherapy; *DFS*, Disease-free survival

of 99 months for patients in stage T1 and T2, and of 12 months in T3 [9]. In his experience, all the patients with a survival longer than 5 years had early stage disease (T1 and T2) without lymph-node involvement (Stage I and II according to TNM UICC). In 25 patients, Pichlmayr observed a median survival of 37 months for stage I and II patients, of 20 months for stage III patients and only 5.8 months for stages IVa and IVb. In his experience, only the patients in stages I and II had a survival longer than 3 years. The univariate and multivariate analyses have confirmed the prognostic value of TNM staging system with a RR of 4.5 [8]. Another prognostic factor is vascular invasion; Robles reports a survival of 0 and 63% in the patients with and without vascular invasion, respectively [3]. The same author has also considered the prognostic value of perineural invasion, with a median survival of 37 months in the presence and 78 months in absence of invasion, and lymphatic invasion with a median survival of 28 months in the presence and 65 months in absence of invasion, respectively. Other authors have underlined the importance of lymphatic invasion as prognostic factor as well; Iwatsuki reports a 5-year survival of 0% in N+ patients vs. 27% in N- patients [9]. Recurrence of disease is quite common, with frequency that varies from 40 to 60% [2,3,7,9,17–19]. Recurrences are usually early; Meyer observed 84% of recurrences in the first two years, localized in the hepatic hilum, transplanted liver and peripancreatic area [2,3,9]. The prognosis of the patients with recurrence is fairly poor, with a median survival after recurrence not longer than 3 months [3].

Combined Transplantation

As recurrence is more frequent at the hepatic and pancreatic area, some authors have proposed alternative surgical strategies, extending resection to the entire biliary tract and combining hepatic transplantation with pancreatoduodenectomy [20]. This approach increases the margins of resection, does not necessitate dissecting the structures adjacent to the neoplasm and allows an extended lymphadenectomy. In 14 patients, Neuhaus obtained a curative resection in more than 90% of the cases, with an operative mortality of 14%. Unfortunately, the long-term results are not satisfactory, with a 4-year survival of 30%. The most frequent cause of death is neoplastic recurrence, with implantation metastases in half of the cases [10].

Other authors have described similar approaches, but despites the significant increase of surgical radicality compared to resective surgery, long-term outcome is unsatisfactory [21,22].

Starzl has proposed a more aggressive operation combining the resection of all the organs derived from the foregut (liver, stomach, spleen, pancreaticoduodenal complex) with subsequent cluster transplantation (liver, pancreas, duodenum) or with isolated hepatic transplantation [1]. This type of operation has been defined as upper abdominal exenteration. The experience of the Pittsburg group in 11 patients showed a high postoperative mortality (18%); in spite of the higher oncologic radicality of cluster transplantation, with clear margins in more than 90% of the operations, the long-term results were poor, with 3-year and 5-year survival of 9.1% [9].

Transplantation with Adjuvant and Neoadjuvant Treatments

In hopes of improving the poor results of transplantation different protocols of adjuvant and neoadjuvant therapy with chemo- and radiation therapy have been proposed.

In 1998 Iwatsuki reported the results in 18 patients of adjuvant therapy with different protocols combining 5-FU chemotherapy with external radiotherapy; he showed a better long-term survival in the patients who underwent adjuvant treatment with median survival of 16.7 months vs 12.3 months in the group without adjuvant therapy [9].

The studies in the literature fail to show a clear utility of adjuvant treatment and do not support evidence that the treatment is useful to modify the prognosis after transplantation [19,23].

Even the experiences of intraoperative radiotherapy (IORT) are limited to isolated cases; Sotiropoulos reports a survival longer than 10 years in a patient who underwent hepatic transplantation with IORT for hilar cholangiocarcinoma. In literature no other significant experiences of such treatment associated with transplantation are reported.

More recently two protocols that combined neoadjuvant chemotherapy with radiotherapy in transplantation have been proposed.

The protocol proposed by the University of Nebraska implies neoadjuvant treatment with Ir-192 biliary catheters brachytherapy for a total dose of 6000cGy associated with chemotherapy with continuous infusion of 5-FU (daily dose 300 mg/m^2). The treatment is continued until transplantation. In this initial experience only patients who were excluded from surgical resection due to the stage of the disease or presence of cirrhosis were included in this study. Six of the 17 recruited patients (35%) were excluded from transplantation since the onset of complications or neoplasm progression while on the waiting list. The 11 patients who underwent transplantation showed a mortality rate of 27% and 3-year survival of 45%; two patients (18%) presented recurrence of disease during follow-up [12].

The second trial proposed by the Mayo Clinic includes patients who were unresectable due to the stage of the disease or concomitant cirrhosis, and is based on external and intraluminal radiation therapy associated with chemotherapy. External beam-irradiation is delivered in a total dose of 4000–4500 cGy in 27–30 fractions and to complete the radiation therapy a boost with trans-catheter irradiation is performed after 2–3 weeks. Brachytherapy is delivered using iridium-192 wire with a total dose of 2000–3000 cGy. During radiotherapy and before transplantation 5-FU chemotherapy is administered (daily dose of 225/500 mg/m^2); more recently chemotherapy in patients on the waiting list has been modified using capecitabine orally (2000 mg/m^2/die, twice every three weeks). All the patients included in the study undergo exploratory laparotomy to verify the absence of local contraindications (peritoneal carcinomatosis, lymph-node metastases) for transplantation after completion of radiation therapy and just before admittance in the waiting list [13–15]. In a recent experience in 106 patients, only 65 (61%) underwent transplantation while 11 patients were excluded from the protocol during neoadjuvant treatment because of progression of disease or onset of severe complications, and 18 were excluded during laparotomy due to the advanced stage of the disease [16]. In the group of patients who underwent operations the prognosis is good, with a 5-year survival of 76% and recurrence rate of 17% of the cases. Many factors have been identified as related to relapse: preoperative serum Ca19-9 level >100, size of residual tumour >2 cm, and presence of perineural invasion [16].

The results of both the series are encouraging and are the only two examples of good long-term results with a low recurrence rate in the literature. On the other hand, some authors have underlined that these experiences are not comparable with the data on surgical resections. In the two series, the frequency of patients with PSC is very high (65% in the Mayo Clinic series [16]). It has been hypothesized that patients with PSC who routinely undergo an accurate follow-up would have an earlier stage of disease, compared to the surgical resection series [24].

Conclusions

At present, studies on transplantation for hilar cholangiocarcinoma are limited and there are no current indications regarding the use of this therapeutic option in clinical practice; only the preliminary experiences on neoadjuvant aggressive treatment seem to improve long-term outcome significantly.

References

1. Alessiani M, Tzakis A, Todo S et al (1995) Assessment of five-year experience with abdominal organ cluster transplantation. J Am Coll Surg 180(1):1–9
2. Meyer CG, Penn I, James L (2000) Liver transplantation for cholangiocarcinoma: results in 207 patients. Transplantation 69(8):1633–1637
3. Robles R, Figueras J, Turrion VS et al (2004) Spanish experience in liver transplantation for hilar and peripheral cholangiocarcinoma. Ann Surg 239(2):265–271
4. Goss JA, Shackleton CR, Farmer DG et al (1997) Orthotopic liver transplantation for primary sclerosing cholangitis. A 12-year single center experience. Ann Surg 225(5):472–481; discussion 481–483
5. Shimoda M, Farmer DG, Colquhoun SD et al (2001) Liver transplantation for cholangiocellular carcinoma: analysis of a single-center experience and review of the literature. Liver Transpl 7(12):1023–1033

6. Abu-Elmagd KM, Selby R, Iwatsuki S et al (1993) Cholangiocarcinoma and sclerosing cholangitis: clinical characteristics and effect on survival after liver transplantation. Transplant Proc 25(1 Pt 2):1124–1125

7. O'Grady JG, Polson RJ, Rolles K et al (1988) Liver transplantation for malignant disease. Results in 93 consecutive patients. Ann Surg 207(4):373–379

8. Pichlmayr R, Weimann A, Klempnauer J et al (1996) Surgical treatment in proximal bile duct cancer. A single-center experience. Ann Surg 224(5):628–638

9. Iwatsuki S, Todo S, Marsh JW et al (1998) Treatment of hilar cholangiocarcinoma (Klatskin tumours) with hepatic resection or transplantation. J Am Coll Surg 187(4):358–364

10. Neuhaus P, Jonas S (2000) Surgery for hilar cholangiocarcinoma—the German experience. J Hepatobiliary Pancreat Surg 7(2):142–147

11. Zheng SS, Huang DS, Wang WL et al (2002) Orthotopic liver transplantation in treatment of 77 patients with end-stage hepatic disease. Hepatobiliary Pancreat Dis Int 1(1):8–13

12. Sudan D, DeRoover A, Chinnakotla S et al (2002) Radiochemotherapy and transplantation allow long-term survival for nonresectable hilar cholangiocarcinoma. Am J Transplant 2(8):774–779

13. De Vreede I, Steers JL, Burch PA et al (2000) Prolonged disease-free survival after orthotopic liver transplantation plus adjuvant chemoirradiation for cholangiocarcinoma. Liver Transpl 6(3):309–316

14. Heimbach JK, Gores GJ, Haddock MG et al (2004) Liver transplantation for unresectable perihilar cholangiocarcinoma. Semin Liver Dis 24(2):201–207

15. Rea DJ, Heimbach JK, Rosen CB et al (2005) Liver transplantation with neoadjuvant chemoradiation is more effective than resection for hilar cholangiocarcinoma. Ann Surg 242(3):451–458; discussion 458–461

16. Heimbach JK, Gores GJ, Haddock MG et al (2006) Predictors of disease recurrence following neoadjuvant chemoradiotherapy and liver transplantation for unresectable perihilar cholangiocarcinoma. Transplantation 82(12):1703–1707

17. Ringe B, Wittekind C, Bechstein WO et al (1989) The role of liver transplantation in hepatobiliary malignancy. A retrospective analysis of 95 patients with particular regard to tumour stage and recurrence. Ann Surg 209(1):88–98

18. Penn I (1991) Hepatic transplantation for primary and metastatic cancers of the liver. Surgery 110(4):726–734; discussion 734–735

19. Goldstein RM, Stone M, Tillery GW et al (1993) Is liver transplantation indicated for cholangiocarcinoma? Am J Surg 166(6):768–771; discussion 771–772

20. Neuhaus P, Blumhardt G (1994) Extended bile duct resection—a new oncological approach to the treatment of central bile duct carcinomas? Description of method and early results. Langenbecks Arch Chir 379(2):123–128

21. Cherqui D, Alon R, Piedbois P et al (1995) Combined liver transplantation and pancreato-duodenectomy for irresectable hilar bile duct carcinoma. Br J Surg 82(3):397–398

22. Anthuber M, Schauer R, Jauch KW et al (1996) Experiences with liver transplantation and liver transplantation combined with Whipple's operation in Klatskin tumour. Langenbecks Arch Chir Suppl kongressbd 113:413–415

23. Pitt HA, Nakeeb A, Abrams RA et al (1995) Perihilar cholangiocarcinoma. Postoperative radiotherapy does not improve survival. Ann Surg 221(6):788–797; discussion 797–798

24. Lang H, Sotiropoulos GC, Kaiser GM et al (2005) The role of liver transplantation in the treatment of hilar cholangiocarcinoma. J Hepatobiliary Pancreat Surg 7:268–272

Adjuvant and Neoadjuvant Therapies

Local recurrence is a frequent event after surgical resection for cholangiocarcinoma; to achieve better control radiotherapy has been proposed, alone or associated with chemotherapy [1], although other authors have suggested applying chemotherapy alone after surgical resection. However, the role of these treatments is not standardized throughout the various centers that manage biliary neoplasms.

Pitt has conducted a study among the members of the IHPBA, AHPBA and the Oncology Group of the American College of Surgeons, and has found out that radiotherapy is applied as adjuvant therapy by 70% of American surgeons compared to 40% of Asian/Pacific surgeons and 29% of European surgeons, that chemotherapy is employed with a similar distribution between different geographic areas (66%, 79% and 68%, respectively) and that the combination radiotherapy-chemotherapy is applied more by American and Asian/Pacific than European surgeons (71%, 55% and 29%, respectively) [2].

Chemotherapy

The role of adjuvant chemotherapy alone after resection for hilar cholangiocarcinoma is still unclear and, according to some authors, it is indicated in resected patients with positive lymph nodes [3]. The most commonly used drug is 5-FU, alone or in combination with others such as methotrexate, leucovorin, cisplatin, mitomycin C or IFN-α. Injection routes aside from the systemic are locoregional, intra-arterial and intraductal. However, most of the studies report small series, retrospective single group experiences with data that are not comparable.

A recent controlled randomized phase-III study by Takada [4] reports data on adjuvant treatment after resection of bilio-pancreatic tumours in 158 pancreatic cancers, 118 extrahepatic biliary tract neoplasms, 112 gallbladder cancers, and 48 carcinomas of the papilla of Vater. Comparison between a group of patients who underwent adjuvant chemotherapy with two cycles of mitomycin C plus 5-FU, followed by oral long-term uptake of 5-FU until the likely recurrence, vs. a

A. Guglielmi, A. Ruzzenente, C. Iacono (eds.) *Surgical Treatment of Hilar and ICC.*
© Springer 2008

group of patients treated by surgical resection alone did not show significant differences considering stage and positive lymph nodes (84 vs. 88%), curative resection (59 vs. 63%) and 5-year survival (26.7 vs. 24%), respectively. The author has observed analogous results in pancreatic and papilla of Vater cancers, while in patients with carcinoma of the gallbladder survival was significantly better in treated vs. non-treated patients (5-year survival: 26 vs. 14.4%; $p=0.0367$).

Data on the use of new drugs such as gemcitabine and oxaliplatin have not yet been reported in literature. At present chemotherapy does not have any role as adjuvant therapy in these tumours apart from controlled clinical trials [5].

Radiotherapy

In the 1990s, non-randomized studies at John Hopkins [6,7] did not show any benefits with radiotherapy alone, external or intramural; conversely, Kamada [8] reports a better survival in resected patients and with positive microscopic margin of resection (R1 resection).

More recently, two studies demonstrated the efficacy of radiotherapy in increasing survival in patients with hilar cholangiocarcinoma. The Japanese study compared four groups of patients who underwent: (1) only surgery (21 cases); (2) surgery associated with external radiotherapy (8 cases, mean dose 43.6 Gy); (3) surgery associated with intraoperative radiotheraphy (IORT) (12 cases, mean dose 21 Gy); (4) surgery associated with external and intraoperative radiotherapy (22 cases). The data showed a better local control of the disease (in 80% of the combined treatment vs. 31% of surgery alone) and a better survival in patients who underwent double radiotherapy (External Beam + IORT) (5-year survival 39.2 vs. 13.5% in patients who underwent surgery alone) [9].

The European study [10] compared a group of patients who underwent surgical treatment alone (20 cases) vs. a group of patients who were subjected to two different types of adjuvant radiotherapy, the former only external (30 cases, mean dose 46 Gy) and the latter (41 cases) external radiotherapy (mean dose 42.3 Gy) associated with brachytherapy with iridium (mean dose 10.4 Gy). Also this study shows a better survival in the patients who underwent adjuvant treatment, with a median survival of 24 months vs. 8 months; but no significant differences were observed between the two types of radiotherapy treatment (median survival 21 vs. 30 months).

Chemoradiation Therapy

Considering the radiosensitivity of some drugs such as 5-FU and gemcitabine, combining both therapies would appear hypothetically more efficient than single treatment. However the data in the literature are divergent even for this therapeutic combination. In a group of 84 patients with cholangiocarcinoma (30 stages I and II, 54 stage III) who submitted to surgery alone and surgery associated with chemoradiation therapy (40 Gy + bolus 5-FU) Kim et al. [11] showed a 5-year survival of 36% in the 47 patients with R0 resection, 35% in the 25 patients with R1 resection and 0% in the 12 patients with R2 resection, showing the value of this combined therapy in the R1 resected patients; similar results have been reported by others [12,13], principally in patients with microscopic infiltrated margins [11,14]. On the other hand Figueras did not show any advantages of chemoradiation vs. radiation therapy alone [15].

By comparing retrospectively two groups with different types of chemoradiation (RT + 5-FU vs. RT + 5-FU + gemcitabine) Nakeeb showed a significantly higher survival in the group with the association of 5-FU + gemcitabine vs. 5-FU alone ($p<0.05$) [16].

Neoadjuvant Therapy

This approach, which in other oncological fields has changed the therapeutic strategy and long-term results, is not indicated in patients with cholangiocarcinoma since nearly all of them present jaundice.

At the end of the 1990s a study reported encouraging data regarding this type of approach, even though the main limit of this paper was the small number (only 9) of treated patients, 5 with hilar and 4 with peripheral cholangiocarcinoma [17]. The authors used an association of chemo-radiation therapy with the following scheme: 5-FU 300mg/m^2/day from Monday to Friday associated with external radiotherapy (45–50 Gy). The results showed a complete pathological response in the specimen in three cases (33%), negative margin of resection in 100% of the cases compared to 54% of non-treated cases; moreover the treatment was well tolerated, without postoperative major complications.

With the exception of this study no other papers report the application of neoadjuvant therapy; however at present there are two ongoing trials regarding neoadjuvant chemoradiation and liver transplantation.

The protocol of the University of Nebraska entails the use of brachytherapy (60 Gy) with iridium 192, through a bilateral PTBD, associated with infusion of 5-FU in a dose of 300 mg/m^2/day until transplantation. The authors observed in 5 of 17 patients a progression of disease that precludes transplantation and in another 5 catheter-related complications (4 perforation of biliary ducts and 1 bilio-portal fistula) that led to death in all 5 patients [18].

The Mayo Clinic group in Rochester, Minnesota, utilizes a chemoradiation protocol similar to the previous one: external RT (45 Gy) associated with infusion of 5-FU in a dose of 500 mg/m^2/day for 3 days, followed by intraductal treatment with brachytherapy (20-30 Gy) associated with infusion of 5-FU in a dose of 225 mg/m^2/day; the patients then undergo explorative laparotomy to evaluate the extension of the disease. Patients who fulfill the criteria of inclusion for transplantation continue the infusion of 5-FU until transplantation. In a more recent study 5-FU was replaced with capecitabine [19,20].

The authors report catheter-related complications in four patients (cholangitis, hepatic abscess, sepsis) and mortality in one patient due to hepatic abscess.

Recently Wiedmann et al. [21] have investigated photodynamic therapy in a phase-II pilot study as a neoadjuvant treatment in seven patients with advanced cholangiocarcinoma. The study, although limited by the low number of patients, has shown a good local control of disease allowing resection with negative margin; nevertheless, at 1 year 17% of the patients had relapsed.

Conclusions

At present no data support the efficacy of adjuvant and neoadjuvant treatment. Data in the literature in fact are somewhat contradictory: despite studies showing an acceptable effectiveness, others do not report any advantages. However all these studies are limited by the small number of cases, and by the fact that the disease is not very frequent; each center recruits small series with few cases treated and long-term surveillance, and often the series includes heterogeneous disease. Therefore, at the present time these therapies have no role in the treatment of cholangiocarcinoma and should be used only in controlled studies and referral centers.

References

1. Chari RS, Anderson CA, Bavarese DMF (2003) Treatment of cholangiocarcinoma. I. In: Rose BD (ed) UpToDate. UpToDate, Wellesley, MA, pp [AQ3]
2. Pitt HA, Broelsch C, Fong Y et al (2003) Adjuvant therapy for biliary malignancies: international trends and possibilities. J Gastrointest Surg 7:309A
3. Nagino M, Nimura Y (2006) Perihilar cholangiocarcinoma with emphasis on presurgical management. In: Blumgart LH (ed) Surgery of the liver, biliary tract, and pancreas. 4 edn. Saunders Elsevier, Philadelphia, pp 804–814
4. Takada T, Amano H, Yasuda H et al; Study Group of Surgical Adjuvant Therapy for Carcinomas of the Pancreas and Biliary Tract (2002) Is postoperative adjuvant chemotherapy useful for gallbladder carcinoma? A phase III multicenter prospective randomized controlled trial in patients with resected pancreaticobiliary carcinoma. Cancer 95(8):1685–1695
5. Khan SA, Thomas HC, Davidson BR, Taylor-Robinson SD (2005) Cholangiocarcinoma. Lancet 366(9493):1303–1314
6. Cameron JL, Pitt HA, Zinner MJ et al (1990) Management of proximal cholangiocarcinomas by surgical resection and radiotherapy. Am J Surg 159(1):91–97; discussion 97–98
7. Pitt HA, Nakeeb A, Abrams RA et al (1995) Perihilar cholangiocarcinoma. Postoperative radiotherapy does not improbe survival. Ann Surg 221(6):788–797; discussion 797–798

8.   Kamada T, Saitou H, Takamura A et al (1996) The role of radiotherapy in the management of extrahepatic bile duct cancer: an analysis of 145 consecutive patients treated with intraluminal and/or external beam radiotherapy. Int J Radiat Oncol Biol Phys 34(4):767–774

9.   Todoroki T, Ohara K, Kawamoto T et al (2000) Benefits of adjuvant radiotherapy after radical resection of locally advanced main hepatic duct carcinoma. Int J Radiat Oncol Biol Phys 46(3):581–587

10. Gerhards MF, van Gulik TM, Gonzalez D et al (2003) Results of postoperative radiotherapy for resectable hilar cholangiocarcinoma. World J Surg 27(2):173–179

11. Kim S, Kim SW, Bang YJ et al (2002) Role of postoperative radiotherapy in the management of extrahepatic bile duct cancer. Int J Radiat Oncol Biol Phys 54(2):414–419

12. Robertson JM, Lawrence TS, Andrews JC et al (1997) Long-term results of hepatic artery fluorodeoxyuridine and conformal radiation therapy for primary hepatobiliary cancers. Int J Radiat Oncol Biol Phys 37(2):325–330

13. Whittington R, Neuberg D, Tester WJ et al (1995) Protracted intravenous fluorouracil infusion with radiation therapy in the management of localized pancreaticobiliary carcinoma: a phase I Eastern Cooperative Oncology Group Trial. J Clin Oncol 13:227–232

14. Serafini FM, Sachs D, Bloomston M et al (2001) Location, not staging, of cholangiocarcinoma determines the role for adjuvant chemoradiation therapy. Am Surg 67(9):839–843; discussion 843–844

15. Figueras J, Llado L, Valls C et al (2000) Changing strategies in diagnosis and management of hilar cholangiocarcinoma. Liver Transpl 6(6):786–794

16. Nakeeb A, Tran KQ, Black MJ et al (2002) Improved survival in resected biliary malignancies. Surgery 132(4):555–563; discussion 563–564

17. McMasters KM, Tuttle TM, Leach SD et al (1997) Neoadjuvant chemoradiation for extrahepatic cholangiocarcinoma. Am J Surg 174(6):605–608; discussion 608–609

18. Sudan D, DeRoover A, Chinnakotla S et al (2002) Radiochemotherapy and transplantation allow long-term survival for nonresectable hilar cholangiocarcinoma. Am J Transplant 2(8):774–779

19. De Vreede I, Steers JL, Burch PA et al (2000) Prolonged disease-free survival after orthotopic liver transplantation plus adjuvant chemoirradiation for cholangiocarcinoma. Liver Transpl 6(3):309–316

20. Heimbach JK, Gores GJ, Nagorney DM, Rosen CB (2006) Liver transplantation for perihilar cholangiocarcinoma after aggressive neoadjuvant therapy: a new paradigm for liver and biliary malignancies? Surgery 140(3):331–334

21. Wiedmann M, Caca K, Berr F et al (2003) Neoadjuvant photodynamic therapy as a new approach to treating hilar cholangiocarcinoma: a phase II pilot study. Cancer 97(11):2783–2790

Palliative Treatments

Palliation of Jaundice

The principal end-point of treatment of cholangiocarcinoma is resection with negative margins, but this goal fails in one-half to two-thirds of cases [1,2]. Only Nimura's group reports a resectability rate of 80% [1–3]. Therefore most patients with cholangiocarcinoma need palliative treatment of jaundice; moreover, local recurrence with relapse of jaundice, which is the most frequent problem after surgery, also requires palliation.

Indications for jaundice palliation are:
- Intractable pruritus
- Cholangitis
- Access for intramural radiotherapy (brachytherapy)
- To increase hepatic function in patient candidates for chemotherapy and/or radiotherapy
- Treatment of recurrence after surgical resection

Although histological diagnosis is not indispensable in presence of resectable neoplasm, it is essential for all patients who undergo palliative treatment [4].

Choice of Treatment

The palliation strategy depends on when the diagnosis of unresectability is made; in fact, when it is obtained preoperatively or at preliminary laparoscopy there are two options: the endoscopic and the percutaneous route. Instead, when the condition of unresectability is verified intraoperatively there are different options: surgical management, maintenance of the biliary drainage, if already positioned, intraoperative trans-tumoral catheterization or postoperative positioning of endoscopic or percutaneous drainage.

The choice of palliative treatment must consider the cost/benefit of each palliation modality and the patient's life expectancy (more or less than 6 months) (Fig. 1).

As previously stated it is sufficient to drain a hepatic volume of 25–50% to resolve jaundice and pruritus [5–7]. However, to plan a correct therapeutic

A. Guglielmi, A. Ruzzenente, C. Iacono (eds.) *Surgical Treatment of Hilar and ICC.*
© Springer 2008

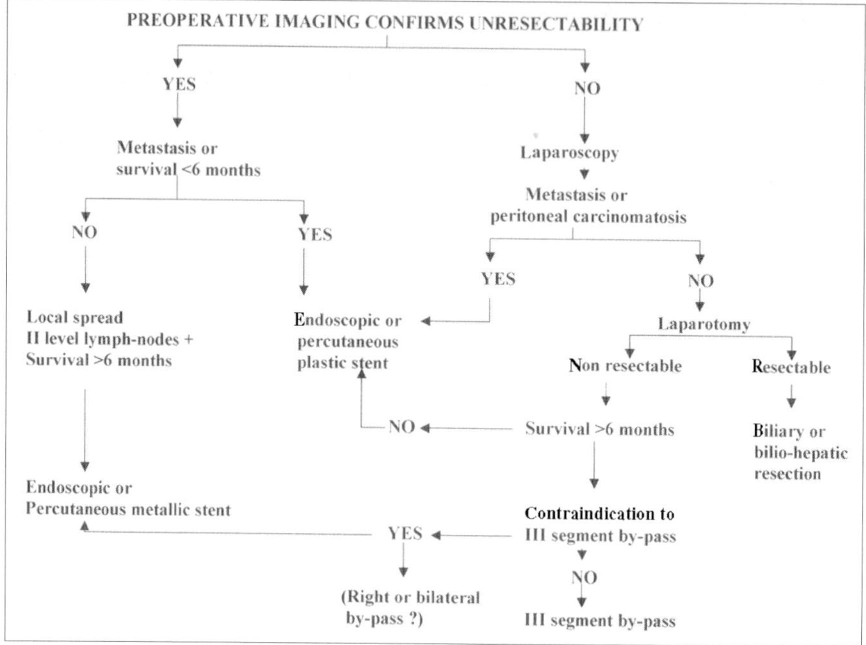

Fig. 1 Decisional flow chart for palliative treatment in unresectable hilar cholangiocarcinoma

approach it is mandatory to know the anatomy of the biliary confluence and intrahepatic branches, the presence of probable anatomical variants of first and second order confluences, the intraductal diffusion of the tumour and the presence or absence of atrophic segments.

Endoscopic or Percutaneous Drainage

As with evaluation of intraductal (longitudinal) diffusion of the tumour and of preoperative drainage of jaundice, there is no unanimous point of view on whether the endoscopic or the percutaneous route is the better approach. In contrast to authors who consider endoscopic drainage the treatment of choice in patients with unresectable cholangiocarcinoma documented by preoperative work-up [8–10], and even intraoperatively in the place of surgical palliation [11], other authors [4,12–17] believe that percutaneous drainage is the treatment of choice. Nevertheless in some cases biliary decompression needs to be performed through a combined endoscopic/percutaneous approach and in a few cases with a simple external drainage.

Plastic or Metallic Stents

Regarding the type of drainage there are two possibilities: a plastic or a metallic stent. The advantages of a plastic stent are low cost, easy placement and medium-lasting patency (about 3 months); disadvantages are the small caliber of the lumen (10 F) which often leads to occlusion by biliary sludge and the risk of determining obstruction of the second order ducts. Both factors can provoke cholangitis, which occurs in 20–40% of cases after placement of these stents [11,18,19].

Metallic stents have a larger caliber (30 F) and this allows long-lasting functioning, sometimes for the rest of the patient's life, and it does not present the risk of obstructing the adjacent segmental ducts since it is fenestrated; disadvantages are the high initial cost and the impossibility of removing the stent itself [20]. Controlled studies comparing the two types of stents [21–24] have confirmed that metallic stents present a longer functionality (median duration 6 months) [19,25,26], a percentage of cholangitis of 4.9–6% [19,26], and late occlusion of the stent in 23% of the cases. All these factors determine less need to substitute the stent, rehospitalization and reduced antibiotic use, with an overall lowering of final costs and a better quality of life for the patients. However, no significant differences on survival have been noted.

Based on previous considerations, for choosing the right stent it is essential to consider the life expectancy of the patient. Patients with unresectable carcinoma without signs of distant metastases and with a life expectancy of 6 months or more benefit more from a metallic stent; conversely, in patients with unresectable disease and hepatic or distant metastases with a short prognosis (<3 months) the placement of a plastic stent is sufficient [22].

Another point still under debate is the number of stents required to obtain adequate palliation: if the disease is in stage I according to Bismuth-Corlette classification a single drain is clearly sufficient; in stage II–IV there is no consensus on how many drains must be employed.

Various studies in the literature have compared unilateral vs. bilateral drainage; Deviere [27] and Cheng [26] show better survival (178 vs. 118 days) and a smaller incidence of complications in patients who underwent double drainage; Abu-Hamda also demonstrates better results compared to unilateral, particularly when the contrast medium is distributed in both hemisystems [9]. De Palma's controlled prospective randomized study [19] which compares the different treatment modalities, unilateral vs. bilateral, shows a greater success rate in placement of the stent (89 vs. 77%), biliary drainage (81 vs. 73%), and fewer complications (19 vs. 27%) in unilateral vs. bilateral stents; related mortality, late complications and survival are similar. The study by Inal et al. [28] does not show significant differences in clinical response to treatment or stent patency rate with unilobar vs. bilateral drainage.

Watanapa, studying hepatic alterations in jaundiced patients who underwent monolateral or complete surgical decompression of jaundice, concludes that unilobar drainage allows resumption of hepatic function after 6 weeks, as with bilateral drainage [29].

The better preoperative classification with non-invasive techniques provided by MRCP will permit more frequent use of selective monolateral drainage; in fact the excellent staging possibility of this imaging technique allows reduced medium contrast injection, decreasing the risk of contaminating biliary segments which otherwise would need to be drained.

Bilateral or multiple drainages are indicated exclusively for patients with cholangitis of the contralateral lobe or of segmental ducts.

Surgical Palliation

When unresectability is determined intraoperatively different therapeutic chances are achievable, represented by surgical palliation by means of bilio-enteric bypasses with peripheral intrahepatic anastomosis.

The commonest operation is segment 3 intrahepatic hepato-jejunostomy, called B3 cholangio-jejunostomy. The technique was described originally by Hepp-Couinaud, and requires complete or partial resection of the third hepatic segment, identification of the biliary duct and latero-lateral bilio-enteric anastomosis performed with a Roux-en-Y jejunal limb. Subsequently, in 1957, Soupault and Couinaud changed this technique using a direct approach to the duct of the three segments through a hepatotomy, avoiding hepatic resection as well. The isolation of the biliary duct is performed through the umbilical scissura. This maneuver permits identification of the portal branch for segment 3, which can reach a diameter of 4–6 mm in the jaundiced patient; cholangio-jejunostomy is then performed on a Roux-en-Y loop with interrupted stitches. An anastomotic stent can be positioned with the egress site on the loop with Vitzel technique or on the liver (Volker) for postoperative control of the anastomosis. This technique was diffused in the 1970s by Bismuth and Corlette [30] and in the 1980s by Blumgart and Kelly [31].

Contraindications to intrahepatic B3 cholangio-jejunostomy are the presence of an atrophic left lobe, the presence of a PTBD on the right lobe, the presence of cholangitis on the right lobe, a percentage of hepatic parenchyma to be drained less than 30% or less than two segments and presence of portal hypertension [8,32].

The surgical decompression on the right lobe can be performed on the ducts of segments 5 and 6 by means of wedge resections or hepatotomies; differently from intrahepatic B3 cholangio-jejunostomy, the isolation of the duct is more difficult and demanding with major risk of complications (fistula) and lesser efficacy of the biliary decompression.

Mortality after segment 3 intrahepatic cholangio-jejunostomy ranges from 3 to 12% [7,32–36] and morbidity from 17 to 51%. In the experience of MSKCC [33] no mortality after intrahepatic B3 cholangio-jejunostomy has been reported in patients with cholangiocarcinoma while it was 21.4% in patients with carcinoma of the gallbladder; mortality rate after right segmental duct anastomosis in patients with cholangiocarcinoma was 14.3% [33].

The most frequent complication of this type of surgery is biliary leak and its related complications, and it ranges from 6 to 21% [33,34,36]; the frequency is higher for right surgical decompression as is the percentage of patients who require re-operation due to failure of the procedure (55 vs. 15%, p=0.06) [33].

Also, the patency rate of the anastomosis at 1 year is higher in segment III intrahepatic cholangio-jejunostomy than right ducts (80 vs. 60%) even if the difference is not statistically significant (p=0.1) [33].

There are no controlled prospective randomized studies that compare surgical vs. endoscopic or percutaneous palliation for hilar cholangiocarcinoma in the literature; for this reason, based on our previous considerations, we can conclude that bypass on segment 3 is an operation that entails acceptable risks of mortality and morbidity, similar to those observed after percutaneous and endoscopic stents, and allows an excellent palliation of jaundice, with a good duration over time and few later complications. Conversely the right intrahepatic cholangio-jejunostomy is associated with high percentage of morbidity and mortality both early and late, and therefore is not competitive vs. non-surgical biliary decompression.

Other possibilities for surgical palliation are:
– *Transtumoral intubation*. This procedure is associated with a high mortality rate (27%) [37] and the disadvantages of an external biliary catheter (dislocation, obstruction, cholangitis); consequently their application is not attractive.
– *Palliative resection of extrahepatic biliary tract*. This operation has the same mortality and morbidity rates as surgical by-pass [38] and allows bilateral drainage [39]; however recurrence rate is very high and for this reason its indication is limited.

Chemotherapy, Radiotherapy and Photodynamic Therapy

The indications for palliative treatment with chemotherapy and/or radiotherapy are limited to patients with unresectable hilar cholangiocarcinoma, with recurrence after resection or with metastatic disease.

Radiotherapy alone or associated with chemotherapy is indicated in patients with local advanced disease without distant metastasis; instead, in presence of this condition chemotherapy is the only possible treatment.

Chemotherapy

Response to chemotherapy is very poor [10,40–43]; in fact at present no chemotherapeutic agent is effective enough to change the natural history of the disease. The most frequently utilized and studied agent is 5-FU alone or associated with other agents. Some studies do not report benefits in the treated patients compared to patients who underwent biliary drainage alone [44,45]. The percentage of response varies in literature from 0% (obtained with 5-FU alone [41]) to 40% (in a group of patients treated with a combination of 5-FU, epirubicine and cisplatin [46]). This last datum shows that the combination of 5-FU with other drugs gives better results. The agents used were leucovorin, otoposide, streptozocin, mitomycin C, doxorubicin and IFN-α. The number of treated patients, however, is low in all the series and ranges from a minimum of 18 to a maximum of 37 patients; median survival ranges from 8 weeks to 12 months. Another important limit of these studies is that most report data on heterogeneous groups of patients with intra- and extrahepatic cholangiocarcinoma, carcinoma of the gallbladder and in some cases pancreatic carcinoma.

Nevertheless there is a study [47] that reports improvement and a positive trend in quality of life in a group of patients with a Karnosfy index greater than 70% and treated with 5-FU, leucovorin and etoposide, compared with patients treated with supportive care alone (6.5 months vs. 2.5 months, p=0.10).

A recent phase-II study [48] has utilized intra-arterial infusion, with Seldinger technique, of epirubicine and cisplatin in combination to systemic 5-FU administration in a group of 30 patients with unresectable carcinoma of biliary tract; a positive response was observed in 40% of the patients (12/30)–one case of complete response and 11 cases of partial response. The median progression-free and overall survival time were 7.1 and 13.2 months, respectively; 1- and 2-year survival were 54 and 20%, respectively. The improvement of performance status was observed in 30% of the patients.

Recently gemcitabine was introduced in clinical practice for treatment of biliary tract neoplasm; it can be used alone in different doses with a response rate that ranges from 8% [49] to 60% [50], with median survival 6.3–16 months, or in combination with other agents such as 5-FU, cisplatin, oxaliplatin, docetaxel, irinotecan and capecitabine, with response rate varying from 9% (combination gemcitabine–docetaxel) [51] to 50% in the combination gemcitabine–cisplatin [52] and with median survival between 20 weeks [53] and 15.4 months [54], with an acceptable toxicity.

The more efficient combinations are those that utilized gemcitabine and cisplatin in the patients with good performance status and hepatic function [43] (response from 27.5 to 50% with median survival 5–11.3 months) and with gemcitabine and oxaliplatin (response in 35% of the patients with good performance status and 22% of the patients with poor performance status). Conversely, combinations with capecitabine, irinotecan and docetaxel do not seem effective [43].

In conclusion, until now there has been no evidence of the utility of these treatments in the palliation of cholangiocarcinoma but results are more encouraging than the past; controlled randomized phase-III multicentric studies are advisable to recruit larger series that compare more promising agents.

Radiotherapy

The types of radiation therapy are different: external, brachytherapy and the association of both; the positioning of the radioactive source can be either endoscopic or percutaneous.

The results of radiation therapy in studies in the literature are contradictory; compared with authors [55–57] who consider this kind of treatment useful for biliary decompression and pain control with a better quality of life, others [58] do not report advantages with external radiotherapy, even using different doses of radiation (from 30 to 85 Gy). Even the results of brachytherapy alone or associated with external radiotherapy are divergent; in fact some authors report favorable results [1,56,59–61] while others do not recognize its usefulness [11] but report a high rate of complications, especially cholangitis (40–50%), and gastroduodenal toxicity ranging from 8 to 42% [11,56,60,61].

Photodynamic Therapy

Photodynamic therapy is indicated for local control of unresectable disease in absence of distant metastases; similarly to other types of tumour such as oesophagus, colon, stomach, bronchi, urinary bladder and brain, photodynamic therapy has been introduced in the treatment of cholangiocarcinoma [62]. The procedure requires the infusion of a photosensitizing drug (sodium porfimer) that accumulates electively in tumoral cells 24–48 h after administration; subsequently cytotoxic free radicals such as singlet oxygen, develop through cholangioscopic photoactivation and determine the death of neoplastic cells. Different phase-II studies report median of survival of 330–439 days with 1-year survival that varies from 45% to 78% [39,62]. A recent prospective randomized study by Ortner's group [63] performed on 39 patients with cholangiocarcinoma stages III and IV, and treated with biliary stent with or without photodynamic therapy, showed a better survival of the treated group (493 vs. 98 days), lower cholestasis rate, and a better quality of life and performance status. The authors believe that the real difference is due to a better biliary decompression following the reduction of the neoplastic mass that the procedure provides.

Witzigmann [64] reports a median survival of 12 months vs. 6.4 months ($p<0.01$), lower bilirubinemia values ($p<0.05$) and higher Karnofsky index ($p<0.01$) in the patients treated with stent and photodynamic therapy vs. patients with biliary stent alone when evaluating the results of his own experience of surgical resection and palliative treatment in 184 cases of hilar cholangiocarcinoma (60 resected: 42 R0, 18 R1-2; 56 treated with biliary stent; 68 with biliary stent combined with photodynamic therapy); in addition, the median survival of patients who underwent photodynamic therapy is similar to that of R1-2 resected patients.

Evaluating the 150 patients reported in the literature, photodynamic therapy associated with biliary stent is shown to improve survival with a range from 9.3 to 16.3 months.

These promising results require further verification and new studies to evaluate the worth of photodynamic therapy with novel chemotherapeutic agents which show more encouraging possibilities as well.

References

1. Chari RS, Anderson CA, Saverese DMF (2003) Treatment of cholangiocarcinoma II. In: Rose BD (ed) UpToDate. UpToDate, Wellesley, MA
2. Vauthey JN, Blumgart LH (1994) Recent advances in the management of cholangiocarcinomas. Semin Liver Dis 14(2):109–114
3. Nimura Y, Kamiya J, Kondo S et al (2000) Aggressive preoperative management and extended surgery for hilar cholangiocarcinoma: Nagoya experience. J Hepatobiliary Pancreat Surg 7(2):155–162
4. Abraham NS, Barkun JS, Barkun AN (2002) Palliation of malignant biliary obstruction: a prospective trial examining impact on quality of life. Gastrointest Endosc 56(6):835–841
5. Bismuth H, Malt RA (1979) Current concepts in cancer: carcinoma of the biliary tract. N Engl J Med 301(13):704–706
6. Dowsett JF, Vaira D, Hatfield AR et al (1989) Endoscopic biliary therapy using the combined percutaneous and endoscopic technique. Gastroenterology 96(4):1180–1186
7. Traynor O, Castaing D, Bismuth H (1987) Left intrahepatic cholangio-enteric anastomosis (round ligament approach): an effective palliative treatment for hilar cancers. Br J Surg 74(10):952–954
8. Singhal D, van Gulik TM, Gouma DJ (2005) Palliative management of hilar cholangiocarcinoma. Surg Oncol 14(2):59–74
9. Abu-Hamda EM, Baron TH (2004) Endoscopic management of cholangiocarcinoma. Semin Liver Dis 24(2):165–175
10. Anderson CD, Pinson CW, Berlin J, Chari RS (2004) Diagnosis and treatment of cholangiocarcinoma. Oncologist 9(1):43–57
11. Gerhards MF, van Gulik TM, Gonzalez Gonzalez D et al (2003) Results of postoperative radiotherapy for resectable hilar cholangiocarcinoma. World J Surg 27(2):173–179
12. Khan SA, Thomas HC, Davidson BR, Taylor-Robinson SD (2005) Cholangiocarcinoma. Lancet 366(9493):1303–1314
13. Shapiro MJ (1995) Management of malignant biliary obstruction: nonoperative and palliative techniques. Oncology 9(6):493–496, discussion 499–500, 503
14. England RE, Martin DF (1996) Endoscopic and percutaneous intervention in malignant obstructive jaundice. Cardiovasc Intervent Radiol 19(6):381–387
15. Nelsen KM, Kastan DJ, Shetty PC et al (1996) Utilization pattern and efficacy of nonsurgical techniques to establish drainage for high biliary obstruction. J Vasc Interv Radiol 7(5):751–756
16. Cowling MG, Adam AN (2001) Internal stenting in malignant biliary obstruction. World J Surg 25(3):355–359; discussion 359–361
17. Lillemoe KD, Cameron JL (2000) Surgery for hilar cholangiocarcinoma: the Johns Hopkins approach. J Hepatobiliary Pancreat Surg 7(2):115–121
18. Liu CL, Lo CM, Lai EC, Fan ST (1998) Endoscopic retrograde cholangiopancreatography and endoscopic endoprosthesis insertion in patients with Klatskin tumours. Arch Surg 133(3):293–296
19. De Palma GD, Galloro G, Siciliano S et al (2001) Unilateral versus bilateral endoscopic hepatic duct drainage in patients with malignant hilar biliary obstruction: results of a prospective, randomized, and controlled study. Gastrointest Endosc 53(6):547–553
20. Venbrux AC (2001) Current status of endoscopic pancreaticobiliary interventions. J Vasc Interv Radiol 12:155–162
21. Davids PH, Groen AK, Rauws EA et al (1992) Randomised trial of self-expanding metal stents versus polyethylene stents for distal malignant biliary obstruction. Lancet 340(8834–8835):1488–1492
22. Kaassis M, Boyer J, Dumas R et al (2003) Plastic or metal stents for malignant stricture of the common bile duct? Results of a randomized prospective study. Gastrointest Endosc 57(2):178–182

23. Prat F, Chapat O, Ducot B et al (1998) A randomized trial of endoscopic drainage methods for inoperable malignant strictures of the common bile duct. Gastrointest Endosc 47(1):1–7

24. Wagner HJ, Knyrim K, Vakil N, Klose KJ (1993) Plastic endoprostheses versus metal stents in the palliative treatment of malignant hilar biliary obstruction. A prospective and randomized trial. Endoscopy 25(3):213–218

25. Glattli A, Stain SC, Baer HU et al (1993) Unresectable malignant biliary obstruction: treatment by self-expandable biliary endoprostheses. HPB Surg 6(3):175–184

26. Cheng JL, Bruno MJ, Bergman JJ et al (2002) Endoscopic palliation of patients with biliary obstruction caused by nonresectable hilar cholangiocarcinoma: efficacy of self-expandable metallic Wallstents. Gastrointest Endosc 56(1):33–39

27. Deviere J, Baize M, de Toeuf J, Cremer M (1988) Long-term follow-up of patients with hilar malignant stricture treated by endoscopic internal biliary drainage. Gastrointest Endosc 34(2):95–101

28. Inal M, Akgul E, Aksungur E, Seydaoglu G (2003) Percutaneous placement of biliary metallic stents in patients with malignant hilar obstruction: unilobar versus bilobar drainage. J Vasc Interv Radiol 14(11):1409–1416

29. Watanapa P (1996) Recovery patterns of liver function after complete and partial surgical biliary decompression. Am J Surg 171(2):230–234

30. Bismuth H, Corlette MB (1975) Intrahepatic cholangioenteric anastomosis in carcinoma of the hilus of the liver. Surg Gynecol Obstet 140(2):170–178

31. Blumgart LH, Kelley CJ (1984) Hepaticojejunostomy in benign and malignant high bile duct stricture: approaches to the left hepatic ducts. Br J Surg 71(4):257–261

32. Connors S, Wigmore SJ, Madhavan KK et al (2005) Surgical palliation for unresectable hilar cholangiocarcinoma. HPB Surg 7:273–277

33. Jarnagin WR, Burke E, Powers C et al (1998) Intrahepatic biliary enteric bypass provides effective palliation in selected patients with malignant obstruction at the hepatic duct confluence. Am J Surg 175(6):453–460

34. Chaudhary A, Dhar P, Tomey S et al (1997) Segment III cholangiojejunostomy for carcinoma of the gallbladder. World J Surg 21(8):866–870; discussion 870–871

35. Guthrie CM, Banting SW, Garden OJ, Carter DC (1994) Segment III cholangiojejunostomy for palliation of malignant hilar obstruction. Br J Surg 81(11):1639–1641

36. Kapoor VK, Pradeep R, Haribhakti SP et al (1996) Intrahepatic segment III cholangiojejunostomy in advanced carcinoma of the gallbladder. Br J Surg 83(12):1709–1711

37. Launois B, Reding R, Lebeau G, Buard JL (2000) Surgery for hilar cholangiocarcinoma: French experience in a collective survey of 552 extrahepatic bile duct cancers. J Hepatobiliary Pancreat Surg 7(2):128–134

38. Jarnagin WR, Fong Y, DeMatteo RP et al (2001) Staging, resectability, and outcome in 225 patients with hilar cholangiocarcinoma. Ann Surg 234(4):507–517; discussion 517–519

39. Berr F, Wiedmann M, Tannapfel A et al (2000) Photodynamic therapy for advanced bile duct cancer: evidence for improved palliation and extended survival. Hepatology 31(2):291–298

40. Kajanti M, Pyrhonen S (1994) Epirubicin-sequential methotrexate-5-fluorouracil-leucovorin treatment in advanced cancer of the extrahepatic biliary system. A phase II study. Am J Clin Oncol 17(3):223–226

41. Takada T, Kato H, Matsushiro T et al (1994) Comparison of 5-fluorouracil, doxorubicin and mitomycin C with 5-fluorouracil alone in the treatment of pancreatic-biliary carcinomas. Oncology 51(5):396–400

42. Mazhar D, Stebbing J, Bower M (2006) Chemotherapy for advanced cholangiocarcinoma: what is standard treatment? Future Oncol 2(4):509–514

43. Thongprasert S (2005) The role of chemotherapy in cholangiocarcinoma. Ann Oncol 16(Suppl 2):ii93–ii96

44. Patt YZ, Hassan MM, Lozano RD et al (2001) Phase II trial of cisplatin, interferon alpha-2b, doxorubicin, and 5-fluorouracil for biliary tract cancer. Clin Cancer Res 7(11):3375–3380

45. Patt YZ, Jones DV Jr, Hoque A et al (1996) Phase II trial of intravenous flourouracil and sub-

cutaneous interferon alfa-2b for biliary tract cancer. J Clin Oncol 14(8):2311–2315

46. Ellis PA, Norman A, Hill A et al (1995) Epirubicin, cisplatin and infusional 5-fluorouracil (5-FU) (ECF) in hepatobiliary tumours. Eur J Cancer 31A(10):1594–1598

47. Glimelius B, Hoffman K, Sjoden PO et al (1996) Chemotherapy improves survival and quality of life in advanced pancreatic and biliary cancer. Ann Oncol 7(6):593–600

48. Cantore M, Mambrini A, Fiorentini G et al (2005) Phase II study of hepatic intraarterial epirubicin and cisplatin, with systemic 5-fluorouracil in patients with unresectable biliary tract tumours. Cancer 103(7):1402–1407

49. Mezger J, Sauerbruch T, Ko Y et al (1998) Phase II trial of gemcitabine in gallbladder and biliary tract carcinomas. Onkologie 21:232–234

50. Dobrila-Dintinjana R, Kovac D, Depolo A et al (2000) Gemcitabine in patients with nonresectable cancer of the biliary system or advanced gallbladder cancer. Am J Gastroenterol 95:2476

51. Kuhn R, Hribaschek A, Eichelmann K et al (2002) Outpatient therapy with gemcitabine and docetaxel for gallbladder, biliary, and cholangio-carcinomas. Invest New Drugs 20(3):351–356

52. Carraro S, Servienti PJ, Bruno MF (2001) Gemcitabine and cisplatin in locally advanced or metastatic gallbladder and bile duct adenocancer. Proc Am Soc Clin Oncol 20:146B (abs 2333)

53. Doval DC, Sekhon JS, Gupta SK et al (2004) A phase II study of gemcitabine and cisplatin in chemotherapy-naive, unresectable gall bladder cancer. Br J Cancer 90(8):1516–1520

54. Andre T, Tournigand C, Rosmorduc O et al; GERCOR Group (2004) Gemcitabine combined with oxaliplatin (GEMOX) in advanced biliary tract adenocarcinoma: a GERCOR study. Ann Oncol 15(9):1339–1343

55. Shinchi H, Takao S, Nishida H, Aikou T (2000) Length and quality of survival following external beam radiotherapy combined with expandable metallic stent for unresectable hilar cholangiocarcinoma. J Surg Oncol 75(2):89–94

56. Ishii H, Furuse J, Nagase M et al (2004) Relief of jaundice by external beam radiotherapy and intraluminal brachytherapy in patients with extrahepatic cholangiocarcinoma: results without stenting. Hepatogastroenterology 51(58):954–957

57. Ohnishi H, Asada M, Shichijo Y et al (1995) External radiotherapy for biliary decompression of hilar cholangiocarcinoma. Hepatogastroenterology 42(3):265–268

58. Crane CH, Macdonald KO, Vauthey JN et al (2002) Limitations of conventional doses of chemoradiation for unresectable biliary cancer. Int J Radiat Oncol Biol Phys 53(4):969–974

59. Kuvshinoff BW, Armstrong JG, Fong Y et al (1995) Palliation of irresectable hilar cholangiocarcinoma with biliary drainage and radiotherapy. Br J Surg 82(11):1522–1525

60. Vallis KA, Benjamin IS, Munro AJ et al (1996) External beam and intraluminal radiotherapy for locally advanced bile duct cancer: role and tolerability. Radiother Oncol 41(1):61–66

61. Foo ML, Gunderson LL, Bender CE, Buskirk SJ (1997) External radiation therapy and transcatheter iridium in the treatment of extrahepatic bile duct carcinoma. Int J Radiat Oncol Biol Phys 39(4):929–935

62. Ortner MA, Liebetruth J, Schreiber S et al (1998) Photodynamic therapy of nonresectable cholangiocarcinoma. Gastroenterology 114(3):536–542

63. Ortner ME, Caca K, Berr F et al (2003) Successful photodynamic therapy for nonresectable cholangiocarcinoma: a randomized prospective study. Gastroenterology 125(5):1355–1363

64. Witzigmann H, Berr F, Ringel U et al (2006) Surgical and palliative management and outcome in 184 patients with hilar cholangiocarcinoma: palliative photodynamic therapy plus stenting is comparable to r1/r2 resection. Ann Surg 244(2):230–239

Part 2
Intrahepatic Cholangiocarcinoma

Diagnosis

About 20–30% of cholangiocarcinomas appear as nodular intrahepatic mass [1,2]; however, intrahepatic cholangiocarcinomas may also be polypoid or focally stenotic. Excluding the nodular intrahepatic type, about three-fourths of cholangiocarcinomas manifest as a focal stricture and one-fourth are polypoid or diffusely stenotic [3].

Ultrasound

The nodular pattern is more frequent (94.4%) than the infiltrative pattern (5.6%). In the former, there is often a single mass that is predominantly located in the posterior segments of the liver parenchyma. Small nodules (<3 cm) most commonly appear as hypo- or isoechoic areas, whereas nodules >3 cm are predominantly hyperechoic. When multiple lesions are present, the echogenicity of the larger mass is higher than that of the daughter nodules. A hypoechoic halo is observed in one-third of patients.

Due to the peripheral location of the mass, bile-duct obstruction is quite rare and, when present, is a helpful sign in the differential diagnosis with hepatocellular carcinoma. Sometimes, the central portion of the tumour may appear hypoechoic, because of the presence of necrosis, or hyperechoic with acoustic shadowing indicating the presence of calcification. The infiltrative growth pattern of cholangiocarcinoma determines the diffuse architectural changes of the hepatic lobe (Figs. 1,2).

The hypovascularity of cholangiocarcinoma manifests as scant color signals at colour Doppler ultrasound; this is a helpful sign in the differential diagnosis with hepatocellular carcinoma, which is typically hypervascular.

A. Guglielmi, A. Ruzzenente, C. Iacono (eds.) *Surgical Treatment of Hilar and ICC.*
© Springer 2008

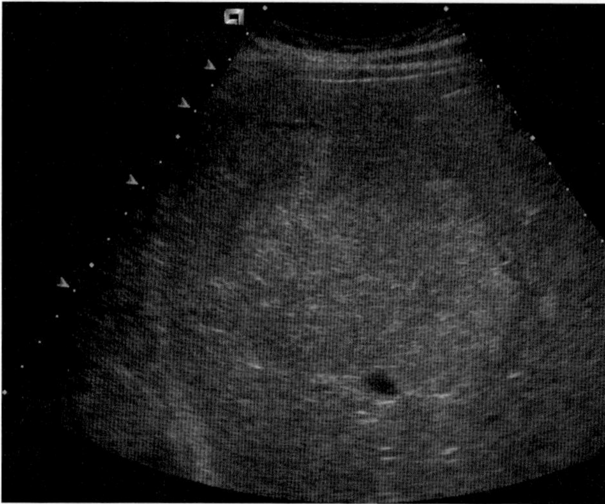

Fig. 1 Ultrasound of a large intrahepatic cholangiocarcinoma of the mass-forming type in the right lobe

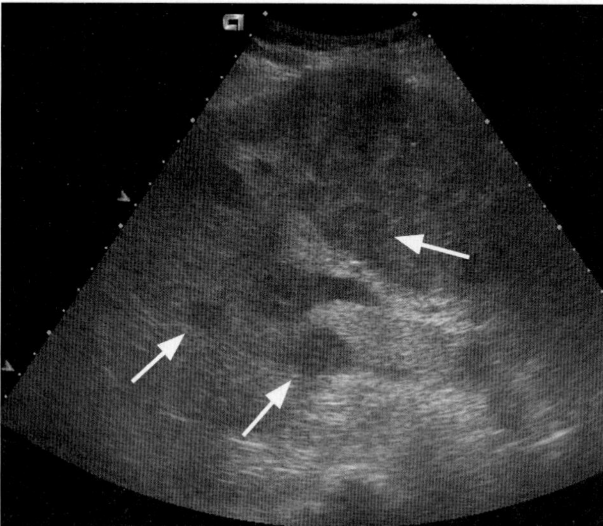

Fig. 2 Ultrasound of an intrahepatic cholangiocarcinoma of the mass-forming type with intrahepatic metastasis (*white arrows*)

Computed Tomography

Unenhanced CT scan shows a hypodense mass, either solitary or with multiple satellite nodules. In mucin-secreting cholangiocarcinomas examined by unenhanced CT, calcifications may be present in the central portion of the lesions. The most common pattern of contrast enhancement in peripheral cholangiocarcinoma is a peripheral area of thin, mild, incomplete, rim-like contrast enhancement on CT scans obtained at the hepatic arterial and portal venous phases [4] (Fig. 3).

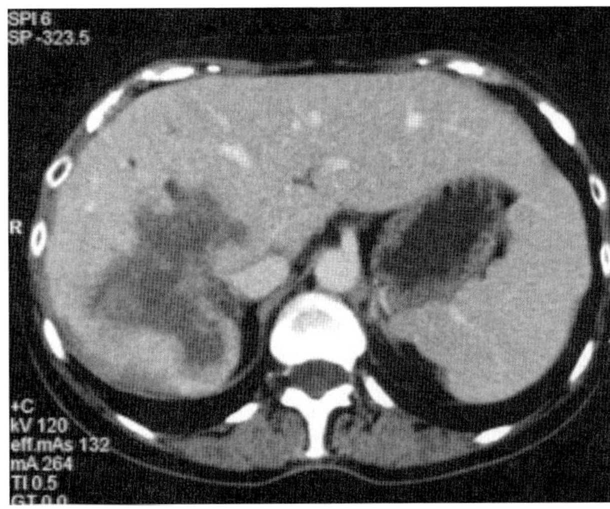

Fig. 3 Hypoattenuating mass in the right hepatic lobe with capsular retraction

Markedly low attenuation mixed with amorphous areas of slightly high attenuation during the arterial and the portal venous phases represents the distinctive intratumoral appearance of peripheral cholangiocarcinoma on two-phase spiral CT scans [4]. Areas of markedly low attenuation in peripheral cholangiocarcinoma correspond to diffuse, microcystic changes of necrosis of the comedo type. Areas of slightly high attenuation in the masses probably correspond to the presence of mucin, which may appear hyperdense on CT scans [4].

Intrahepatic cholangiocarcinomas show an enhancement greater than the normal liver parenchyma on equilibrium-phase contrast-enhanced images. This occurs in 74% of patients undergoing delayed imaging [5]. This approach is therefore useful in detecting intrahepatic cholangiocarcinoma nodules, differentiating them from dilated bile ducts or fatty infiltration of the liver and better defining the tumour margins. In addition, although not necessary for diagnosis, delayed enhancement can be helpful as a target for CT-guided biopsy. It has been suggested that the typical delayed enhancement of cholangiocarcinoma may be due to the retention of contrast material within the fibrous stroma, which represents the essential element of these tumours [6,7].

Besides fibrosis, other factors affect delayed enhancement, e.g. the distribution of fibrosis [5] and tumour grading, since better-differentiated tumours are more likely to show delayed contrast-agent retention than poorly differentiated ones [5]. The contrast-enhancement pattern of cholangiocarcinoma differs from that of hepatocellular carcinoma or other hypervascular tumours, which most commonly show a predominantly high attenuation during the hepatic arterial phase and isoattenuation or low attenuation during the portal venous phase. Furthermore, most cholangiocarcinomas occur in non-cirrhotic livers and frequently cause bile duct dilatation; other characteristic are the absence of a pseudocapsule, the presence of intratumoral calcifications and, rarely, vessel invasion. Extension through the hepatic capsule and invasion of adjacent organs are common in intrahepatic cholangiocarcinoma but rare in hepatocellular carcinoma. The invasion of nearby vascular structures is rare in peripheral cholangiocarcinoma. All these criteria are helpful for the differential diagnosis between cholangiocarcinoma and hepatocellular carcinoma—the two most common primary liver neoplasms.

Hypovascular metastases, especially from adenocarcinoma of the gastrointestinal tract, may have a pattern similar to that of peripheral cholangiocarcinoma, making the differential diagnosis very difficult [8]. Clues for the differential diagnosis between metastases and intrahepatic cholangiocarcinoma are unknown primary tumour, a relatively large tumour size and other, ancillary findings such as segmentary or subsegmentary bile-duct dilatation, and retraction of the liver capsule [4].

Sometimes, a papillary intrahepatic cholangiocarcinoma produces abundant mucin, that may calcify, resulting in a well-marginated cystic mass resembling biliary cystoadenocarcinoma. The mucin may also obstruct the duct lumen distal to the carcinoma [9] (Fig. 4).

Magnetic Resonance Imaging

The MRI appearance of cholangiocarcinoma is that of a non-capsulated tumour, hypointense on T1-weighted images and hyperintense on T2-weighted images. The signal intensity of the tumour varies according to the amount of fibrosis, necrosis, and mucinous material within it. Central hypointensity may be seen on

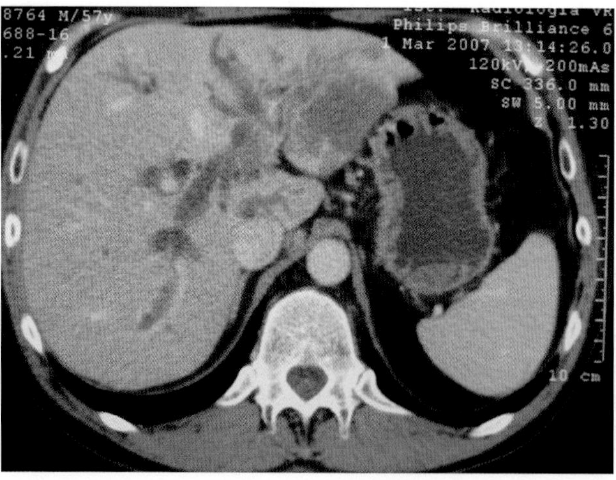

Fig. 4 Axial CT image during the arterial phase shows a hypodense-centred mass on the left hepatic duct infiltrating the left hepatic artery

T2-weighted images, corresponding to fibrosis (central scar). Importantly, a central scar can be a reliable feature for differentiating primary liver neoplasm from metastases on MRI evaluation [10,11]. The central scar may enhance with gadolinium chelates on delayed images, but become isointense with the tumour rather than hyperintense as is seen in focal nodular hyperplasia [13].

Mucinous cholangiocarcinoma is one of the subtypes of cholangiocarcinomas. Depending on its predominant features, it can be extremely hypointense on T1-weighted images and hyperintense on T2-weighted images, due to the presence of large mucinous lakes within the tumour.

On dynamic MRI studies, the size of the tumour influences the enhancement pattern. Small tumours (2–4 cm) may enhance homogeneously and simulate a hepatocellular carcinoma [12]; in larger tumours, minimal to moderate peripheral enhancement is evident followed by progressive and concentric filling of the tumour with contrast medium [13]. Pooling of contrast within the tumour on delayed MRI can be a distinctive finding, diagnostic of peripheral cholangiocarcinoma; however, incomplete central filling is also noted on delayed images. This characteristic enhancement pattern may reflect the large amount of fibrous tissue and neovascularity at the periphery of the lesion.

Although some authors have stressed that the portal and hepatic veins are not commonly invaded in cholangiocarcinoma and make this a differentiating point from hepatocellular carcinoma [14], most authors report that the portal vein is commonly involved by tumour and they emphasise the role of MRI in making the correct diagnosis [13] (Fig. 5).

Dilatation of the peripheral portion of the intrahepatic biliary ducts is occasionally seen in peripheral cholangiocarcinomas, especially in patients with associated clonorchiasis [16].

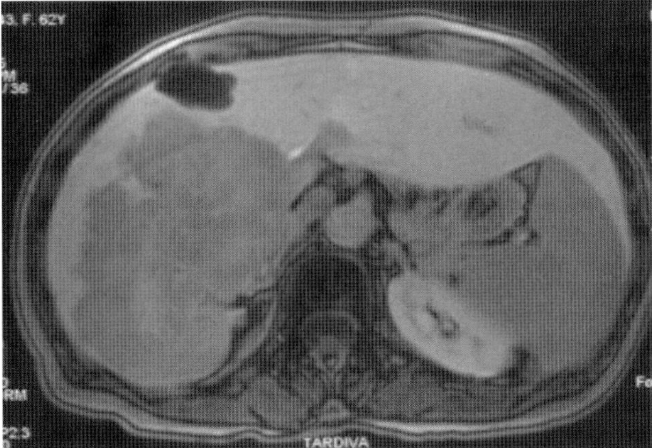

Fig. 5 Delayed contrast-enhanced T1-weighted image shows a hypointense mass in the right hepatic lobe

Angiography

Angiographically, intrahepatic cholangiocarcinoma is predominantly hypovascular, and the appearance of thin vessels is pathognomonic of its fibrous nature [17]. Encasement of hepatic arteries and other major vessels is associated with the degree of sclerosis resulting from the tumour.

References

1. Thorsen MK, Quiroz F, Lawson TL et al (1984) Primary biliary carcinoma: CT evaluation. Radiology 152(2):479–483
2. Nesbit GM, Johnson CD, James EM et al (1988) Cholangiocarcinoma: diagnosis and evaluation of resectability by CT and sonography as procedures complementary to cholangiography. AJR Am J Roentgenol 151(5):933–938
3. Kokubo T, Itai Y, Ohtomo K et al (1988) Mucin-hypersecreting intrahepatic biliary neoplasms. Radiology 168(3):609–614
4. Kim TK, Choi BI, Han JK et al (1997) Peripheral cholangiocarcinoma of the liver: two-phase spiral CT findings. Radiology 204(2):539–543
5. Lacomis JM, Baron RL, Oliver JH 3rd et al (1997) Cholangiocarcinoma: delayed CT contrast enhancement patterns. Radiology 203(1):98–104
6. Takayasu K, Ikeya S, Mukai K et al (1990) CT of hilar cholangiocarcinoma: late contrast enhancement in six patients. AJR Am J Roentgenol 154(6):1203–1206
7. Honda H, Onitsuka H, Yasumori K et al (1993) Intrahepatic peripheral cholangiocarcinoma: two-phased dynamic incremental CT and pathologic correlation. J Comput Assist Tomogr 17(3):397–402
8. Choi BI, Han JK, Shin YM et al (1995) Peripheral cholangiocarcinoma: comparison of MRI with CT. Abdom Imaging 20(4):357–360
9. Itai Y, Araki T, Furui S et al (1983) Computed tomography of primary intrahepatic biliary malignancy. Radiology 147(2):485–490
10. Ishak KG, Sesterhenn IA, Goodman ZD et al (1984) Epithelioid hemangioendothelioma of the liver: a clinicopathologic and follow-up study of 32 cases. Hum Pathol 15(9):839–852
11. Rummeny E, Weissleder R, Stark DD et al (1989) Primary liver tumours: diagnosis by MR imaging. AJR Am J Roentgenol 152(1):63–72
12. Adjei ON, Tamura S, Sugimura H et al (1995) Contrast-enhanced MR imaging of intrahepatic cholangiocarcinoma. Clin Radiol 50(1):6–10
13. Soyer P, Bluemke DA, Reichle R et al (1995) Imaging of intrahepatic cholangiocarcinoma: 1. Peripheral cholangiocarcinoma. AJR Am J Roentgenol 165(6):1427–1431
14. Ros PR, Buck JL, Goodman ZD et al (1988) Intrahepatic cholangiocarcinoma: radiologic-pathologic correlation. Radiology 167(3):689–693
15. Tani K, Kubota Y, Yamaguchi T et al (1991) MR imaging of peripheral cholangiocarcinoma. J Comput Assist Tomogr 15(6):975–978
16. Choi BI, Kim TK, Han JK (1998) MRI of clonorchiasis and cholangiocarcinoma. J Magn Reson Imaging 8(2):359–366
17. Kaude J, Rian R (1971) Cholangiocarcinoma. Radiology 100(3):573–580

Prognostic Factors

The main prognostic factors of intrahepatic cholangiocarcinoma (ICC) are: gross type (size, multifocality, vascular, serosal and biliary involvement), local extent, lymph-node involvement and microscopic and molecular biological patterns.

Gross Type

The classification proposed by the Liver Cancer Study Group of Japan (LCSGJ) distinguishes three different macroscopic types: mass forming (MF), periductal-infiltrating (PI), and intraductal growth (IG) [1]. These three macroscopic forms reflect different biological behaviours and neoplastic diffusion. MF cholangiocarcinoma is associated with early portal invasion and intra hepatic metastases; the PI type is characterised by invasion of the biliary tree and of Glisson's sheath, with preferential spread to the lymph nodes of the hepatic hilum [2–4].

The IG type represents 8–29% of the resected ICC [5–7]. This papillary form is well-differentiated in the majority of cases and shows a low rate of vascular, lymphatic and perineural invasion [5]. Radial diffusion of the neoplasm is limited to the wall of the small bile ducts, without invasion of the surrounding parenchyma in 31–36% of cases [5,8]. In more than 40% of patients with IG-type cholangiocarcinoma, the neoplasm reveals feature of superficial mucosal spread extending far from the tumour along the duct; these are the so-called "superficially spreading tumours" [8]. Long-term survival after surgical resection of IG cholangiocarcinoma is good, with a 5-year survival ranging from 41 to 80% [5,7,8]. The survival of patients with IG-type disease is significantly longer than that of patients with MF and PI types even in patients with lymph-node metastases [9]. Relapse after R0 resection is not very frequent and has a reported rate of <20% [5,8].

A. Guglielmi, A. Ruzzenente, C. Iacono (eds.) *Surgical Treatment of Hilar and ICC.*
© Springer 2008

MF cholangiocarcinoma is the most frequent type and represents 60–70% of all cases [10,11]; vascular invasion occurs in 47% of patients, intrahepatic metastases in 36% and lymph-node metastases in 31% [12]. The 5-year survival rate reported in the literature varies from 25 to 47% (Table 1). In 63%, patients with MF-type disease have histological evidence of bile-duct invasion. These lesions more frequently have a microscopic pattern that is prognostically negative, associated with an increased rate of vascular, perineural and lymphatic invasion (65, 69 and 80%) compared to neoplasms without ductal infiltration (33, 6 and 33%) [13]. The long-term prognosis is significantly worse for patients with ductal-invasive MF than for those without ductal invasion with a 5-years survival rate of 11 vs. 62%, respectively [13].

The prognosis of PI-type cholangiocarcinoma is worse than that of the other two types. The prevalence of this form ranges between 15 and 35% [9,11,14]. PI-type disease is associated with biliary-duct infiltration at the hepatic hilum; vascular and lymphatic involvement are frequent at this same site. Conversely, the rates of portal invasion and intrahepatic metastases are lower [2]. Five-year survival in patients with PI-type cholangiocarcinoma ranges from 0 to 49% [4,9,15].

The MF+PI mixed type of cholangiocarcinoma is observed in 25–46% of patients and has the worst prognosis [4,16,17]. This form correlates with a more advanced stage of disease, with a higher frequency of lymph-node metastases, gross vascular invasion and intrahepatic metastases (80, 80 and 46%, respectively) [17]. The long-term outcome is poor, with a 5-year survival rate <10% (Table 1).

Table 1 Intrahepatic cholangiocarcinoma, survival according to gross type

Author	Year	5-Year survival		5-Year survival		5-Year survival	
		MF	MF (%)	PI	PI (%)	MF +PI	MF +PI (%)
Nozaki [16]	1998	30	36	2	0	13	7
Yamamoto [4]	1998	28	39	14	17	18	0
Isaji [17]	1999	15	25	3	33	15	7
Isa [9]	2001	12	33	7	0	-	-
Suzuki [15]	2002	12	47	-	-	7	0
Morimoto [14]	2003	29[a]	0	13	49	-	-
Nakagawa [18]	2005	17	51[c]	11[b]	36[c]	-	-
Miwa [19]	2006	25	44	-	-	16	7

MF, Mass forming; *PI*, periductal infiltrating
[a]PI and MF+PI
[b]Eight cases of MF+PI were included in this group
[c]Three-years survival

The site of the neoplasm is significantly related to gross type and prognosis. The peripheral ones are mainly MF type while the central neoplasms show a higher prevalence of PI type associated or not with MF-type neoplasms. Isaji noted that 67% of the central neoplasms are MF+PI type, compared to 29% for peripheral lesions [17]. Central neoplasms are more aggressive than peripheral ones and have a significantly higher percentage of macroscopic portal invasion (66 vs. 37%) and of nodal metastases (75 vs. 45%) [17]. Long-term outcome is significantly better in patients with peripheral cholangiocarcinomas than in those with central variants. The 5-year survival rate is 37–43% vs. 0–4% [17,20].

T Category

The most important prognostic factors related to local extent, as identified in the literature, are size, multifocality, vascular invasion, serosal invasion and biliary tract invasion.

Tumour size represents the principal prognostic factor and it correlates with prognosis. The 5-year survival rates in patients with neoplasm <3 cm, between 3 and 6 cm, and >6 cm are 42, 15 and 0%, respectively (p=0.02) [9].

The presence of intrahepatic metastases is another negative prognostic factor that has been noted in approximately 20–33% of patients who underwent surgical resection, and it is more frequently associated with the MF type of disease [4,9,15]. The occurrence of intrahepatic metastases is directly associated with tumour size and the presence of vascular involvement [21,22].

The presence of intrahepatic metastases worsens the prognosis compared to patients with single lesion, with 5-year survival rates between 0 and 7% vs. 35 and 57% (Table 2).

Table 2 Survival after surgical resection according to the presence of intrahepatic metastases

Author	Year	Patients numbers	Single 5-year surv.	Multiple (%)	Multiple 5-year surv.
Casavilla [23]	1997	34	77[a]	44	10[a]
Okabayashi [24]	2001	60	45	46	10[a]
Isa [9]	2001	27	35	19	0
Suzuki [15]	2002	19	41	31	0
Nakagawa 18]	2005	28	55 (3-year)	21	0 (3-year)
Ikai [10][b]	2005	1364	41	21	7.5–22
Lang [25]	2006	54	57	53	7

[a]Median survival (months)
[b]Japanese nationwide follow-up survey

Portal invasion is an important prognostic factor for peripheral ICC. Survival is significantly longer in patients without portal-vein involvement than in those with macroscopic portal infiltration (3-year survival rates of 46.1 and 0%, respectively). The type of vascular involvement has a prognostic significance too: 5-year survival of patients with invasion of the peripheral portal branches is significantly higher than that of patients with invasion of the major branches or the main portal trunk (5-year survival of 25 vs. 0%, respectively [24]).

The prognostic significance of serosal invasion is still unclear. Uenishi reported a 5-year survival rate of 24 vs. 39% in patients with or without serosal invasion—a difference that was not statistically significant [12]. Conversely, other authors found a relationship between prognosis and serosal involvement, with a relative risk for survival of 3.94 at univariate analysis [26].

N Category

The presence of lymph-node metastases in ICC is a major negative prognostic factor. The prevalence of nodal metastases is high and varies from 7 to 73% [2,17,18,27,28]. Long-term prognosis in patients with lymph-node metastases is poor (5-year survival of 0–17%; Table 3).

Table 3 Survival according to lymph-node status

Author	Year	Patients numbers	Frequency N+ (%)	5-Year survival N+	5-Year survival N-
Casavilla [23]	1997	34	17	6.5 (months)	22.4*(months)
Nozaki [16]	1998	47	31	7	38*
Yamamoto [29]	1999	51	45	0	51*
Valverde [22]	1999	30	27	0	46*
Isa [9]	2001	27	55	7	45*
Okabayashi [24]	2001	60	36	0	40*
Suzuki [15]	2002	19	73	(33 single, 0 ≥2)	80
Morimoto [14]	2003	51	32	0	40*
Huang [30]	2004	31	22	0	35 (overall)
Ikai [10][a]	2005	1364	31	17	43
Nakagawa [18]	2005	30	46	25 (3-year)[b]	62 (3-year)*
Uenishi [12]	2005	63	33	5	47*
Miwa [19]	2006	41	39	0	49*
Lang [25]	2006	54	37	22 (3-year)	47 (3-year)*

* $p<0.05$

[a]Japanese nationwide follow-up survey

[b]Survival for patients with <3 positive lymph nodes was 50%, whereas it was 0% for >3 positive lymph nodes

The distinction between regional and non-regional lymph nodes and their prognostic significance in ICC are still debated. Moreover, as already underlined, the subdivision into regional and non-regional lymph nodes according to UICC/AJCC and LCSGJ definitions does not seem to have prognostic value [10,29].

The routes of diffusion of ICC to lymph nodes also remain matters of study and are influenced by gross type, stage and site of the neoplasm.

The frequency of lymph-node involvement in IG neoplasm is significantly lower than in the other macroscopic types and does not exceed 20%. The difference in the occurrence of lymph-node involvement in MF and PI types is less clear; however, it is evident that the rate of lymph-node metastases of the combined type (PF+MF), is significantly higher than the rate of the other gross types (Table 4).

Table 4 Gross type and frequency of lymph-node involvement

Author	Year	Patients (number)	IG (% N+)	MF (% N+)	PI (% N+)	MF+PI (% N+)
Yamamoto [29]	1999	51	20	42	33	73*
Isaji [17]	1999	36	0	33	100	80
Tsuji [31]	2001	39	0	69	0	-*
Hirohashi [13]	2002	41	-	33	-	80*
Morimoto [14]	2003	51	14	41	15	-*
Miwa [19]	2006	41	-	42	-	50

*$p<0.05$; *IG*, intraductal growth; *MF*, mass forming; *PI*, periductal infiltrating

The stage of the neoplasm significantly determines the occurrence of lymph-node metastases (Table 5). In particular, Miwa observed that N+ patients more frequently presented with larger tumours and involvement of hepatic hilus [19].

The location of the neoplasms determines both the frequency and the distribution of nodal involvement. Central cholangiocarcinomas have a higher frequency of nodal metastases than peripheral ones (75 vs. 46%) [17].

Studies on nodal diffusion of ICC have evidenced that the major lymphatic spreading routes of intrahepatic cholangiocarcinoma are (1) through the hepatoduodenal ligament, (2) through the paracardial, lesser-curvature or left-gastric nodes and (3) through the inferior phrenic artery or directly from the right liver to the lateral para-aortic group. In addition, neoplasms of the left lobe exhibit nodal spreading not only to the hepatoduodenal ligament but also to right paracardial stations, along the lesser curvature and left gastric artery [16].

Table 5 Rate of lymph-node involvement according to clinicopathologic findings. Adapted from [31]

Characteristic	Patients (number)	Patients with N+ (%)	p
Tumour location			0.49
Hilar	16	11 (69)	
Right peripheral	7	3 (43)	
Left peripheral	16	10 (63)	
Tumour extent			0.02
T2	15	5 (33)	
T3	10	8 (80)	
T4	14	11 (79)	
Macroscopic types			0.03
Mass-forming	35	24 (69)	
Periductal infiltrating	3	0	
Intraductal growth	1	0	
Growth type			0.04
Expansive	9	3 (33)	
Infiltrative	30	21 (70)	
Serosal invasion			0.80
S0	9	5 (56)	
S1	18	12 (67)	
S2	12	7 (58)	
Total	39	24 (62)	

The preferential lymphatic drainage of right-lobe ICCs is through the right pathway, with involvement of the hepatoduodenal ligament lymph nodes. In contrast, left-lobe neoplasms involve the lesser gastric-curvature nodes (left pathway) in 25–31% of patients [3,32]. Yamamoto observed that hepatoduodenal positive lymph nodes were present in all left-lobe ICC with lesser-curvature nodal involvement. However, Okami found that lesser-curvature nodal metastases were not associated with hepatoduodenal metastases in 29% of patients [32].

The prognostic value of metastatic lymph nodes was studied by Nakagawa, who reported a 3-year survival of 61% for NO patients, of 7% for patients with less than three positive lymph nodes, and of 0% for patients with more than three positive lymph nodes ($p<0.0001$). Patients with more than three positive nodes had advanced disease with the presence of intrahepatic multiple nodules and positive resection margins. Patients with intrahepatic and >3 positive lymph nodes metastases presented with early intrahepatic recurrences even though they underwent curative resection (within 4 months) [18].

Microscopic Pattern

The main histologic patterns related to prognosis are: cellular differentiation, perineural, vascular and lymphatic invasion.

Concerning cellular differentiation, well or moderately differentiated neoplasms have a better prognosis than poorly differentiated ones. Five-year survival rates of 50, 39 and 0% respectively, were reported in patients with well, moderate and poorly differentiated tumours [16].

Perineural invasion is a negative prognostic factor and is associated with a high frequency of nodal metastases and vascular invasion. Suzuki reported 5-year survival rate of 83% in patients with MF cholangiocarcinoma without perineural infiltration vs. 8% in patients with perineural infiltration [13]. Nakagohri confirmed these data, reporting a 5-year survival rate of 50 vs. 7% [20].

Lymphatic invasion represents a further negative independent prognostic factor for survival. In one study, patients without lymphatic invasion had a 5-year survival rate of 71% while none of the patients with lymphatic invasion survived more than 3 years [33].

Biological and Molecular Factors

Many biological and molecular prognostic factors have been identified in ICC including interleukin (IL)-6, hepatocyte growth factors (HGFs), c-met, transforming growth factor (TGF)-β, epidermal growth factor (EGF), c-erb-2, lymphocyte inhibitory factor, k-ras and p53 [34–37].

The expression of IL-6 is inversely related with cellular proliferation and directly correlated with cholangiocarcinoma differentiation. Increase levels of IL-6 are frequently found in well-differentiated cholangiocarcinoma whereas decreased levels of this cytokine are observed in moderately or poorly differentiated ICC.

A mutation in the oncogene k-ras is a frequent finding in ICC; the prevalence is related to the gross type: MF types rarely show k-ras mutations in contrast to periductal infiltrating cholangiocarcinoma. According to Isa, such mutations are related to a poor prognosis, although the difference did not reach statistical significance (p=0.0898). Nevertheless in that study none of the patients with a survival longer than 5 years had tumours with k-ras mutations.

The incidence of p53 mutation in intrahepatic cholangiocarcinoma ranges between 3 and 35%, and occurs especially in the MF type. MDM2 (inhibitory oncoprotein of p53) expression increases in intrahepatic cholangiocarcinoma. This amplified expression of p53 is related to tumour stage and to the presence of metastases. It represents a late event in tumour progression and is related with a poor prognosis.

Cholangiocarcinomas with increased expression of *N*-myristoyltransferase (NMT), a signal modulator of intracellular transduction, and p53 are more aggressive and have a higher number of metastases.

Cholangiocarcinomas with a decrease in the expression of the cycle-dependent kinase inhibitor p27kip1 are poorly differentiated. These tumours are characterised by increased T-stage as well as lymphatic and lymph-node invasion. Patients with this type of cholangiocarcinoma have a lower survival.

Alterations of E-caderin, α-catenin and β-catenin regulation in intrahepatic cholangiocarcinomas are associated with high tumour grade and stage, and rapid disease progression.

Vascular endothelial growth factor (VEGF-C) is an important lympho-angiogenic factor. Park reported that the association of VEGF-C expression with the development of lymph-node metastases is statistically significant ($p=0.032$). This is also the case for positive resection margins ($p=0.03$). The increased expression of VEGF-C represented a negative independent prognostic factor also for survival [38].

Many studies have demostrated a role for mucins in complex biological processes, such as differentiation, epithelial cell renewal, cellular adhesion and carcinogenesis. Tissue expression of the mucin proteins MUC 1 and 2 in ICC is related with gross type; high-level expression of MUC 1 is observed in MF and PI types compared to IG type, in which MUC 1 expression is usually low [39].

Recent studies have suggested that the serum concentration of MUC 5AC represents negative prognostic marker in patients with ICC. Conclusive data on biological and molecular prognostic factors are still lacking and under evalutaion.

References

1. The Liver Cancer Study Group of Japan (2003). General rules for the clinical and pathological study of primary liver cancer, 2nd edn. Kanehara, Tokyo
2. Sasaki A, Aramaki M, Kawano K et al (1998) Intrahepatic peripheral cholangiocarcinoma: mode of spread and choice of surgical treatment. Br J Surg 85(9):1206–1209
3. Yamamoto M, Takasaki K, Yoshikawa T (1999) Extended resection for intrahepatic cholangiocarcinoma in Japan. J Hepatobiliary Pancreat Surg 6(2):117–121
4. Yamamoto M, Takasaki K, Yoshikawa T et al (1998) Does gross appearance indicate prognosis in intrahepatic cholangiocarcinoma? J Surg Oncol 69(3):162-167
5. Suh KS, Roh HR, Koh YT et al (2000) Clinicopathologic features of the intraductal growth type of peripheral cholangiocarcinoma. Hepatology 31(1):12–17
6. Ohashi K, Nakajima Y, Kanehiro H et al (1995) Ki-ras mutations and p53 protein expressions in intrahepatic cholangiocarcinomas: relation to gross tumour morphology. Gastroenterology 109(5):1612–1617
7. Yeh CN, Jan YY, Yeh TS et al (2004) Hepatic resection of the intraductal papillary type of peripheral cholangiocarcinoma. Ann Surg Oncol 11(6):606–611
8. Sakamoto E, Hayakawa N, Kamiya J et al (1999) Treatment strategy for mucin-producing intrahepatic cholangiocarcinoma: value of percutaneous transhepatic biliary drainage and cholangioscopy. World J Surg 23(10):1038–1043
9. Isa T, Kusano T, Shimoji H et al (2001) Predictive factors for long-term survival in patients with intrahepatic cholangiocarcinoma. Am J Surg 181(6):507–511
10. Ikai I, Arii S, Ichida T et al (2005) Report of the 16th follow-up survey of primary liver cancer. Hepatol Res 32(3):163–172

11. Yamasaki S (2003) Intrahepatic cholangiocarcinoma: macroscopic type and stage classification. J Hepatobiliary Pancreat Surg 10(4):288–291

12. Uenishi T, Yamazaki O, Yamamoto T et al (2005) Serosal invasion in TNM staging of mass-forming intrahepatic cholangiocarcinoma. J Hepatobiliary Pancreat Surg 12(6):479–483

13. Hirohashi K, Uenishi T, Kubo S et al (2002) Histologic bile duct invasion by a mass-forming intrahepatic cholangiocarcinoma. J Hepatobiliary Pancreat Surg 9(2):233–236

14. Morimoto Y, Tanaka Y, Ito T et al (2003) Long-term survival and prognostic factors in the surgical treatment for intrahepatic cholangiocarcinoma. J Hepatobiliary Pancreat Surg 10(6):432–440

15. Suzuki S, Sakaguchi T, Yokoi Y et al (2002) Clinicopathological prognostic factors and impact of surgical treatment of mass-forming intrahepatic cholangiocarcinoma. World J Surg 26(6):687–693

16. Nozaki Y, Yamamoto M, Ikai I et al (1998) Reconsideration of the lymph-node metastasis pattern (N factor) from intrahepatic cholangiocarcinoma using the International Union Against Cancer TNM staging system for primary liver carcinoma. Cancer 83(9):1923–1929

17. Isaji S, Kawarada Y, Taoka H et al (1999) Clinicopathological features and outcome of hepatic resection for intrahepatic cholangiocarcinoma in Japan. J Hepatobiliary Pancreat Surg 6(2):108–116

18. Nakagawa T, Kamiyama T, Kurauchi N et al (2005) Number of lymph-node metastases is a significant prognostic factor in intrahepatic cholangiocarcinoma. World J Surg 29(6):728–733

19. Miwa S, Miyagawa S, Kobayashi A et al (2006) Predictive factors for intrahepatic cholangiocarcinoma recurrence in the liver following surgery. J Gastroenterol 41(9):893–900

20. Nakagohri T, Asano T, Kinoshita H et al (2003) Aggressive surgical resection for hilar-invasive and peripheral intrahepatic cholangiocarcinoma. World J Surg 27(3):289–293

21. Nakajima T, Kondo Y, Miyazaki M, Okui K (1988) A histopathologic study of 102 cases of intrahepatic cholangiocarcinoma: histologic classification and modes of spreading. Hum Pathol 19(10):1228–1234

22. Valverde A, Bonhomme N, Farges O et al (1999) Resection of intrahepatic cholangiocarcinoma: a Western experience. J Hepatobiliary Pancreat Surg 6(2):122–127

23. Casavilla FA, Marsh JW, Iwatsuki S et al (1997) Hepatic resection and transplantation for peripheral cholangiocarcinoma. J Am Coll Surg 185(5):429–436

24. Okabayashi T, Yamamoto J, Kosuge T et al (2001) A new staging system for mass-forming intrahepatic cholangiocarcinoma: analysis of preoperative and postoperative variables. Cancer 92(9):2374–2383

25. Lang H, Kaiser GM, Zopf T et al (2006) Surgical therapy of hilar cholangiocarcinoma. Chirurg 77(4):325–334

26. Ohtsuka M, Ito H, Kimura F et al (2002) Results of surgical treatment for intrahepatic cholangiocarcinoma and clinicopathological factors influencing survival. Br J Surg 89(12):1525–1531

27. Yamanaka N, Okamoto E, Ando T et al (1995) Clinicopathologic spectrum of resected extraductal mass-forming intrahepatic cholangiocarcinoma. Cancer 76(12):2449–2456

28. Cherqui D, Tantawi B, Alon R et al (1995) Intrahepatic cholangiocarcinoma. Results of aggressive surgical management. Arch Surg 130(10):1073–1078

29. Yamamoto M, Takasaki K, Yoshikawa T (1999) Lymph-node metastasis in intrahepatic cholangiocarcinoma. Jpn J Clin Oncol 29(3):147–150

30. Huang JL, Biehl TR, Lee FT et al (2004) Outcomes after resection of cholangiocellular carcinoma. Am J Surg 187(5):612–617

31. Tsuji T, Hiraoka T, Kanemitsu K et al (2001) Lymphatic spreading pattern of intrahepatic cholangiocarcinoma. Surgery 129(4):401–407

32. Okami J, Dono K, Sakon M et al (2003) Patterns of regional lymph-node involvement in intrahepatic cholangiocarcinoma of the left lobe. J Gastrointest Surg 7(7):850–856

33. Uenishi T, Hirohashi K, Kubo S et al (2001) Clinicopathological factors predicting outcome after resection of mass-forming intrahepatic cholangiocarcinoma. Br J Surg 88(7):969–974

34. Abdalla EK, Vauthey JN (2001) Biliary tract cancer. Curr Opin Gastroenterol 17(5):450–457
35. Rashid A, Ueki T, Gao YT et al (2002) K-ras mutation, p53 overexpression, and microsatellite instability in biliary tract cancers: a population-based study in China. Clin Cancer Res 8(10):3156–3163
36. Malhi H, Gores GJ (2006) Cholangiocarcinoma: modern advances in understanding a deadly old disease. J Hepatol 45(6):856–867
37. Nakanuma Y, Harada K, Ishikawa A et al (2003) Anatomic and molecular pathology of intrahepatic cholangiocarcinoma. J Hepatobiliary Pancreat Surg 10(4):265–281
38. Park BK, Paik YH, Park JY et al (2006) The clinicopathologic significance of the expression of vascular endothelial growth factor-C in intrahepatic cholangiocarcinoma. Am J Clin Oncol 29(2):138–142
39. Andrianifahanana M, Moniaux N, Batra SK (2006) Regulation of mucin expression: mechanistic aspects and implications for cancer and inflammatory diseases. Biochim Biophys Acta 1765(2):189–222

Staging Systems

The staging systems of intrahepatic cholangiocarcinoma (ICC) are based on pathological findings. The most common classification systems are the TNM UICC/AJCC classification (6th edn.) 2002 [1] and the TNM classification of the Liver Cancer Study Group of Japan (LCSGJ) (2nd English edn.) 2003 [2].

TNM Staging System According to UICC/AJCC

The sixth edition of TNM defined by International Union Against Cancer (UICC) is the same as that of the American Joint Committee on Cancer (AJCC). This edition, same as the previous one, uses the classification criteria developed for hepatocellular carcinoma. Subdivision in stages is obtained through definition of T, N, and M categories.

T Category

T category values the extent of disease based on size of neoplasm, focality, vascular invasion and extension to adjacent organs. It divides the neoplasms into four categories (Table 1).

Although there are few reports on the validation of T-staging, the components that define T category (size, number, vascular invasion) have shown a close correlation with prognosis in several studies [3–8]. Miwa et al. have observed that the size of the tumour significantly determined the prognosis; in 41 patients, 5-year survival was 47% for those with lesions <4.5 cm vs. 16% for patients whose lesions were larger (p=0.01). The same author underlined that portal involvement represents a negative prognostic factor: 5-year survival was 24% in patients with portal involvement vs. 47% in those without (p=0.07) [7].

In a series of 1,364 surgical resections for ICC, the 16th national follow-up survey of Japan reported a 5-year survival of 66% for tumours <2 cm, 36% for

A. Guglielmi, A. Ruzzenente, C. Iacono (eds.) *Surgical Treatment of Hilar and ICC.*
© Springer 2008

Table 1 T category according to the TNM system of the UICC/AJCC

T1	Solitary tumour without vascular invasion
T2	Solitary tumour with vascular invasion or multiple tumours, none >5 cm in the greatest dimension
T3	Multiple tumours >5 cm or tumour involving a major branch of the portal or hepatic vein(s)
T4	Tumour(s) with direct invasion of adjacent organs other than the gallbladder or with perforation of visceral peritoneum

tumours between 2 and 5 cm and 30% for tumours between 5 and 10 cm. Five-year survival was 41% in patients with a single lesion, 22% in patients with two lesions and 7.5% in patients with more than two lesions [9].

N Category

According to the IUCC/AJCC classification, regional lymph nodes are located at the hepatic hilum, along the proper hepatic artery, along the portal vein and along the vena cava above the renal veins (except the inferior phrenic nodes). Two classes are defined: N0 and N1 on the basis of positive and negative regional nodes; involvement of non-regional nodes is considered indicative of distant metastasis (M1) (Table 2).

Table 2 N category according to the TNM system of the UICC/AJCC

N0	Absence of nodal involvement
N1	Presence of regional lymph-node involvement

The pathways of lymph-node spreading of ICC are still argued and conclusive data are lacking. Lymph nodes of the hepatoduodenal ligament are considered regional lymph nodes by the UICC classification. Prognostic significance of lymph-node involvement has been determined in many studies, with 5-year survival of 45% in N0 patients vs. 7–17% in N+ patients [10]. More controversial is the significance of regional and non-regional lymph-node involvement. Nozaki did not find any survival differences between N+ patients with lymph-node metastases classified as N1 and patients with non regional lymph-node metastases (M1). The 5-year survival was 0 and 8.3%, respectively [11].

M Category

Evaluation of M category is based on the presence of metastases to other organs or non-regional lymph nodes. Two categories are therefore identified: M0 and M1 (Table 3).

Table 3 M category according to the TNM system of the UICC/AJCC

M0	Absence of metastases
M1	Presence of metastases

Stage Grouping

The three categories T, N and M, are combined to subdivide patients in homogeneous prognostic groups. In the sixth edition of the UICC/AJCC classification, six stages have been defined (Table 4).

Table 4 Stage grouping according to the TNM system of the UICC/AJCC

	T	N	M
Stage I	T1	N0	M0
Stage II	T2	N0	M0
Stage IIIA	T3	N0	M0
Stage IIIB	T4	N0	M0
Stage IIIC	Any T	N1	M0
Stage IV	Any T	Any N	M1

The staging system proposed by UICC/AJCC has been formulated for hepatocellular carcinoma, as previously stated. This is the main limit of this classification in that two diseases with completely different biological behaviours (i.e. vascular invasion, limph-nodes involvement) are joined.

The literature contains very few validation experiences regarding the 6th TNM UICC/AJCC classification. Lang identified a correlation between TNM stages, curative resection survival and recurrence. In this clinical study of 27 patients who underwent surgical resection all stage I and II patients underwent a R0 resection vs. 42% of stage III patients [12]. Several published studies did, however, confirm the 5th edition of TNM UICC. These demonstrated that TNM stage is related to long-term outcome. In 27 patients, Isa reported a 5-year survival of 42% for stage I and II patients, 25% for those with stage III and 0% for those with stage IV (p=0.001) [11].

Similar results were obtained by Fu in 79 patients in whom median survival after surgical resection was 20 months in stage I, 16 months in stage II, 15 months in stage IIIa, 9 months in stage IIIb and 5 months in stage IVa [5].

TNM Classification According to the LCSGJ

In 1992, the LCSGJ convened a research group to formulate a new staging system specific for ICC. This group carried out a multicentric study with nine Japanese surgical institutions and analysed 173 patients who underwent resection with curative intent for ICC. In 1997, the first edition of this new classification was published and it was revised in 2003 [2].

The Japanese classification of cholangiocarcinoma defines intrahepatic neoplasm as originating from the peripheral branches of biliary ducts (beyond second-order divisions). Based on the gross appearance of the tumour, three patterns of growth are defined. that can be present alone or in combination: mass-forming type (MF), periductal infiltrating type (PI) and intraductal growth (IG) type cholangiocarcinoma (Fig. 1).

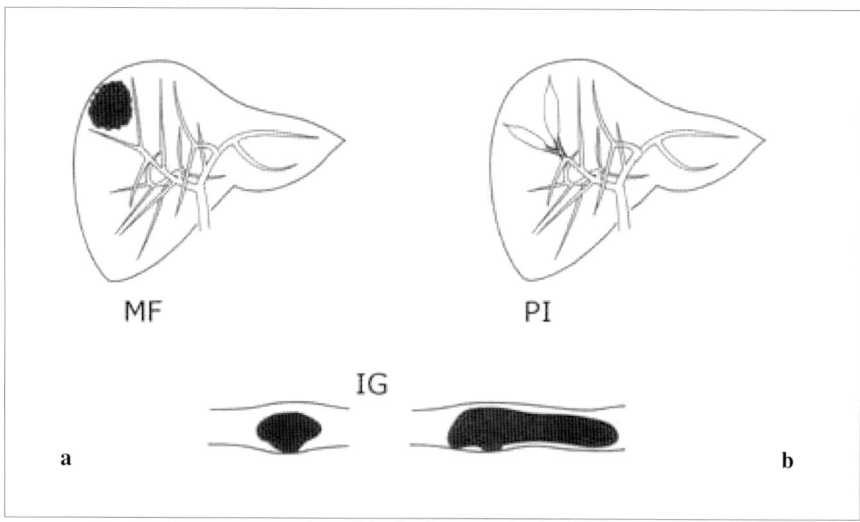

Fig. 1. Growth patterns of cholagiocarcinoma: mass-forming (*MF*), periductal infiltrating (*PI*) and intraductal growth (*IG*) types. **a** Intraductal papillary growth; **b** intraduct, growth forming a tumour thrombus

The MF type is characterised by a distinct, round-shaped mass localised inside the liver, with a well-defined margin between cancer and the surrounding parenchyma.

The PI type is characterised by diffuse infiltration along the major axis of the portal tract, with involvement of the biliary tract, vessels and periductal connective tissue.

The IG type is characterised by a papillary and/or granular growth within a dilated duct; sporadically a superficial spread or the formation of intraductal tumoral nodules is seen. Dilatation of the cystic duct due to mucin, produced by an intraductal tumour, that collects inside the ducts should not be misdiagnosed as cystadenocarcinoma of the biliary duct.

Macroscopic type is determined by the most representative type inside the lesion; thus, when more than one type is present the neoplasm, is classified by the more prevalent form and the other types are described with a + symbol (i.e. MF+PI).

A LCSGJ staging system for MF type or forms in which the MF type is prevalent had been formulated. A staging classification for the PI and IG forms has not been formulated yet, as there are very few data. The staging system considers the local extent of disease (T), nodal diffusion (N) and distant metastases (M).

T Category

Valuation of the extent of neoplasm (T) is assessed by one or more of three different parameters: (1) focality (single or multifocal), (2) size of the lesion (≤ 2 or >2 cm) and (3) vascular (portal vein or hepatic vein) and/or serosal involvement.

Four T categories with prognostic value are defined (Table 5).This division in T categories comes from the multicentric experience of the LCSGJ. In that study of 136 patients with MF cholangiocarcinoma, univariate analysis identified the following prognostic factors correlated with survival: size ≥ 2 cm (HR 2.39), lymph nodes metastases (HR 2.36), serosal invasion (HR 2.19), portal-vein invasion (HR 1.68) multiple nodules (HR 1.95) and hepatic-vein invasion (HR 1.18) [6]. These factors have been identified also in other clinical studies that highlight among

Table 5 T category according to the LCSGJ

Criteria	
	1: Unifocal lesion
	2: Size ≤ 2 cm
	3: No vascular or serosal involvement
T1	All criteria are satisfied
T2	Two out of three criteria are satisfied
T3	One out of three criteria is satisfied
T4	No criterion is satisfied

the most important prognostic factors size, focality and vascular invasion [13–17]. More controversial is the prognostic significance of serosal invasion; some authors emphasised its value, such as Ohtsuka [8] who identified the prognostic value of this factor in univariate analysis, whereas other authors, such as Uenishi, did not find any significant differences in survival between patients with or without serosal invasion, with a 5-year survival of 24 and 39% ($p=0.16$), respectively [8,13].

N Category

The lymphatic system of the liver can be divided into a superficial and a deep system. The lymph of the upper portions of the liver (diaphragmatic side) drains to lymphatic stations situated at the confluence of the hepatic veins and near the falciform, coronary and triangular ligaments. Then the lymph passes through the diaphragm and enters into the mediastinal lymphatic system. Inferior portions of the liver (visceral side), in contrast, drain to lymphatic stations of the hepatic hilum, lesser omentum and subsequently to abdominal lymphatic system.

According to the Japanese classification, lymph nodes are numbered as shown in Table 6.

Unlike the first English edition, in the second classification of the LCSGJ N category is no longer subdivided as a function of the site of the neoplasm.

Table 6 Japanese classification of lymph-nodes stations

Number	Site
1	Right cardial
2	Left cardial
3	Lesser gastric curvature
4	Greater curvature
5	Suprapyloric
6	Infrapyloric
7	Left gastric artery
8	Hepatic artery
9	Celiac trunk
10	Splenic hilum
11	Splenic artery
12	Hepatoduodenal ligament
13	Retropancreatic
14	Superior mesenteric artery
15	Middle colic
16	Para-aortic
17	Superior pancreatic
18	Inferior pancreatic
19	Subdiaphragmatic
20	Para-oesophageal
110	Intrathoracic para-oesophageal
111	Supradiaphragmatic

Clinical studies in patients with ICC have found different lymphatic drainage patterns depending on the site of the tumour. Nozaki observed that neoplasms situated in the left lobe show lymph-node involvement along the lesser gastric curvature in up to 30% of N+ patients [11]. In left lobe cholangiocarcinoma, diffusion to the lymph nodes of the lesser curvature can be present even in the absence of a hepatoduodenal ligament localisation in up to 29% of patients [18].

Since these observations in the first English edition of the LCSGJ classification, lymphatic stations for cholangiocarcinoma have been differentiated depending on the site of the tumour. Regional lymph nodes for lesions of the right lobe are those of the hepatoduodenal ligament (12), whereas for left-lobe tumours hepatoduodenal ligament (12), lesser gastric curvature (3) and right cardial (1) nodes are involved. Other lymph-node localisations have been defined as non-regional (N2 and N3).

The simplification of the second English edition is the product of many clinical studies that did not show a significant difference of prognosis in patients with regional (N1) positive lymph nodes versus those with non-regional positive lymph nodes (N2 and N3). Yamamoto, in a study of 51 patients with ICC, did not observe significant differences in survival between patients with N1, N2 and N3 positive lymph nodes according to the first LCSGJ classification [19]. These data were confirmed in a nation-wide survey comprising 791 Japanese institutions. The results of 1,087 patients with ICC did not show significant differences in the 3-year survival of N1, N2 and N3 patients: 29, 22 and 12%, respectively [20].

The second edition of the LCGSJ classification subdivides N category only according to lymph-node involvement, without providing a proposal for further lymph-node grouping at the first or second level for this type of neoplasm. N category is therefore divided in two categories: N1 and N0 (Table 7).

Table 7 N category according to the LCSGJ

N0	No lymph-node metastases
N1	Lymph-node metastases

M Category

Evaluation of M category is based on the presence of metastases to other organs or non-regional lymph nodes. Two categories are defined: M0 and M1 (Table 8).

Table 8 M category according to the LCSGJ

M0	Absence of metastases
M1	Presence of metastases

Stage Grouping

As noted previously, the staging system proposed by the LCSGJ can be applied only to the MF type of ICC and to tumours in which the MF type is prevalent. It cannot be applied to PI and IG neoplasms. The stage defined by the T, N and M categories determines four subdivisions having different prognoses (Table 9).

Table 9 Stage grouping according to the LCSGJ

	T	N	M
Stage I	T1	N0	M0
Stage II	T2	N0	M0
Stage III	T3	N0	M0
Stage IVA	T4	N0	M0
Stage IVB	T1–T4	N1	M0
	T1–T4	N0, N1	M1

The survival of patients is significantly related to different stages: the 5-year survival for stage I was 100%, for stage II it was 70%, for stage III 40% and for stage IV 10% [6].

Other experiences in the literature have confirmed the prognostic significance of the LCGSJ staging system. Uenishi reported that the 5-year survival of 63 patients was 100% for those with stage I, 54% for patients with stage II, 44% for those with stage III and 7% for stage IV patients [13].

Conclusions

Correct staging of ICC is still a subject of debate. However, the differences between ICC and hepatocellular carcinoma are clear. For these reasons, the staging system proposed by the UICC/AJCC, which was mainly developed to stage hepatocarcinoma, is quite limited when it is applied to ICC. The UICC/AJCC classification does not differentiate neoplasms on the basis of type of tumoral growth and provides a limited differentiation of the criteria of local disease and disease involving lymph-node diffusion. In contrast, the classification proposed by the LCSGJ is specific for ICC. In addition, it differentiates these neoplasms as a function of tumoral growth. Unfortunately LCSGJ classification refers only to MF-type, whereas there is not staging system for PI- and IG-types. Nonetheless the classification proposed by the LCSGJ will eventually become the most useful to assess the prognosis of ICC.

References

1. Sobin LH, Wittekind C (eds) (2002) TNM classification of malignant tumours, 6th edn. Wiley, New York
2. Liver Cancer Study Group of Japan (2003) General rules for clinical and pathological study of primary liver cancer, 2nd English Edition. Kanehara, Tokyo
3. Roayaie S, Guarrera JV, Ye MQ et al (1998) Aggressive surgical treatment of intrahepatic cholangiocarcinoma: predictors of outcomes. J Am Coll Surg 187(4):365–372
4. Kinoshita H, Tanimura H, Uchiyama K et al (2002) Prognostic factors of intrahepatic cholangiocarcinoma after surgical treatment. Oncol Rep 9(1):97–101
5. Fu XH, Tang ZH, Zong M et al (2004) Clinicopathologic features, diagnosis and surgical treatment of intrahepatic cholangiocarcinoma in 104 patients. Hepatobiliary Pancreat Dis Int 3(2):279–283
6. Yamasaki S (2003) Intrahepatic cholangiocarcinoma: macroscopic type and stage classification. J Hepatobiliary Pancreat Surg 10(4):288–91
7. Miwa S, Miyagawa S, Kobayashi A et al (2006) Predictive factors for intrahepatic cholangiocarcinoma recurrence in the liver following surgery. J Gastroenterol 41(9):893–900
8. Ohtsuka M, Ito H, Kimura F et al (2002) Results of surgical treatment for intrahepatic cholangiocarcinoma and clinicopathological factors influencing survival. Br J Surg 89(12):1525–1531
9. Ikai I, Arii S, Ichida T et al (2005) Report of the 16th follow-up survey of primary liver cancer. Hepatol Res 32(3):163–172
10. Isa T, Kusano T, Shimoji H et al (2001) Predictive factors for long-term survival in patients with intrahepatic cholangiocarcinoma. Am J Surg 181(6):507–511
11. Nozaki Y, Yamamoto M, Ikai I et al (1998) Reconsideration of the lymph-node metastasis pattern (N factor) from intrahepatic cholangiocarcinoma using the International Union Against Cancer TNM staging system for primary liver carcinoma. Cancer 83(9):1923–1929
12. Lang H, Sotiropoulos GC, Fruhauf NR et al (2005) Extended hepatectomy for intrahepatic cholangiocellular carcinoma (ICC): when is it worthwhile? Single center experience with 27 resections in 50 patients over a 5-year period. Ann Surg 241(1):134–143
13. Uenishi T, Yamazaki O, Yamamoto T et al (2005) Serosal invasion in TNM staging of mass-forming intrahepatic cholangiocarcinoma. J Hepatobiliary Pancreat Surg 12(6):479–483
14. Uenishi T, Hirohashi K, Kubo S et al (2001) Clinicopathological factors predicting outcome after resection of mass-forming intrahepatic cholangiocarcinoma. Br J Surg 88(7):969–974
15. Morimoto Y, Tanaka Y, Ito T et al (2003) Long-term survival and prognostic factors in the surgical treatment for intrahepatic cholangiocarcinoma. J Hepatobiliary Pancreat Surg 10(6):432–440
16. Inoue K, Makuuchi M, Takayama T et al (2000) Long-term survival and prognostic factors in the surgical treatment of mass-forming type cholangiocarcinoma. Surgery 127(5):498–505
17. Shimada M, Yamashita Y, Aishima S et al (2001) Value of lymph node dissection during resection of intrahepatic cholangiocarcinoma. Br J Surg 88(11):1463–1466
18. Okami J, Dono K, Sakon M et al (2003) Patterns of regional lymph-node involvement in intrahepatic cholangiocarcinoma of the left lobe. J Gastrointest Surg 7(7):850–856
19. Yamamoto M, Takasaki K, Yoshikawa T (1999) Lymph-node metastasis in intrahepatic cholangiocarcinoma. Jpn J Clin Oncol 29(3):147–150
20. Ikai J, Itai Y, Okita K et al (2004) Report of the 15th follow-up survey of primary liver cancer. Hepatol Res 28:21–29

Surgical Treatment

Intraoperative Assessment of Resectability

At the time of diagnosis, patients with intrahepatic cholangiocarcinoma (ICC) are frequently found to have disease beyond the limits of surgical therapy, such the presence of intrahepatic satellite nodules, vascular invasion, or regional lymph-nodes metastases. In such patients, the resectability rate varies from 19 to 74% [1–4]. Moreover, exploratory laparotomy or R1 resection has a poor prognosis, with median patient survival of 5 months and postoperative complications of 17% [4]. Consequently, palliative resection is not justified; instead, there is clearly a need to improve the assessment of resectability, in order to avoid unnecessary laparotomy and to develop an aggressive approach to obtain complete resection (R0).

Both of these aims can be achieved by laparoscopy with laparoscopic ultrasound that showed a reduction in exploratory laparotomy from 27 to 36% [5,6].

As previously described for hilar cholangiocarcinoma, in ICC after laparotomy the abdominal cavity has to be carefully inspected to identify peritoneal metastases and loco-regional or distantly involved lymph nodes. The liver is explored with the aid of intraoperative ultrasound to determine the extent and site of the neoplasm as well as the number and localisation of metastatic nodules. All doubtful lesions, either peritoneal or intrahepatic, and lymph nodes that appear increased in size or consistency must be sent for frozen sectioning.

In a considerable number of patients (36–41% [4,7]), hepatic resection, considered curative, showed involvement of the liver margins, mostly because of infiltration by small satellite lesions. Intraoperative ultrasound allows the detection of intrahepatic metastases <1 cm. It remains to be investigated whether intraoperative ultrasound with contrast agent can reduce the number of incomplete resections by providing better visualisation of small, otherwise undetectable lesions [8,9].

It is also important to carefully evaluate the condition of the hepatic parenchyma, especially in the presence of chronic hepatopathy or cirrhosis,

A. Guglielmi, A. Ruzzenente, C. Iacono (eds.) *Surgical Treatment of Hilar and ICC.*
© Springer 2008

either of which could limit or contraindicate surgical resection. This situation is not exceptional: Isaji [10] reported that 30% of patients with peripheral ICC have HBsAg- or HCV-positive hepatitis, and this rate reaches 42% in patients with mass-forming ICC.

Indications for Surgical Resection

As with extrahepatic cholangiocarcinoma, R0 of ICC is the most effective treatment and the only therapy associated with prolonged disease-free survival. Nonetheless, there is currently little agreement on the indications for surgical resection. According to some authors curative resection (R0) of ICC is feasible only in patients with a single lesion, negative lymph nodes and resectable hepatic margins of >1 cm [7], or in patients without gross intrahepatic biliary infiltration; all patients with stage III and IV disease are therefore excluded from surgical resection [11]. Following these indications the results are good, with 2- and 5-year survival rates of 100 and 42%, respectively [7,11].

Unfortunately, according to these highly selective criteria, patients who present with one or more negative prognostic factors will not undergo surgical resection but only palliative treatment. The survival rate of such patients is between 6 and 12 months. It has also been suggested that, even in the presence of negative prognostic factors, better results can be achieved with surgical resection than with palliative therapy alone, with some reports of long-term survival of these patients. It is therefore evident that the precise indications for surgical resection require an analysis of the value of each prognostic factor, and a comparison of the results with the limited benefits of palliative therapy with respect to morbidity and mortality.

Type of Surgical Resection

Surgical resection of cholangiocarcinoma is represented by anatomic hepatic resection. Advanced-stage neoplasms must often be treated by extended hepatectomy, with extension of the resection to the extrahepatic biliary tract, vascular hilar structures, vena cava and diaphragm. Usually, this type of neoplasm develops in a non-cirrhotic liver, which allows the surgeon to perform extended resection without the need of portal-vein embolisation. The mortality and morbidity rates in these cases vary from 3–9% and 30–40%, respectively [4,12–15].

The surgical approach has to be tailored in consideration of the gross type of neoplasm, the presence of multifocal lesions (perilesional satellitosis and distant metastases), vascular, biliary and serosal involvement and lymph-nodes metastases. However, even after aggressive resections the prognosis remains unsatisfactory, with a 5-year survival rate of 21–42% [11,15–19].

The intraductal growth (IG) type of ICC shows intraductal and/or granular growth and is sometimes associated with carcinoma that spreads over the superficial mucosa or with intraductal tumour thrombus. This type of biliary epithelial neoplasia is frequently associated with gastrointestinal metaplasia and overproduction of mucin and mucobilia, i.e. biliary intraductal growth mucin-producing cholangiocarcinoma [20]. In these patients, in order to obtain correct preoperative staging of the tumour Sakamoto [20] recommended preoperative percutaneous biliary drainage and percutaneous cholangioscopy with biopsy in order to accurately assess the extent of the tumour into the intrahepatic segmental duct. This type of staging can be also achieved non invasively through the endoscopic route with peroral cholangioscopy.

After anatomic hepatic resection, the biliary duct margins should be evaluated by frozen sectioning. If neoplastic infiltration of the proximal biliary margin is diagnosed, the resection must be extended to the biliary confluence (Fig. 1). If the distal intrapancreatic margin is positive, pancreaticoduodenectomy is indicated.

Because of the high percentage of satellite nodules in mass-forming-type (MF) neoplasms, from 26 to 58% of patients treated surgically [1,2,7,10,21], an accurate intraoperative sonographic study is mandatory, both near the main lesion and of all the liver in order to identify metastatic nodules and verify the plane and radicality of resection. All suspicious nodules should be verified with intraoperative frozen sectioning. Anatomic resection with a section parenchymal margin at least 5–10 mm (R0) is adequate for MF neoplasms located peripherally (Fig. 2).

In cases of MF lesions either with biliary duct infiltration or located centrally near the biliary confluence, frozen section is always indicated to assess the margins of the biliary resection; if the results are positive, the resection has to be extended.

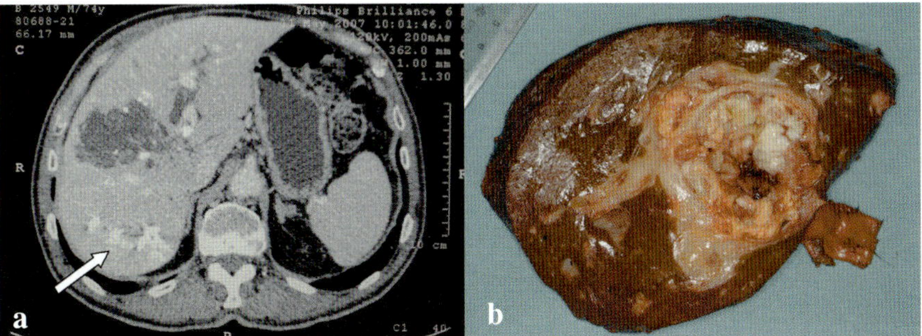

Fig. 1a,b A centrally located, intraductal-growth type of cholangiocarcinoma , treated with right portal-vein embolisation (*white arrow*) and right trisectionectomy with extrahepatic bile duct resection, **a** CT scan; **b** surgical specimen

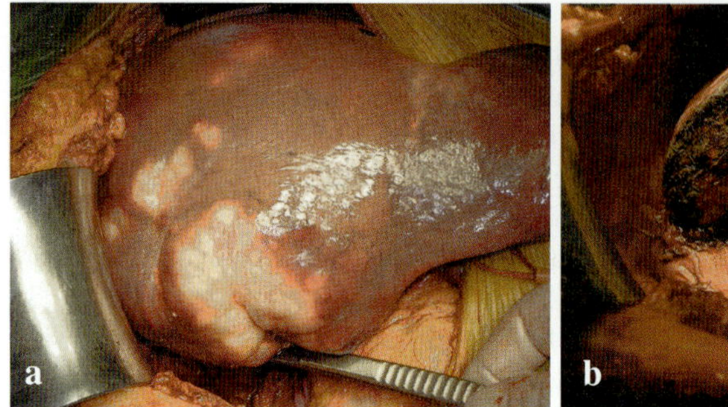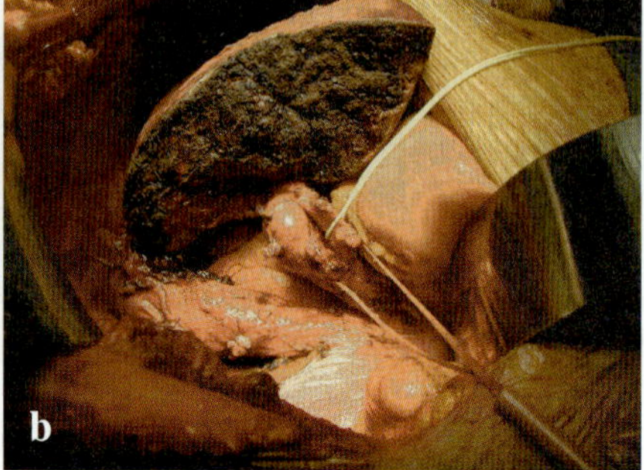

Fig. 2a,b Mass-forming type of cholangiocarcinoma with satellite lesions (**a**) treated with right hepatectomy and lymph-node dissection. Intraoperative field after resection (**b**)

The presence of intrahepatic metastases represents a negative independent factor that is always associated with very low survival similar to those of palliative treatment: Madariaga [1] reported a 3-year survival that is nil and no survivors after 14 months; Isa [22] found a median survival of 19 months; in the series of Nakagawa [15], none of the patients with multiple lesions and extended lymph-node involvement reached a survival of 3 years, although Uenishi [23] published a 3-year survival rate in such cases of 6%.

In the light of these results, surgical indications for multifocal lesions are the subject of debate. We believe that multifocal lesions with unilobar satellite nodules or located in the same segmental area of the main lesion can be resected if the programmed operation is of low risk and no other negative prognostic factors, such as nodal metastases, are present.

Multiple bilobar lesions or lymph-node metastases contraindicate surgical resection, since R0 resection is not possible. In these patients with lymph-node and intrahepatic metastases, the prognosis is as poor as that of non-resected patients, and adjuvant or neoadjuvant therapies must be considered.

Periductal-infiltrating-type (PI) neoplasms that spread along Glisson's sheath through lymphatic vessels, with a low incidence of spreading in the portal system, frequently show nodal involvement as well as perineural and vascular invasion. In these cases, the surgical approach is the same as for MF neoplasms and necessitates anatomic hepatic resection always in association with biliary-duct sampling and extrahepatic biliary resection, if the margins are positive. Lymph-node dissection is also indicated with the modalities described below.

Ultimately, mixed forms (MF+PI) of neoplasms are characterised by considerable biological aggressiveness, with vascular and lymph-node infiltration in 80% of the cases, intrahepatic metastases in 46% [10] and a worse prognosis than either MF or PI neoplasms. The 5-year survival rate is between 0 and 7% [16,22]. These poor results are the consequences of early intrahepatic and extrahepatic diffusion of the neoplasm, which makes it difficult to achieve R0 resection (Fig. 3).

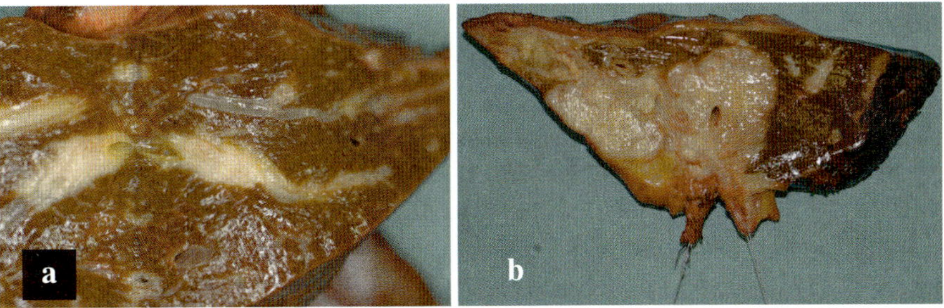

Fig. 3a,b Intrahepatic cholangiocarcinoma of the periductal infiltrating type (**a**). Intrahepatic cholangiocarcinoma of the combined mass-forming and periductal-infiltrating types (MF+PI) (**b**)

In these cases, the surgical approach is the same as for the PI type, i.e. anatomic hepatic resection and biliary-duct sampling with likely extrahepatic biliary resection. It must be kept in mind that patients with advanced PI or mixed form (MF+PI) of cholangiocarcinoma have not benefited from extended surgery (hepatic and biliary resection, extended lymphadenectomy) in terms of improved surgical outcome compared to conventional resection (hepatic resection alone), with increased rates of mortality and morbidity. The surgical indications are controversial in these cases and must be limited to patients without other negative prognostic factors (intrahepatic metastases and positive lymph nodes).

The size of the neoplasm does not represent a prognostic factor that limits surgical indication, even if small tumours show a better prognosis than large ones. This suggests that if radical removal of the tumour is technically feasible and can be accomplished safely, it should be performed independently of the size of the intrahepatic tumour [17].

Vascular involvement is present in 27–85% of patients [24] and represents a negative prognostic factor. Casavilla [25], in a series of 39 patients, found that those with vascular infiltration did not reach 5-year survival. However, Inoue [17] reported 5-year survival rates of 60 and 22% in patients without and with vascular infiltration, respectively; survival in the latter group was significantly better than in non-resected patients. Therefore vascular invasion, even if it is a negative prognostic factor, does not represent an absolute contraindication to surgery.

Indications for Lymphadenectomy

The rational extent of radical lymphadenectomy for ICC has not been clearly defined and there is no consensus on the role of lymph-node dissection [18,26]. The incidence of lymph-node metastasis in ICC is 43–62% [1,2,7,10,15,21].

Several series have shown that one of the strongest prognostic factors in ICC is lymph-node involvement [17,25,27,28]. All of these studies reported that no patients with lymph-node involvement survived for more than 3 years after surgery. Inoue [17] stated that lymph-node metastasis in MF neoplasms is a sign of non-curative disseminated disease, and therefore hepatectomy is contraindicated if metastatic involvement is observed at the time of lymph-node sampling. Nonetheless, Murakami [29] and Weber [5] reported long-term survivors (more than 5 years) with lymph-node metastasis. Ohtsuka [12] did not consider lymph-node involvement to be a significant prognostic factor in patients who underwent lymph-node dissection, with a few patients who survived more than 3 years.

Isa [22] reported 3-year survival rate in N+ patients of 6.7%, with a median survival of 10 months. Some authors have underlined the prognostic importance of the number of positive lymph nodes, analogous to gastric and colonic cancers: Suzuki [30] reported that 5-year survival in patients with a single lymph-node metastasis is 33%, and that patients with two or more lymph-node metastases do not survive beyond 2 years; Nakagawa [15] series had 3-year survival rates of 62, 50 and 0% in patients with N0 tumours, with one or two nodes and with more than three nodes, respectively.

These results suggest that, although lymph-node involvement may generally be associated with an unfavourable prognosis, long-term survival might be expected following aggressive surgical resection, including lymph-node dissection, in highly selected patients, providing that nodal diffusion, as confirmed by intraoperative sampling, is not beyond regional station.

In the presence of extensive nodal diffusion or in association with other negative prognostic factors, such as multifocal involvement, resection does not guarantee better results than palliative therapy and is therefore not recommended.

Major lymphatic spreading of ICC follows three routes: (1) through the hepatoduodenal ligament; (2) through the paracardial, lesser curvature and left gastric artery and (3) through the inferior phrenic artery or directly from the right liver to the lateral para-aortic group. Neoplasms located in the left lobe present either a right pathway of diffusion to the hepatoduodenal ligament (with N+ in 38% of patients) or a left pathway to the right paracardial stations, along the lesser curvature and left gastric artery (with N+ in 31% of patients) [31]. Consequently, the rational extent of radical lymphadenectomy should include not only the hepatoduodenal ligament with the hepatic artery, para-aortic, retro-pancreatic and mesenteric nodes but also the left gastric nodes, the perigastric nodes along the lesser curvature, and the right paracardial nodes, especially in left-located lesions [26].

Before surgical resection we always submit hepatoduodenal ligament nodes or grossly suspected nodes to frozen section. If more than three nodes or distant-station nodes are positive, the indication for hepatic resection becomes controversial and might be considered only in selected patients with low surgical risk and single lesion. In these cases, combination with adjuvant therapy must be considered.

Extrahepatic Metastases

The presence of peritoneal metastases detected with laparoscopy or laparotomy is an absolute contraindication to surgical operation. Isaji [10] reported that the outcome in 17 patients who underwent resection for stage IV B neoplasms was as poor as that in 12 patients who did not undergo resection, with no survivors after 2 years. In these cases, adjuvant therapy may be considered, even if satisfactory results have not been reported until now.

References

1. Madariaga JR, Iwatsuki S, Todo S et al (1998) Liver resection for hilar and peripheral cholangiocarcinomas: a study of 62 cases. Ann Surg 227(1):70–79
2. Yamanaka N, Okamoto E, Ando T et al (1995) Clinicopathologic spectrum of resected extraductal mass-forming intrahepatic cholangiocarcinoma. Cancer 76(12):2449–2456
3. Lieser MJ, Barry MK, Rowland C et al (1998) Surgical management of intrahepatic cholangiocarcinoma: a 31-year experience. J Hepatobiliary Pancreat Surg 5(1):41–47
4. Lang H, Sotiropoulos GC, Fruhauf NR (2005) Extended hepatectomy for intrahepatic cholangiocellular carcinoma (ICC): when is it worthwhile? Single center experience with 27 resections in 50 patients over a 5-year period. Ann Surg. Jan 241(1):134–143
5. Weber SM, Jarnagin WR, Klimstra D (2001) Intrahepatic cholangiocarcinoma: resectability, recurrence pattern, and outcomes. J Am Coll Surg 193(4):384–391
6. Goere D, Wagholikar GD, Pessaux P et al (2006) Utility of staging laparoscopy in subsets of biliary cancers : laparoscopy is a powerful diagnostic tool in patients with intrahepatic and gallbladder carcinoma. Surg Endosc 20(5):721–725
7. Cherqui D, Tantawi B, Alon R et al (1995) Intrahepatic cholangiocarcinoma. Results of aggressive surgical management. Arch Surg 130(10):1073–1078
8. Harvey CJ, Blomley MJ, Eckersley RJ et al (2000) Pulse-inversion mode imaging of liver specific microbubbles: improved detection of subcentimetre metastases. Lancet 355(9206):807–808
9. Skjoldbye B, Pedersen MH, Struckmann J et al (2002) Improved detection and biopsy of solid liver lesions using pulse-inversion ultrasound scanning and contrast agent infusion. Ultrasound Med Biol 28(4):439–444
10. Isaji S, Kawarada Y, Taoka H et al (1999) Clinicopathological features and outcome of hepatic resection for intrahepatic cholangiocarcinoma in Japan. J Hepatobiliary Pancreat Surg 6(2):108–116
11. Harrison LE, Fong Y, Klimstra DS et al (1998) Surgical treatment of 32 patients with peripheral intrahepatic cholangiocarcinoma. Br J Surg 85(8):1068–1070
12. Ohtsuka M, Ito H, Kimura F et al (2002) Results of surgical treatment for intrahepatic cholangiocarcinoma and clinicopathological factors influencing survival. Br J Surg 89(12):1525–1531
13. Morimoto Y, Tanaka Y, Ito T et al (2003) Long-term survival and prognostic factors in the surgical treatment for intrahepatic cholangiocarcinoma. J Hepatobiliary Pancreat Surg 10(6):432–440
14. Huang JL, Biehl TR, Lee FT et al (2004) Outcomes after resection of cholangiocellular carcinoma. Am J Surg 187(5):612–617
15. Nakagawa T, Kamiyama T, Kurauchi N et al (2005) Number of lymph-node metastases is a significant prognostic factor in intrahepatic cholangiocarcinoma. World J Surg 29(6):728–733

16. Yamamoto M, Takasaki K, Yoshikawa T et al (1998) Does gross appearance indicate prognosis in intrahepatic cholangiocarcinoma? J Surg Oncol 69(3):162–167

17. Inoue K, Makuuchi M, Takayama T et al (2000) Long-term survival and prognostic factors in the surgical treatment of mass-forming type cholangiocarcinoma. Surgery 127(5):498–505

18. Shimada M, Yamashita Y, Aishima S et al (2001) Value of lymph node dissection during resection of intrahepatic cholangiocarcinoma. Br J Surg 88(11):1463–1466

19. Shirabe K, Shimada M, Harimoto N et al (2002) Intrahepatic cholangiocarcinoma: its mode of spreading and therapeutic modalities. Surgery 131(1 Suppl):S159-S164

20. Sakamoto E, Hayakawa N, Kamiya J et al (1999) Treatment strategy for mucin-producing intrahepatic cholangiocarcinoma: value of percutaneous transhepatic biliary drainage and cholangioscopy. World J Surg 23(10):1038–1043; discussion 1043–1044

21. Sasaki A, Aramaki M, Kawano K et al (1998) Intrahepatic peripheral cholangiocarcinoma: mode of spread and choice of surgical treatment. Br J Surg 85(9):1206–1209

22. Isa T, Kusano T, Shimoji H et al (2001) Predictive factors for long-term survival in patients with intrahepatic cholangiocarcinoma. Am. J. Surg 181(6):507–511

23. Uenishi T, Yamazaki O, Yamamoto T et al (2005) Serosal invasion in TNM staging of mass-forming intrahepatic cholangiocarcinoma. J Hepatobiliary Pancreat Surg 12(6):479–483

24. Weinbren K, Mutum SS (1983) Pathological aspects of cholangiocarcinoma. J Pathol 139(2):217–238

25. Casavilla FA, Marsh JW, Iwatsuki S et al (1997) Hepatic resection and transplantation for peripheral cholangiocarcinoma. J Am Coll Surg 185(5):429–436

26. Tsuji T, Hiraoka T, Kanemitsu K et al (2001) Lymphatic spreading pattern of intrahepatic cholangiocarcinoma. Surgery 129(4):401–407

27. Uenishi T, Hirohashi K, Kubo S et al (2001) Clinicopathological factors predicting outcome after resection of mass-forming intrahepatic cholangiocarcinoma. Br J Surg 88(7):969–974

28. Chu KM, Lai EC, Al-Hadeedi S et al (1997) Intrahepatic cholangiocarcinoma. World J Surg 21(3):301–305

29. Murakami Y, Yokoyama T, Takesue Y (2000) Long-term survival of peripheral intrahepatic cholangiocarcinoma with metastasis to the para-aortic lymph nodes. Surgery 127(1):105–106

30. Suzuki S, Sakaguchi T, Yokoi Y et al (2002) Clinicopathological prognostic factors and impact of surgical treatment of mass-forming intrahepatic cholangiocarcinoma. World J Surg 26(6):687–693

31. Okami J, Dono K, Sakon M et al (2003) Patterns of regional lymph-node involvement in intrahepatic cholangiocarcinoma of the left lobe. J Gastrointest Surg 7(7):850–856

Results of Surgery

An analysis of the results of surgery for intrahepatic cholangiocarcinoma (ICC), as reported in the literature is difficult, because the patient-selection criteria are not homogeneous, and the series of cases are limited by the rarity of the disease and the prolonged amount of time needed for data collection. Prognostic factors related to the characteristics of the neoplasm were analysed previously. Herein, only the early and late results of surgical operation are considered.

Morbidity and Mortality

Surgery of ICC is often carried out in advanced neoplasms, with the need to perform extended hepatic resection in 21–100% of such patients [1]. Hepatic resection is associated with extrahepatic biliary resection in 60–74% of the cases and with portal (4–26%) or arterial (0–10%) resection and reconstruction. Resection of the diaphragm (10%) and vein cava (7%) occur less frequently [2–6]. Even with improvements in surgical technique and perioperative management, extended hepatectomies still entail significant mortality and morbidity. In the majority of studies, mortality was <5% and some authors reported no mortality at all (Table 1). Mortality is often related to extended hepatic resection or to associated procedures, such as vascular and biliary reconstruction or hepato-pancreatectomy: in these cases, mortality increases to 7–9.5% [1,3].

The complications after surgical exeresis of ICC range from 20 to 50% (Table 1) and are comparable to those following common hepatic resection of a non-cirrhotic liver. Postoperative hepatic failure is less frequent than after resection for hilar neoplasms and occurs in about 10% of patients. Other complications are subphrenic collections (4–8%), biliary leakage (8–12%), pulmonary embolism (6%) and respiratory complications (4%) [1,4,7,8].

The complication rate is also related to the type of operation: 45% in simple hepatectomy and 56% in patients who underwent extended hepatectomy with vascular, diaphragmatic or hilar resection. Exploratory laparotomy has a relevant complication rate of 17% [1].

A. Guglielmi, A. Ruzzenente, C. Iacono (eds.) *Surgical Treatment of Hilar and ICC*.
© Springer 2008

Table 1 Hepatic resection for intrahepatic cholangiocarcinoma: morbidity and mortality

Author	Year	Patients	Morbidity (%)	30-Day mortality (%)
Valverde [7]	1999	30	36	0
Isaji [9]	1999	36	8	0
Kawarada [10]	2002	37	21.6	0
Suzuki [3]	2002	19	33	9.5
Morimoto [4]	2003	49	35	3.8
Ohtsuka [11]	2003	50	50	8
Lang [1]	2005	27	52	6
DeOliveira [12]	2007	44	35	4

Long-Term Survival

The prognosis after ICC resection is still unsatisfactory. The 5-year overall survival rate varies from 14 to 36% and does not exceed 40% in the majority of series, even in the more recent ones (Table 2). The main reasons for these results are the late diagnosis of disease in the absence of specific symptoms and in the absence of risk categories for patients with cirrhosis who undergo screening for hepatocellular carcinoma. Spreading of disease through intrahepatic metastases or diffusion in lymphatic and perineural structures occurs in the early stages and lesions located near the hepatic hilum show early infiltration of vascular and biliary structures. For these reasons, curative resection is often difficult to achieve. The resectability rate of ICC is variable, ranging between 19 and 74% [1,13–15]. In attempts to obtain significant improvements in patient survival, many authors have applied the criteria of extended surgery in 21–100% of patients. However, at present, there are not clear survival advantages that support this surgical approach (Table 3).

The percentage of radical hepatic resection (R0) reported in the literature varies from 30 to 80%. The radicality of the operation depends on the gross tumour type and its location; in fact, Isajii reported a surgical radicality of 46% for mass-forming (MF) type, 33% for periductal-infiltrating (PI) type and 6% for the combined (MF+PI) type of neoplasm. The same author noted 50% radicality in peripheral lesions and 0% in central ones [9]. The site determines long-term outcome too, with a survival rate for peripheral cholangiocarcinoma of 48% and 37% at 3 and 5 years, respectively, while all patients with central cholangiocarcinoma died within 2 years; in this latter group, a high percentage had undergone R1 resection.

Very frequently, the resected margins contain microscopic infiltrations that were not detected either at surgery or by intraoperative ultrasound. This occurs even after surgery with curative intent and has been reported in 36–41% of the

Table 2 Outcome after surgery for primary intrahepatic cholangiocarcinoma

Author	Year	Patients	N+ (%)	IM (%)	Median survival (months)	Survival		
						1-Year	3-Year	5-Year
Yamamoto [16]	1992	20	25	35	-	66	36	36
Cherqui [17]	1995	14	14	29	14	58	-	-
Chou [18]	1995	19	58	-	9	49	37	-
Yamanaka [14]	1995	26	58	46	-	41	14	14
Pichlmayr [19]	1995	32	22	41	13	-	25	21
Berdah [20]	1996	19	37	26	15	67	-	32
Casavilla [21]	1997	34	17	44	-	60	37	31
Madariaga [13]	1998	34	18	47	19	67	40	35
Nozaki [22]	1998	47	32	36	-	59	30	27
Isaji [9]	1999	36	46	54	-	44	24	24
Valverde [7]	1999	30	37	26	15	67	-	32
Isa [23]	2001	27	55	19	-	52	33	22
Okabayashi [24]	2001	60	36	46	20	68	35	29
Suzuki [3]	2002	19	74	32	18	63	35	28
Ohtsuka [11]	2002	48	36	-	25	62	38	23
Morimoto [4]	2003	49	32	-	-	68	44	32
Uenishi [25]	2005	63	33	36	18	61	40	33
Lang [6]	2006	54	37	54	25	64	37	28

IM, Intrahepatic metastases

cases, mainly in patients with advanced lesions and/or centro-hepatic disease [1,17].

R0 resection is the only approach that can offer acceptable long-term results, with 5-year survival rates 36–54%; in contrast, R1 non-radical resections offer a 5-year survival rate of 0–21% (Table 4). The prognostic significance of determining TNM stage, according to the sixth edition of the UICC/AJCC manual, is

Table 3 Survival according to rate of extended hepatic resection

Author	Year	Patients	Extended resection (%)	3-Year survival	5-Year survival
Yamamoto [16]	1992	20	45	37.6	37.6
Casavilla [21]	1997	34	44	37	31
Chu [26]	1997	39	21	24	16
Chou [18]	1998	23	0	20	-
Harrison [27]	1998	32	50	56	42
Lieser [15]	1998	28	0	60	-
Madariaga [13]	1998	34	53	40	35
Roayaie [28]	1998	16	69	64	21
Weimann [29]	2000	95	-	31	21
Inoue [30]	2000	52	44	36	36
Weber [31]	2001	33	45	55	31
Kawarada [19]	2002	37	51	34	24
Lang [1]	2005	27	100	55	-

still under evaluation. Huang reported a median survival of 57 months for stage I patients, 33 months for those stage II, 26 months for those with stage IIIA and 14 months for patients with stage IIIC. The author underlined the negative prognostic significance of lymph-node metastases (stage IIIC UICC/AJCC), in that none of the stage IIIC patients had survived at 5 years [8].

Conclusive data of validation are also lacking for the Japanese staging system proposed by the Liver Cancer Study Group of Japan. Uenishi observed a significant difference in survival between stage I, II and III patients, with 5-year survival rate of 100, 54 and 44%, respectively [25]. The author proposed a new classification that omits the parameter "serosal invasion" from the formulation of T-stage. With this novel grouping, he obtained survival curves that showed statistical differences between the different stages: 5-year survival in stage I was 100%, in stage II 62%, in stage III 25%, and in stage IV 7% [25].

Since the number of long-term survivors (>5 years) is very small (13–26%), the prognostic factors pertaining to these patients have been analyzed [3,23,32]. Comprehensively, 25% of the long-term survivors were those who present with intraductal growth (IG)- or MF-type neoplasms, have no lymph-node metastasis (but in two cases with only one positive lymph node), no portal or biliary invasion and perineural invasion [3]. All patients underwent curative R0 resection.

Table 4 Long-term survival according to the presence of residual tumour after surgery

Author	Year	Patients	R0 (%)	3-Year survival following R0 (%)	5-Year survival following R1 (%)
Casavilla [21]	1997	34	58	38 months	7 months
Harrison [27]	1998	32	81	63 months	9 months
Yamamoto [2]	1998	70	50	53	4
Isaji [12]	1999	36	33	61 (3-year)	5 (3-year)
Isa [23]	2001	27	67	43	0
Okabayashi [24]	2001	60	45	39	16
Morimoto [4]	2003	49	67	40–58	0
Nakagawa [33]	2005	30	82	55 (3-year)	0 (3-year)
Uenishi [25]	2005	63	81	39	0
Ikai [5][a]	2005	1364	59	43	21
Lang [6]	2006	54	55	48	0
Miwa [34]	2006	41	76	36	0

[a]Japanese nationwide follow-up survey

Table 5 Mean time to recurrence of intrahepatic cholangiocarcinoma after surgery, as reported in the literature

Author	Year	Patients	Recurrence (%)	Mean time to recurrence
Valverde [7]	1999	30	82	2–56 months
Okabayashi [24]	2001	60	71	<6 months
Huang [8]	2004	31	58	13 months
Suzuki [3]	2002	19	78	-
Lang [1]	2005	27	38	4–36 months

Recurrence

Recurrence after R0 resection is frequent, ranging from 38 to 82%; it is usually early and most often occurs within 2 years postoperatively. Huang reported a median time of disease relapse of 13 months [8].

The most frequent sites of recurrence are: intrahepatic (74%), peritoneal (22%), bone (11%), lymph node (11%) and, less frequently, distantly (lung, abdominal wall) [34]. The factors related to the onset of recurrence are many and are associated with gross tumour type and extent of disease. The former determines the site of recurrence, with the MF form particularly associated with an increase frequency of intrahepatic recurrences (68% of all recurrences), while lymph nodal recurrence is more frequent in MF+PI and PI neoplasms (Table 6).

Concerning the extent of disease, Miwa used univariate and multivariate analysis to identify other significant factors: hilar location, size >45 mm, portal-vein involvement, presence of lymph-node metastases, serum Ca19-9 values >37 U/ml; the odds ratios were 2.9, 5.4, 6.7, 15.8 and 22.5, respectively [34].

The treatment of recurrence changes as a function of the site and extent and in the majority of the cases is palliative and non-surgical. In isolated cases, long-term survival was reported after resection of intrahepatic or loco-regional recurrences [3,35]. Cherqui performed three re-resections (including a transplantation) to treat recurrent MF cholangiocarcinoma and reported good long-term outcome [17]. Indications for the most appropriate treatment of recurrence, either surgical resection or a palliative approach, have not been established in the literature. However, in highly selected cases involving recurrences that can be resected radically, surgical treatment can offer an acceptable long-term outcome.

Table 6 Site of first recurrence according to gross tumour type [20]

Gross type	Patients	Recurrence	Liver	Lymph nodes	Peritoneum	Bile duct	Remote organs
MF	21	16	11	1	1	0	3
MF+PI	15	11	4	4	1	1	0
PI	2	2	0	2	0	0	0
IG	9	1	0	0	0	0	1
Total	47	30	15	7	2	1	4

References

1. Lang H, Sotiropoulos GC, Fruhauf NR et al (2005) Extended hepatectomy for intrahepatic cholangiocellular carcinoma (ICC): when is it worthwhile? Single center experience with 27 resections in 50 patients over a 5-year period. Ann Surg 241(1):134–143

2. Yamamoto M, Takasaki K, Yoshikawa T et al (1998) Does gross appearance indicate prognosis in intrahepatic cholangiocarcinoma? J Surg Oncol 69(3):162–167
3. Suzuki S, Sakaguchi T, Yokoi Y et al (2002) Clinicopathological prognostic factors and impact of surgical treatment of mass-forming intrahepatic cholangiocarcinoma. World J Surg 26(6):687–693
4. Morimoto Y, Tanaka Y, Ito T et al (2003) Long-term survival and prognostic factors in the surgical treatment for intrahepatic cholangiocarcinoma. J Hepatobiliary Pancreat Surg 10(6):432–440
5. Ikai I, Arii S, Ichida T et al (2005) Report of the 16th follow-up survey of primary liver cancer. Hepatol Res 32(3):163–172
6. Lang H, Kaiser GM, Zopf T et al (2006) Surgical therapy of hilar cholangiocarcinoma. Chirurg 77(4):325–334
7. Valverde A, Bonhomme N, Farges O et al (1999) Resection of intrahepatic cholangiocarcinoma: a Western experience. J Hepatobiliary Pancreat Surg 6(2):122–127
8. Huang JL, Biehl TR, Lee FT et al (2004) Outcomes after resection of cholangiocellular carcinoma. Am J Surg 187(5):612–617
9. Isaji S, Kawarada Y, Taoka H et al (1999) Clinicopathological features and outcome of hepatic resection for intrahepatic cholangiocarcinoma in Japan. J Hepatobiliary Pancreat Surg 6(2):108–116
10. Kawarada Y, Yamagiwa K, Das BC (2002) Analysis of the relationships between clinico-pathologic factors and survival time in intrahepatic cholangiocarcinoma. Am J Surg 183(6):679–685
11. Ohtsuka M, Ito H, Kimura F et al (2002) Results of surgical treatment for intrahepatic cholangiocarcinoma and clinicopathological factors influencing survival. Br J Surg 89(12):1525–1531
12. DeOliveira ML, Cunningham SC, Cameron JL et al (2007) Cholangiocarcinoma: thirty-one-year experience with 564 patients at a single institution. Ann Surg 245(5):755–762
13. Madariaga JR, Iwatsuki S, Todo S et al (1998) Liver resection for hilar and peripheral cholangiocarcinomas: a study of 62 cases. Ann Surg 227(1):70–79
14. Yamanaka N, Okamoto E, Ando T et al (1995) Clinicopathologic spectrum of resected extraductal mass-forming intrahepatic cholangiocarcinoma. Cancer 76(12):2449–2456
15. Lieser MJ, Barry MK, Rowland C et al (1998) Surgical management of intrahepatic cholangiocarcinoma: a 31-year experience. J Hepatobiliary Pancreat Surg 5(1):41–47
16. Yamamoto J, Kosuge T, Takayama T et al (1992) Surgical treatment of intrahepatic cholangiocarcinoma: four patients surviving more than five years. Surgery 111(6):617–622
17. Cherqui D, Tantawi B, Alon R et al (1995) Intrahepatic cholangiocarcinoma. Results of aggressive surgical management. Arch Surg 130(10):1073–1078
18. Chou FF, Sheen-Chen SM, Chen CL et al (1995) Prognostic factors of resectable intrahepatic cholangiocarcinoma. J Surg Oncol 59(1):40–44
19. Pichlmayr R, Lamesch P, Weimann A et al (1995) Surgical treatment of cholangiocellular carcinoma. World J Surg 19(1):83–88
20. Berdah SV, Delpero JR, Garcia S et al (1996) A western surgical experience of peripheral cholangiocarcinoma. Br J Surg 83(11):1517–1521
21. Casavilla FA, Marsh JW, Iwatsuki S et al (1997) Hepatic resection and transplantation for peripheral cholangiocarcinoma. J Am Coll Surg 185(5):429–436
22. Nozaki Y, Yamamoto M, Ikai I et al (1998) Reconsideration of the lymph-node metastasis pattern (N factor) from intrahepatic cholangiocarcinoma using the International Union Against Cancer TNM staging system for primary liver carcinoma. Cancer 83(9):1923–1929
23. Isa T, Kusano T, Shimoji H et al (2001) Predictive factors for long-term survival in patients with intrahepatic cholangiocarcinoma. Am J Surg 181(6):507–511
24. Okabayashi T, Yamamoto J, Kosuge T et al (2001) A new staging system for mass-forming intrahepatic cholangiocarcinoma: analysis of preoperative and postoperative variables. Cancer 92(9):2374–2383

25. Uenishi T, Yamazaki O, Yamamoto T et al (2005) Serosal invasion in TNM staging of mass-forming intrahepatic cholangiocarcinoma. J Hepatobiliary Pancreat Surg 12(6):479–483
26. Chu KM, Lai EC, Al-Hadeedi S et al (1997) Intrahepatic cholangiocarcinoma. World J Surg 21(3):301–305
27. Harrison LE, Fong Y, Klimstra DS et al (1998) Surgical treatment of 32 patients with peripheral intrahepatic cholangiocarcinoma. Br J Surg 85(8):1068–1070
28. Roayaie S, Guarrera JV, Ye MQ et al (1998) Aggressive surgical treatment of intrahepatic cholangiocarcinoma: predictors of outcomes. J Am Coll Surg 187(4):365–372
29. Weimann A, Varnholt H, Schlitt HJ et al (2000) Retrospective analysis of prognostic factors after liver resection and transplantation for cholangiocellular carcinoma. Br J Surg 87(9):1182–1187
30. Inoue K, Makuuchi M, Takayama T et al (2000) Long-term survival and prognostic factors in the surgical treatment of mass-forming type cholangiocarcinoma. Surgery 127(5):498–505
31. Weber SM, Jarnagin WR, Klimstra D et al (2001) Intrahepatic cholangiocarcinoma: resectability, recurrence pattern, and outcomes. J Am Coll Surg 193(4):384–391
32. Jan YY, Yeh CN, Yeh TS et al (2005) Clinicopathological factors predicting long-term overall survival after hepatectomy for peripheral cholangiocarcinoma. World J Surg 29(7):894–898
33. Nakagawa T, Kamiyama T, Kurauchi N et al (2005) Number of lymph-node metastases is a significant prognostic factor in intrahepatic cholangiocarcinoma. World J Surg 29(6):728–733
34. Miwa S, Miyagawa S, Kobayashi A et al (2006) Predictive factors for intrahepatic cholangiocarcinoma recurrence in the liver following surgery. J Gastroenterol 41(9):893–900
35. Kurosaki I, Hatakeyama K (2005) Repeated hepatectomy for recurrent intrahepatic cholangiocarcinoma: report of two cases. Eur J Gastroenterol Hepatol 17(1):125–130

The Role of Liver Transplantation

Surgical resection is the only therapeutic approach that produces good survival results for patients with intrahepatic cholangiocarcinoma. However, advanced disease stage and infiltration to vascular structures often require extended and complicated hepatic resections, such that curative operation is not always possible.

From an oncologic point of view, transplantation should allow a remarkable increase of surgical radicality and the possibility to obtain curative treatment even in patients who cannot undergo hepatic resection because of the extent of disease and concomitant chronic liver disease. Unfortunately, the results of hepatic transplantation of patients with intrahepatic cholangiocarcinoma are still poor and limited to few tens of cases without homogeneous indications. Some authors reported that the results are even worse than those for extrahepatic cholangiocarcinoma [1,2], whereas others reported a similar outcome [3–5].

Initially, patients who underwent transplantation for intrahepatic cholangiocarcinoma was restricted to those with advanced disease who were excluded from resection. At the end of the 1980s, Ringe reported on 10 patients who had a median survival of 4 months and a 90% recurrence rate [6]. The Pichlmayr group, with a more extensive follow-up time confirmed these results and reported a 3-year survival rate of 0% [7]. More recent experience suggests a slight increase of overall survival and disease-free survival; Casavilla reported 3 and 5-year survival rates of 29 and 18% in 20 patients with unresectable cholangiocarcinoma; nine patients underwent cluster transplantation [5].

Weimann, adopting similar indications in 23 patients, obtained 1- and 3-year survival rates of 21 and 4% and no survivors after 5 years. Robles, in a multicentre Spanish study, reported more promising data, with 3- and 5-year survival rates of 65 and 42%, respectively [8]. Currently, there are no precise indications reported in the literature.

Recurrence after transplantation is quite frequent. In the series of Casavilla, the recurrence rate was 55%, with a disease-free survival rate of 31% at 3- and 5-year [5]. Other authors have reported similar results. Robles determined 3- and 5-year disease-free survival rates of 45 and 27%, with 23% of the patients disease-free at 10 years [8] (Table 1).

A. Guglielmi, A. Ruzzenente, C. Iacono (eds.) *Surgical Treatment of Hilar and ICC.*
© Springer 2008

Table 1 Liver transplantation for intrahepatic cholangiocarcinoma: survival and disease-free survival (DFS)

Author	Year	Institution	N	Survival			DFS		
				1-Year	3-Year	5-Year	1-Year	3-Year	5 Year
O'Grady [4]	1988	King's College	13	38	10	10	-	-	-
Pichlmayr (2) [9]	1995	Hannover	18	13.9	-	-	-	-	-
Yokoyama [10]	1990	Pittsburgh	2	50	0	-	-	-	-
Casavilla [5]	1997	Pittsburgh	20	70	29	18	67	31	31
Meyer [11]	2000	Cincinnati registry[a]	207	72	-	23	-	-	-
Shimoda [12]	2001	UCLA	16	62	39	-	70	35	-
Robles [8]	2004	Spanish surveya	23	77	65	42	68	45	27
Becker N [13]	2007	UNOS[a]	280	74	-	38	-	-	-

[a]Nationwide follow-up survey

The onset of recurrence is usually relatively soon: about two-thirds of recurrences appear within 2 years post-operatively. The median survival of patients with disease relapse is only 6 months [8]. The most common site of recurrences is intra-abdominal, mainly in the transplanted liver [8,14].

Despite the limited number of series, prognostic factors that affect survival and recurrence after transplantation have been identified. Casavilla, in his study of 20 patients, showed that prognostic factors were related to overall survival and to disease-free survival. Multivariate analysis demonstrated a correlation between prognosis and positive margins, multifocality and the presence of lymph-node metastases, with an odds ratio (OR) of 1.74, 1.63 and 1.60, respectively. Median survival was 14.3 months in patients with nodal metastases vs 19.2 months in N0 patients [5]. Conversely, Robles found that the presence after perineural invasion and TNM UICC stage are related to prognosis of transplantation for cholangiocarcinoma. Patients in stage I–II disease had 3- and 5-year survival rates of 80%and 40%, while the rates of those in stage III–IVa were 46 and 31%, respectively ($p<0.05$) [8].

Intrahepatic as well as extrahepatic cholangiocarcinoma can be identified incidentally during transplantation for primary sclerosing cholangitis. Even if definitive results regarding the prognostic advantages of transplantation after incidental cholangiocarcinoma vs preoperatively diagnosed cholangiocarcinoma have not been published, it seems clear that an earlier stage of disease detection ensures better outcome [12].

Hepato-cholangiocarcinoma is a rare variant form. Its histologic patterns resemble both hepatocarcinoma and cholangiocarcinoma. Reports in the literature are few but the prognosis in patients who underwent transplantation is not different from the disappointing results of intrahepatic cholangiocarcinoma [1,11,12,15].

Some authors have reported their experience with cluster transplantation (liver, duodenum-pancreas, part of jejunum) in patients with advanced cholangiocarcinoma infiltrating other organs; however, the results are inadequate, the number of patients is small and the follow-up time is too short to be able to draw conclusions. The University of Pittsburgh reported a 5-year survival of 30% in nine patients with advanced and unresectable cholangiocarcinomas (stage IV and IVa) who underwent to cluster transplantation [5,16].

There are no data in the literature on the results of adjuvant and neoadjuvant treatments in transplantation for intrahepatic cholangiocarcinoma. In the light of the current data, transplantation does not represent a treatment option for intrahepatic cholangiocarcinoma and its use must be restricted to clinical trials.

References

1. Pichlmayr R, Weimann A, Oldhafer KJ et al (1995) Role of liver transplantation in the treatment of unresectable liver cancer. World J Surg 19(6):807–813
2. Penn I (1991) Hepatic transplantation for primary and metastatic cancers of the liver. Surgery 110(4):726–34; discussion 734–735
3. Nakeeb A, Pitt HA, Sohn TA et al (1996) Cholangiocarcinoma. A spectrum of intrahepatic, perihilar, and distal tumours. Ann Surg 224(4):463–473; discussion 473–475
4. O'Grady JG, Polson RJ, Rolles K et al (1988) Liver transplantation for malignant disease. Results in 93 consecutive patients. Ann Surg 207(4):373–379
5. Casavilla FA, Marsh JW, Iwatsuki S et al (1997) Hepatic resection and transplantation for peripheral cholangiocarcinoma. J Am Coll Surg 185(5):429–436
6. Ringe B, Wittekind C, Bechstein WO et al (1989) The role of liver transplantation in hepatobiliary malignancy. A retrospective analysis of 95 patients with particular regard to tumour stage and recurrence. Ann Surg 209(1):88–98
7. Pichlmayr R, Weimann A, Ringe B (1994)Indications for liver transplantation in hepatobiliary malignancy. Hepatology 20(1 Pt 2):33S-40S
8. Robles R, Figueras J, Turrion VS et al (2004) Spanish experience in liver transplantation for hilar and peripheral cholangiocarcinoma. Ann Surg 239(2):265–271

9. Pichlmayr R, Weimann A, Oldhafer KJ et al (1995) Role of liver transplantation in the treatment of unresectable liver cancer. World J Surg 19(6):807–813

10. Yokoyama I, Todo S, Iwatsuki S, Starzl TE (1990) Liver transplantation in the treatment of primary liver cancer. Hepatogastroenterology 37(2):188–193

11. Meyer CG, Penn I, James L (2000) Liver transplantation for cholangiocarcinoma: results in 207 patients. Transplantation 69(8):1633–1637

12. Shimoda M, Farmer DG, Colquhoun SD et al (2001) Liver transplantation for cholangiocellular carcinoma: analysis of a single-center experience and review of the literature. Liver Transpl 7(12):1023–1033

13. Becker N, Rodriguez J, Barshes N et al (2007) Outcome analysis for 280 patients with cholangiocarcinoma treated with liver transplantation over 18-year period. HPB 9(1): 74–75 (abs)

14. Weimann A, Varnholt H, Schlitt HJ et al (2000) Retrospective analysis of prognostic factors after liver resection and transplantation for cholangiocellular carcinoma. Br J Surg 87(9):1182–1187

15. Pichlmayr R, Lamesch P, Weimann A et al (1995) Surgical treatment of cholangiocellular carcinoma. World J Surg 19(1):83–88

16. Alessiani M, Tzakis A, Todo S et al (1995) Assessment of five-year experience with abdominal organ cluster transplantation. J Am Coll Surg 180(1):1–9

Adjuvant and Palliative Treatments

The role of adjuvant and palliative chemo- and radiotherapy in the treatment of intrahepatic cholangiocarcinoma (ICC) is controversial. There are no prospective and randomised studies or large series that provide conclusive indications regarding the efficacy of these therapies in ICC. Moreover, the majority of oncologic papers in the literature that address this topic include intrahepatic and extrahepatic (hilar, middle and distal) cancers and even gallbladder carcinoma. Consequently, specific data for each localisation concerning treatment indication, dosage, type of approach and results are lacking.

Adjuvant Therapy

The different forms of adjuvant therapy are systemic and loco-regional chemotherapy, radiotherapy, transcatheter hepatic arterial chemoembolisation (TACE), immunotherapy and monoclonal-antibody therapies. There is not complete agreement on the parameters that should be used to select those patients who will benefit from adjuvant treatment after surgery. Some investigators have stated that positive margins or local recurrence represent indications to adjuvant treatment [1], others consider positive lymph nodes, particularly second-order and para-aortic [2] nodes, and others base their decision on the presence of UICC stage III and IV disease [3]. Miwa concluded that patients who should receive adjuvant therapy are those with elevated serum Ca19-9 levels and preoperative jaundice [4].

Due to the numerous therapeutic protocols that have been proposed, it is almost impossible to compare data and to evaluate the real efficacy of adjuvant treatment.

A. Guglielmi, A. Ruzzenente, C. Iacono (eds.) *Surgical Treatment of Hilar and ICC.*
© Springer 2008

Chemotherapy

The chemotherapeutic agents most commonly used to treat ICC are 5-FU and gemcitabine alone or in chemotherapeutic association with epirubicin, cisplatin, mitomycin C, doxorubicin, leucovorin, methotrexate and interferon.

If the reports that analysed only intrahepatic cholangiocarcinoma are evaluated [1,5–8], then it can be stated that adjuvant treatment seems to provide advantages for long-term survival compared to patients treated by surgery alone. Yi-Yin Jan reported a relative risk for survival of 1.823 (95% CI: 1.414, 2.353; $p<0.001$) for patients with positive section margins or local recurrence who underwent surgery alone vs. postoperative chemotherapy with a 5-FU-based regimen [1]. Nevertheless other authors have stated that there is insufficient evidence supporting the use of post surgical adjuvant therapy [9–12].

Radiotherapy

Adjuvant radiotherapy is usually indicated in the presence of positive resection margins or local recurrence [1], with better results in treated vs. non-treated patients. Zeng [13] considers adjuvant radiotherapy to be indicated also in patients who undergo resection of ICC with synchronous or metachronous lymph-node metastases. The median total dose of external radiation therapy used by this group was 50 Gy (range 30–60 Gy), administered in daily doses of 2 Gy/fraction, five times a week. A comparison of the results of 16 treated patients vs. 14 patients who underwent hepatectomy alone showed better survival in the radiotherapy group (median survival 468 vs. 211 days, respectively, $p=0.075$). However other authors [10] did not show any patient benefits after adjuvant radiotherapy.

Transcatheter Hepatic Arterial Chemoembolisation

This type of adjuvant approach was used by Xiao-Hui Fu [5], who subsequently evaluated the results in 79 patients with mass-forming (MF) cholangiocarcinoma. Adjuvant therapy with TACE was administered (1–3 times postoperatively) to 29 patients and 50 underwent surgery alone. Median survival was 16 months in the former group vs. 8 months in the latter ($p=0.0389$).

Immunotherapy

Recently, immunotherapy with CD3-activated T cells and tumour lysate- or peptide-pulse dendrite cells has been introduced as adjuvant post-surgical treatment in patients with advanced cholangiocarcinoma. This approach seems to decrease the percentage of recurrences [14].

Radiofrequency Ablation

As for other malignant lesions of the liver, different types of treatments, including those involving chemo/radiotherapy, have been used to treat ICC. In the literature, there are reports describing the treatment of small intrahepatic cholangiocarcinomas [15,16] and of recurrence after resection [17] by means of radiofrequency. Chiou reported data on 10 patients with cholangiocarcinoma who were treated with RFA. The tumour ranged in size between 1.9 and 6.8 cm; complete necrosis was obtained in eight tumours (5 out of 5 tumours with <3 cm in size, 2 out of 3 tumours with sizes between 3.1 and 5 cm, and 1 out of 3 tumours >5 cm) [16]. There are no data on the efficacy of the treatment or on the long-term results regarding local recurrence and survival.

Palliative Therapy

Chemotherapy

Khan [9], in the consensus document of guidelines for the diagnosis and treatment of cholangiocarcinoma, reported: "to date, a review of over 65 disparate studies using chemotherapy and/or radiations suggests that was no strong evidence of survival benefit. However, most studies were small, lacked control groups (phase II) and were difficult to interpret."

Data from a phase II study suggested that gemcitabine monotherapy is an active and well-tolerated treatment. Combinations of gemcitabine with cisplatin, gemcitabine and oxaliplatin have demonstrated promising activity [18].

Other palliative treatments are obtained by intra-arterial injection of chemotherapeutic agents (5-FU, gemcitabine, or cisplatin and epirubicin) into the hepatic artery with a surgically implanted pump, or with percutaneous approach [11,19,20]. This strategy seems to improve the prognosis of patients with unresectable ICC [11]. Mambrini treated 12 patients with unresectable cholangiocarcinoma by bolus infusion in the hepatic artery of epirubicin (50 mg/m^2) plus cisplatin (60 mg/m^2) and capecitabine (1000 mg/m^2) given orally bid from day 2 to day 15. This combined intra-arterial and oral approach was found to be active and safe and produced encouraging survival results [21].

Recently, a German group tested a dose of intra-arterial gemcitabine >1000 mg/m^2 for patients with unresectable ICC who did not respond to systemic chemotherapy. The drug was administered with and without starch microspheres into the hepatic artery [20], with good tolerance and respectable results.

Cholangiocarcinoma cells express the epidermal growth factor receptor (EGFR), which plays an important role in the pathogenesis of these tumours. Thus, an anti-EGFR antibody (cetuximab) was used successfully in combination with radiotherapy [22] or with gemcitabine [23]. The papers about the use of this therapy are case reports on unresectable cholangiocarcinoma [23] or with distant metastases [22]. Other immunotherapeutic agents are a monoclonal antibody against vascular endothelial growth factor receptor (bevacizumab) and tyrosine kinase inhibitors, either alone or in combination with chemotherapeutic agents [18]. The potential benefit of combining regional chemo-embolisation with systemic chemotherapy for the treatment of unresectable ICC was recently suggested [24].

Transcatheter Hepatic Arterial Chemoembolisation

The unresectable ICC has also been treated with TACE [25]. Burger reported 17 patients who underwent one or more cycles of TACE between 1995 and 2004. This form of therapy showed a good tolerance rate (82% of the patients) and median survival was 23 months, with down-staging in two patients who were able to undergo resection after TACE.

Radiotherapy

Radiotherapy has also been used in the palliative treatment of ICC. A retrospective Chinese study [13] reported the results of radiation therapy in 22 patients with unresectable ICC compared with a non-treated group of patients. One- and 2-year survival rates in the treated group were 36.1 and 5.2% vs. 19 and 4.7% in the non-treated group ($p=0.021$).

At present, there is not evidence on the efficacy of these treatments, either as adjuvant or palliative therapy. Nevertheless, recent results are more encouraging than those obtained in the past. Controlled multicentric randomised phase-III studies are still needed to recruit a larger number of patients, which would enable the study of homogeneous patient groups in order to compare the most promising agents.

References

1. Jan YY, Yeh CN, Yeh TS, Chen TC (2005) Prognostic analysis of surgical treatment of peripheral cholangiocarcinoma: two decades of experience at Chang Gung Memorial Hospital. World J Gastroenterol 11(12):1779–1784
2. Asakura H, Ohtsuka M, Ito H et al (2005) Long-term survival after extended surgical resection of intrahepatic cholangiocarcinoma with extensive lymph-node metastasis. Hepatogastroenterology 52(63):722–724
3. Puhalla H, Schuell B, Pokorny H et al (2005) Treatment and outcome of intrahepatic cholangiocellular carcinoma. Am J Surg 189(2):173–177
4. Miwa S, Miyagawa S, Kobayashi A et al (2006) Predictive factors for intrahepatic cholangiocarcinoma recurrence in the liver following surgery. J Gastroenterol 41(9):893–900
5. Fu XH, Tang ZH, Zong M et al (2004) Clinicopathologic features, diagnosis and surgical

treatment of intrahepatic cholangiocarcinoma in 104 patients. Hepatobiliary Pancreat Dis Int 3(2):279–283

6. Knox JJ, Hedley D, Oza A et al (2005) Combining gemcitabine and capecitabine in patients with advanced biliary cancer: a phase II trial. J Clin Oncol 23(10):2332–2338

7. Thongprasert S (2005) The role of chemotherapy in cholangiocarcinoma. Ann Oncol 16(Suppl 2):ii93–ii96

8. Kelley ST, Bloomston M, Serafini F et al (2004) Cholangiocarcinoma: advocate an aggressive operative approach with adjuvant chemotherapy. Am Surg 70(9):743–748; discussion 748–749

9. Khan SA, Davidson BR, Goldin R et al; British Society of Gastroenterology (2002) Guidelines for the diagnosis and treatment of cholangiocarcinoma: consensus document. Gut 51(Suppl 6):VI1-VI9

10. Casavilla FA, Marsh JW, Iwatsuki S et al (1997) Hepatic resection and transplantation for peripheral cholangiocarcinoma. J Am Coll Surg 185(5):429–436

11. Tanaka N, Yamakado K, Nakatsuka A et al (2002) Arterial chemoinfusion therapy through an implanted port system for patients with unresectable intrahepatic cholangiocarcinoma–initial experience. Eur J Radiol 41(1):42–48

12. Valverde A, Bonhomme N, Farges O et al (1999) J Hepatobiliary Pancreat Surg 6(2):122–127

13. Zeng ZC, Tang ZY, Fan J et al (2006) Consideration of the role of radiotherapy for unresectable intrahepatic cholangiocarcinoma: a retrospective analysis of 75 patients. Cancer J 12(2):113–122

14. Higuchi R, Yamamoto M, Hatori T et al (2006) Intrahepatic cholangiocarcinoma with lymph-node metastasis successfully treated by immunotherapy with CD3-activated T cells and dendritic cells after surgery: report of a case. Surg Today 36(6):559–562

15. Zgodzinski W, Espat NJ (2005) Radiofrequency ablation for incidentally identified primary intrahepatic cholangiocarcinoma. World J Gastroenterol 11(33):5239–5240

16. Chiou YY, Hwang JI, Chou YH et al (2005) Percutaneous ultrasound-guided radiofrequency ablation of intrahepatic cholangiocarcinoma. Kaohsiung J Med Sci 21(7):304–309

17. Slakey DP (2002) Radiofrequency ablation of recurrent cholangiocarcinoma. Am Surg 68(4):395–397

18. Mazhar D, Stebbing J, Bower M (2006) Chemotherapy for advanced cholangiocarcinoma: what is standard treatment? Future Oncol 2(4):509–514

19. Cantore M, Mambrini A, Fiorentini G et al (2005) Phase II study of hepatic intraarterial epirubicin and cisplatin, with systemic 5-fluorouracil in patients with unresectable biliary tract tumours. Cancer 103(7):1402–1407

20. Vogl TJ, Schwarz W, Eichler K et al (2006) Hepatic intraarterial chemotherapy with gemcitabine in patients with unresectable cholangiocarcinomas and liver metastases of pancreatic cancer: a clinical study on maximum tolerable dose and treatment efficacy. J Cancer Res Clin Oncol 132(11):745–755

21. Mambrini A, Guglielmi A, Pacetti P et al (2007) Capecitabine plus hepatic intraarterial epirubicin and cisplatin in unresectable biliary cancer: a phase II study. Anticancer Res (in press)

22. Huang TW, Wang CH, Hsieh CB (2007) Effects of the anti-epidermal growth factor receptor antibody cetuximab on cholangiocarcinoma of the liver. Onkologie 30(3):129–131

23. Sprinzl MF, Schimanski CC, Moehler M et al (2006) Gemcitabine in combination with EGF-Receptor antibody (Cetuximab) as a treatment of cholangiocarcinoma: a case report. BMC Cancer 6:190

24. Kirchhoff T, Zender L, Merkesdal S et al (2005) Initial experience from a combination of systemic and regional chemotherapy in the treatment of patients with nonresectable cholangiocellular carcinoma in the liver. World J Gastroenterol 11(8):1091–1095

25. Burger I, Hong K, Schulick R et al (2005) Transcatheter arterial chemoembolization in unresectable cholangiocarcinoma: initial experience in a single institution. J Vasc Interv Radiol 16(3):353–361

Subject Index

Anastomotic leak 155, 156
Anatomic right trisectionectomy 136, 137
Angiography 25, 32, 34
Arterial resection 80, 148
Assessment of resectability 35, 115, 116

Bile duct dilatation 189, 190
Bile duct dysplasia 12
Bile duct margins 5, 7, 12, 122, 136, 159,
    215, 216
Bile duct resection 5, 121, 131, 153, 159,
    160
Biliary anastomosis 59, 123, 129, 134, 144,
    145, 148, 150, 155, 156, 178, 179
Biliary dissection 131
Biliary involvement 7, 11, 29, 30, 87, 88,
    96, 97, 99, 100, 120, 193
Biliary obstruction 24, 30, 49, 50
Biliary stent 181
Biological prognostic factors 76, 77, 199
Bisectionectomy 141–143
Bismuth-Corlette classification 6, 11, 30,
    36, 60, 87, 88, 99, 120, 177
Blood invasion 11
Brachytherapy 166, 170, 171, 175, 180, 181
Brushing 4, 24

Caudate lobectomy 121–125, 132, 133,
    135–142, 157
Central hepatectomy 141
Chemoradiation therapy 170, 171
Chemotherapy 52, 53, 69, 166, 169, 170,
    175, 179, 233–235
Cholangioscopy 18, 24, 25, 32, 215

Cholangitis 4, 23, 24, 38, 49, 50, 58, 60–62,
    153, 155, 163, 172, 175, 177–179, 181,
    213
Combined transplantation 165
Computed tomography (CT) 4, 18–25,
    29–38, 43, 52, 148, 188–190
Curative resection 29, 62, 72, 88, 113, 114,
    119, 143, 158, 159, 163, 165, 170, 198,
    205, 214, 222
Cholangiography 18, 21, 23, 24, 30–32, 35,
    37, 61, 122

Early cancer 78, 96, 97
Endoscopic percutaneous drainage 60, 175,
    176
Endoscopic retrograde cholangiopancreato-
    graphy (ERCP)18–21, 23–25, 30, 31
External drainage 50, 61, 62, 176
Extrahepatic metastases 69, 219

Fine needle aspiration (FNA) 4, 18, 19, 36
Frozen section 5, 44, 114, 116, 131, 134,
    215, 218

Gazzaniga staging system 96, 98
Gross type 8, 75, 78, 157, 193–195, 197,
    199, 200

Hepatic failure 52, 67, 70, 123, 221
Hepatic function 37, 49, 50–53, 58, 59, 61,
    62, 67, 69, 72, 113, 116, 120–122, 175,
    177, 180
Hepatic lobar atrophy 33
Hepatic pedicle dissection 130

Hepatic regeneration 52, 53, 61, 62, 67–69
Hepatopancreatoduodenectomy (HPD) 32,
    120, 149
Histological grade 11
Histological type 10

Immunohistochemistry 13, 14
Immunotherapy 233, 234
Infiltrative type 23, 75
Internal drainage 61–63
Intraductal polypoid growth 8
Intraductal ultrasound 19, 20
Intraoperative exploration 130
Intraoperative radiotherapy (IORT) 166, 170

JSBS staging system 91, 93, 95, 96, 99

K-Ras 76, 199

Laparoscopic ultrasound 45, 213
Laparoscopy 37, 43–46, 175, 213, 219
Left hepatectomy 5, 118, 121, 124, 125,
    138, 139, 146, 149, 159
Left trisectionectomy 121, 125, 139–141
Lymphatic invasion 11, 12, 79, 165, 194,
    199
Lobar atrophy18, 33, 35, 36, 38, 44, 69, 99,
    115, 116, 118, 120
Lobar hypertrophy 61
Lymph-node involvement 36, 46, 75, 78, 81,
    89, 99, 100, 115, 119, 129, 157, 165, 193,
    197, 198–205, 209, 216, 218
Lymph node stations 45, 93–95
Lymphadenectomy 119, 129–131, 157, 165,
    217, 218

Magnetic resonance imaging (MRI) 4, 18,
    22, 25, 29, 33, 34–38, 43, 190, 191
Mass forming type 8, 9, 11, 193, 194, 197,
    206, 215, 217, 222, 234
Microsatellite instability (MSI) 76, 77
Microscopic pattern 76, 194, 199
Minor complications 44, 153, 155
Molecular prognostic factors 76, 77, 199
MR-cholangiography 21
MSKCC staging system 44, 87, 98, 99, 119

Needle biopsy 4, 5
Nodular type 8, 23, 32, 92

No-touch technique 114, 124

Obstructive jaundice 17, 32, 52, 67, 53 76,
    77, 199

Pancreaticoduodenectomy (PD) 57, 58, 154,
    164, 165, 215
Papillary type 32, 75, 92
Papillomatosis 12
Parenchymal margins 13, 215
Percutaneous drainage 57, 59–61, 122, 175,
    176
Perineural invasion 5, 13, 78–80, 157, 165,
    167, 193, 199, 224, 231
Peritoneal carcinomatosis 18, 44, 45, 167
Photodynamic therapy 20, 172, 179, 181
Portal resection 116, 117, 124, 125, 137,
    143, 144, 146
Portal thrombosis 70, 72
Positron emission tomography (PET) 18,
    23, 37, 43
Postoperative mortality 57, 157, 165
Percutaneous transhepatic biliari drainage
    (PTBD) 24, 57–62, 171, 178

Radiofrequency ablation 235
Radiotherapy 164, 166, 169–171, 175,
    179–181, 233–236
Rational cine-cholangiography 32
Recurrence 5, 62, 77, 78, 122, 153, 159,
    160, 163, 165, 167, 169, 175, 179, 205,
    225, 226, 29, 230, 233–235
Regional lymph nodes 10, 90, 91, 159, 204,
    209, 213
Resection rate 114, 158
Right hepatectomy 70, 116, 121, 123, 124,
    133, 135, 144, 148, 159, 216
Right trisectionectomy 102, 116, 121, 124,
    135, 137, 215
Roux-en-Y jejunal loop 129, 132, 134, 136,
    139, 140, 150, 178

Sectionectomy 121, 123, 141, 142
Serosal involvement 196, 207, 214
Sonographic contrast agents 19
Steatosis 52, 53, 69
Surgical indication 53, 217
Surgical margin 6, 7, 134, 135, 146, 159
Surgical resection 23, 29, 81

TNM AJCC/UICC staging system 3, 75–83, 87–91, 96, 99, 130, 197, 203–205, 210, 223, 224
Transabdominal ultrasound 17, 19, 30, 36
Transcatheter hepatic arterial chemoembolisation (TACE) 233, 234, 236
Transparenchymal portography 71
Trasplantation 52, 163–167, 171, 172, 226, 229–231

Vascular involvement 17, 33–36, 87, 99, 115–116, 120, 56, 95, 96, 217
Vessel invasion 8, 11–13

Printed in Italy in October 2007